T0176737

Methodological Developments
in Data Linkage

WILEY SERIES IN PROBABILITY AND STATISTICS

Established by WALTER A. SHEWHART and SAMUEL S. WILKS

Editors: *David J. Balding, Noel A. C. Cressie, Garrett M. Fitzmaurice, Geof H. Givens, Harvey Goldstein, Geert Molenberghs, David W. Scott, Adrian F. M. Smith, Ruey S. Tsay, Sanford Weisberg*
Editors Emeriti: *J. Stuart Hunter, Iain M. Johnstone, Joseph B. Kadane, Jozef L. Teugels*

A complete list of the titles in this series appears at the end of this volume.

Methodological Developments in Data Linkage

Edited by

Katie Harron
London School of Hygiene and Tropical Medicine, UK

Harvey Goldstein
University of Bristol and University College London, UK

Chris Dibben
University of Edinburgh, UK

WILEY

This edition first published 2016
© 2016 John Wiley & Sons, Ltd

Registered Office
John Wiley & Sons, Ltd, The Atrium, Southern Gate, Chichester, West Sussex, PO19 8SQ, United Kingdom

For details of our global editorial offices, for customer services and for information about how to apply for permission to reuse the copyright material in this book please see our website at www.wiley.com.

The right of the author to be identified as the author of this work has been asserted in accordance with the Copyright, Designs and Patents Act 1988.

All rights reserved. No part of this publication may be reproduced, stored in a retrieval system, or transmitted, in any form or by any means, electronic, mechanical, photocopying, recording or otherwise, except as permitted by the UK Copyright, Designs and Patents Act 1988, without the prior permission of the publisher.

Wiley also publishes its books in a variety of electronic formats. Some content that appears in print may not be available in electronic books.

Designations used by companies to distinguish their products are often claimed as trademarks. All brand names and product names used in this book are trade names, service marks, trademarks or registered trademarks of their respective owners. The publisher is not associated with any product or vendor mentioned in this book.

Limit of Liability/Disclaimer of Warranty: While the publisher and author have used their best efforts in preparing this book, they make no representations or warranties with respect to the accuracy or completeness of the contents of this book and specifically disclaim any implied warranties of merchantability or fitness for a particular purpose. It is sold on the understanding that the publisher is not engaged in rendering professional services and neither the publisher nor the author shall be liable for damages arising herefrom. If professional advice or other expert assistance is required, the services of a competent professional should be sought

The advice and strategies contained herein may not be suitable for every situation. In view of ongoing research, equipment modifications, changes in governmental regulations, and the constant flow of information relating to the use of experimental reagents, equipment, and devices, the reader is urged to review and evaluate the information provided in the package insert or instructions for each chemical, piece of equipment, reagent, or device for, among other things, any changes in the instructions or indication of usage and for added warnings and precautions. The fact that an organization or Website is referred to in this work as a citation and/or a potential source of further information does not mean that the author or the publisher endorses the information the organization or Website may provide or recommendations it may make. Further, readers should be aware that Internet Websites listed in this work may have changed or disappeared between when this work was written and when it is read. No warranty may be created or extended by any promotional statements for this work. Neither the publisher nor the author shall be liable for any damages arising herefrom.

Library of Congress Cataloging-in-Publication data applied for

ISBN: 9781118745878

A catalogue record for this book is available from the British Library.

Cover image: Cover photograph courtesy of Harvey Goldstein.

Set in 10/12pt Times by SPi Global, Pondicherry, India
Printed and bound in Singapore by Markono Print Media Pte Ltd

1   2016

Contents

Foreword

The methodology of data linkage is emerging as an important area of scientific endeavour as the opportunities for harnessing big data expand. Linkage of administrative data offers an efficient tool for research to improve understanding of people's lives and for building a stronger evidence base for policy and service development. Linkage between data collected in primary research studies and administrative data could transform the scope, design and efficiency of primary studies such as surveys and clinical trials. To realise these potential advantages, we need to address the core methodological challenge of how to minimise the errors associated with linking imperfect or incomplete personal identifiers while preserving individual privacy. A second challenge is the need for methods to adapt to the widening opportunities for combining 'big data' and developments in computing systems.

A third challenge is for data governance to keep pace with new developments while addressing public concerns and perceived benefits and threats. As research needs public support, strict controls on use of linked data for research are a key tool for allaying public concerns, despite being burdensome and sometimes restricting the scope of research. In contrast, outside of research, linkage of large data sources captured as part of routine administration of services or transactions is fast becoming a normal feature of daily life. Data linkage is now essential for many daily tasks. If we buy a car, take out insurance, apply to university, use a reward card or obtain a driving licence, consent to linkage to additional information is often conditional – no consent, no service. Governance of linkage for these disparate purposes for data linkage, research and running services, could be brought closer together. Moreover, they share a need for methodological developments to reduce the harms of linkage error and minimise threats to privacy.

A fourth challenge for linkage methodology is that opportunities for research into data linkage tend to be restricted to the few analysts or researchers able to access identifiable data. Data linkers and analysts evaluating linkage error are often constrained by commercial or service interests or by Data Protection Regulations. Publication of linkage algorithms or of evaluations demonstrating linkage error may be bad for business, reveal problems in services or threaten security. However, transparency about linkage is essential for users of linked data – governments, businesses, service providers and users – to be able to interpret results from data linkage and take account of potential biases. It has long been recognised that even small amounts of error in the linkage process can produce substantially biased results, particularly when errors are more likely to occur in records belonging to specific groups of people. This book is important because it opens up the black box surrounding data linkage and should encourage more transparency about linkage processes and their potential impacts.

The book draws together methods arising from a range of contexts, including statistical and computer science perspectives, with detailed coverage of novel methods such as graph databases, and of new applications for linkage, such as the Beyond 2011 evaluation of whether the UK census could be replaced by linkage of administrative data sources. It combines excellent coverage of the current state of the science of data linkage methods with discussion of potential future developments.

This book is essential reading for data linkers, for users of linked data and for those who determine governance frameworks within which linkage can take place. There are few settings across the world where administrative data contains complete and wholly accurate identifiers and where linkage error is not a problem. This book should help to develop methods to improve linkage quality and transparency about linkage processes and errors, to ensure that the power of data linkage for services and research is realised.

Professor Ruth Gilbert
Institute of Child Health, University College London, UK

Contributors

Owen Abbott
Office for National Statistics
London, UK

Megan Bohensky
Department of Medicine Melbourne EpiCentre
University of Melbourne
Parkville, Victoria, Australia

Raymond Chambers
National Institute for Applied Statistics Research Australia (NIASRA)
School of Mathematics and Applied Statistics
University of Wollongong
Wollongong, New South Wales, Australia

Chris Dibben
University of Edinburgh
Edinburgh, UK

Mark Elliot
University of Manchester
Manchester, UK

James M. Farrow
SANT Datalink
Adelaide, South Australia, Australia
and
Farrow Norris
Sydney, New South Wales, Australia

Harvey Goldstein
Institute of Child Health
University College London
London, UK
and
Graduate School of Education
University of Bristol
Bristol, UK

Heather Gowans
University of Oxford
Oxford, UK

Katie Harron
London School of Hygiene and Tropical Medicine
London, UK

Peter Jones
Office for National Statistics
London, UK

Gunky Kim
National Institute for Applied Statistics Research Australia (NIASRA)
School of Mathematics and Applied Statistics
University of Wollongong
Wollongong, New South Wales, Australia

Darren Lightfoot
University of St Andrews
St Andrews, UK

Martin Ralphs
Office for National Statistics
London, UK

Rainer Schnell
Research Methodology Group, University Duisburg-Essen
Duisburg, Germany

William E. Winkler
Center for Statistical Research and Methodology
U.S. Bureau of the Census
Suitland, MD, USA

1

Introduction

Katie Harron[1], Harvey Goldstein[2,3] and Chris Dibben[4]

[1] London School of Hygiene and Tropical Medicine, London, UK
[2] Institute of Child Health, University College London, London, UK
[3] Graduate School of Education, University of Bristol, Bristol, UK
[4] University of Edinburgh, Edinburgh, UK

1.1   Introduction: data linkage as it exists

The increasing availability of large administrative databases for research has led to a dramatic rise in the use of data linkage. The speed and accuracy of linkage have much improved over recent decades with developments such as string comparators, coding systems and blocking, yet the methods still underpinning most of the linkage performed today were proposed in the 1950s and 1960s. Linkage and analysis of data across sources remain problematic due to lack of identifiers that are totally accurate as well as being discriminatory, missing data and regulatory issues, especially concerned with privacy.

In this context, recent developments in data linkage methodology have concentrated on bias in the analysis of linked data, novel approaches to organising relationships between databases and privacy-preserving linkage. *Methodological developments in data linkage* bring together a collection of chapters on cutting-edge developments in data linkage methodology, contributed by members of the international data linkage community.

The first section of the book covers the current state of data linkage, methodological issues that are relevant to linkage systems and analyses today and case studies from the United Kingdom, Canada and Australia. In this introduction, we provide a brief background to the development of data linkage methods and introduce common terms. We highlight the most important issues that have emerged in recent years and describe how the remainder of the book attempts to deal with these issues. Chapter 2 summarises the advances in linkage accuracy and speed that have arisen from the traditional probabilistic methods proposed by Fellegi and Sunter. The first section concludes with a description of the data linkage environment as it is today, with

Methodological Developments in Data Linkage, First Edition. Edited by Katie Harron, Harvey Goldstein and Chris Dibben.
© 2016 John Wiley & Sons, Ltd. Published 2016 by John Wiley & Sons, Ltd.

case study examples. Chapter 3 describes the opportunities and challenges provided by data linkage, focussing on legal and security aspects and models for data access and linkage.

The middle section of the book focusses on the immediate future of data linkage, in terms of methods that have been developed and tested and can be put into practice today. It concentrates on analysis of linked data and the difficulties associated with linkage uncertainty, highlighting the problems caused by errors that occur in linkage (false matches and missed matches) and the impact that these errors can have on the reliability of results based on linked data. This section of the book discusses two methods for handling linkage error, the first relating to regression analyses and the second to an extension of the standard multiple imputation framework. Chapter 7 presents an alternative data storage solution compared to relational databases that provides significant benefits for linkage.

The final section of the book tackles an aspect of the potential future of data linkage. Ethical considerations relating to data linkage and research based on linked data are a subject of continued debate. Privacy-preserving data linkage attempts to avoid the controversial release of personal identifiers by providing means of linking and performing analysis on encrypted data. This section of the book describes the debate and provides examples.

The establishment of large-scale linkage systems has provided new opportunities for important and innovative research that, until now, have not been possible but that also present unique methodological and organisational challenges. New linkage methods are now emerging that take a different approach to the traditional methods that have underpinned much of the research performed using linked data in recent years, leading to new possibilities in terms of speed, accuracy and transparency of research.

1.2   Background and issues

A statistical definition of data linkage is 'a merging that brings together information from two or more sources of data with the object of consolidating facts concerning an individual or an event that are not available in any separate record' (Organisation for Economic Co-operation and Development (OECD)). Data linkage has many different synonyms (record linkage, record matching, re-identification, entity heterogeneity, merge/purge) within various fields of application (computer science, marketing, fraud detection, censuses, bibliographic data, insurance data) (Elmagarmid, Ipeirotis and Verykios, 2007).

The term 'record linkage' was first applied to health research in 1946, when Dunn described linkage of vital records from the same individual (birth and death records) and referred to the process as 'assembling the book of life' (Dunn, 1946). Dunn emphasised the importance of such linkage to both the individual and health and other organisations. Since then, data linkage has become increasingly important to the research environment.

The development of computerised data linkage meant that valuable information could be combined efficiently and cost-effectively, avoiding the high cost, time and effort associated with setting up new research studies (Newcombe et al., 1959). This led to a large body of research based on enhanced datasets created through linkage. Internationally, large linkage systems of note are the Western Australia Record Linkage System, which links multiple datasets (over 30) for up to 40 years at a population level, and the Manitoba Population-Based Health Information System (Holman et al., 1999; Roos et al., 1995). In the United Kingdom, several large-scale linkage systems have also been developed, including the Scottish Health Informatics Programme (SHIP), the Secure Anonymised Information Linkage (SAIL) Databank and the Clinical Practice Research Datalink (CPRD). As data linkage becomes a more established part of research relating to health and society, there has been an increasing interest in methodological issues associated with creating and analysing linked datasets (Maggi, 2008).

1.3 Data linkage methods

Data linkage brings together information relating to the same individual that is recorded in different files. A set of linked records is created by comparing records, or parts of records, in different files and applying a set of linkage criteria or rules to determine whether or not records belong to the same individual. These rules utilise the values on 'linking variables' that are common to each file. The aim of linkage is to determine the true **match status** of each comparison pair: a **match** if records belong to the same individual and a **non-match** if records belong to different individuals.

As the true match status is unknown, linkage criteria are used to assign a **link status** for each comparison pair: a **link** if records are classified as belonging to the same individual and a **non-link** if records are classified as belonging to different individuals.

In a perfect linkage, all matches are classified as links, and all non-matches are classified as non-links. If comparison pairs are misclassified (false matches or missed matches), error is introduced. **False matches** occur when records from different individuals link erroneously; **missed matches** occur when records from the same individual fail to link.

1.3.1 Deterministic linkage

In deterministic linkage, a set of predetermined rules are used to classify pairs of records as links and non-links. Typically, deterministic linkage requires exact agreement on a specified set of identifiers or matching variables. For example, two records may be classified as a link if their values of National Insurance number, surname and sex agree exactly. Modifications of strict deterministic linkage include 'stepwise' deterministic linkage, which uses a succession of rules; the '$n-1$' deterministic procedure, which allows a link to be made if all but one of a set of identifiers agree; and ad hoc deterministic procedures, which allow partial identifiers to be combined into a pseudo-identifier (Abrahams and Davy, 2002; Maso, Braga and Franceschi, 2001; Mears et al., 2010). For example, a combination of the first letter of surname, month of birth and postcode area (e.g. H01N19) could form the basis for linkage.

Strict deterministic methods that require identifiers to match exactly often have a high rate of missed matches, as any recording errors or missing values can prevent identifiers from agreeing. Conversely, the rate of false matches is typically low, as the majority of linked pairs are true matches (records are unlikely to agree exactly on a set of identifiers by chance) (Grannis, Overhage and McDonald, 2002). Deterministic linkage is a relatively straightforward and quick linkage method and is useful when records have highly discriminative or unique identifiers that are well completed and accurate. For example, the community health index (CHI) is used for much of the linkage in the Scottish Record Linkage System.

1.3.2 Probabilistic linkage

Newcombe was the first to propose that comparison pairs could be classified using a probabilistic approach (Newcombe et al., 1959). He suggested that a match weight be assigned to each comparison pair, representing the likelihood that two records are a true match, given the agreement of their identifiers. Each identifier contributes separately to an overall match weight. Identifier agreement contributes positively to the weight, and disagreement contributes a penalty. The size of the contribution depends on the discriminatory power of the identifier, so that agreement on name makes a larger contribution than agreement on sex (Zhu et al., 2009). Fellegi and Sunter formalised Newcombe's proposals into the statistical theory underpinning probabilistic linkage today (Fellegi and Sunter, 1969). Chapter 2 provides details on the match calculation.

In probabilistic linkage, link status is determined by comparing match weights to a threshold or cut-off match weight in order to classify as a match or non-match. In addition, manual review of record pairs is often performed to aid choice of threshold and to deal with uncertain links (Krewski et al., 2005). If linkage error rates are known, thresholds can be selected to minimise the total number of errors, so that the number of false matches and missed matches cancels out. However, error rates are usually unknown. The subjective process of choosing probabilistic thresholds is a limitation of probabilistic linkage, as different linkers may choose different thresholds. This can result in multiple possible versions of the linked data.

There are certain problems with the standard probabilistic procedure. The first is the assumption of independence for the probabilities associated with the individual matching variables. For example, observing an individual in any given ethnic group category may be associated with certain surname structures, and hence, the joint probability of agreeing across matching variables may not simply be the product of the separate probabilities. Ways of dealing with this are suggested in Chapters 2 and 6. A second typical problem is that records with match weights that do not reach the threshold are excluded from data analysis, reducing efficiency and introducing bias if this is associated with the characteristics of the variables to be analysed. Chapter 6 suggests a way of dealing with this using missing data methods. A third problem occurs when the errors in one or more matching variables are associated with the values of the secondary data file variables to be transferred for analysis. This non-random linkage error can lead to biases in the estimates from subsequent analyses, and this is discussed in Chapters 4–6. Chapter 4 reviews the literature and sets out the situations where linkage bias of any kind can arise, including the important case when individual consent to linkage may be withheld so leading to incomplete administrative registers. Chapter 5 looks explicitly at regression modelling of linked data files when different kinds of errors are present, and Chapter 6 proposes a Bayesian procedure for handling incomplete linkages.

One of the features of traditional probabilistic methods is that once weights have been computed, the full pattern of similarities that give rise to these weights, based upon the matching variables, is either discarded or stored in a form that requires any future linkage to repeat the whole process. In Chapter 7, a graphical approach to data storage and retrieval is proposed that would give the data linker efficient access to such patterns from a graph database. In particular, it would give the linker the possibility to readily modify her algorithm or update files as further information becomes available. Chapter 7 discusses implementation details.

1.3.3   Data preparation

Quality of data linkage ultimately depends on the quality of the underlying data. If datasets to be linked contained sufficiently accurate, complete and discriminative information, data linkage would be a straightforward database merging process. Unfortunately, many administrative datasets contain messy, inconsistent and missing data. Datasets also vary in structure, format and content. The way in which data are entered can influence data quality. For example, errors may be more likely to occur in identifiers that are copied from handwritten forms, scanned or transcribed from a conversation. These issues mean that techniques to handle complex and imperfect data are required. Although data preparation is an important concern when embarking on a linkage project, we do not attempt to cover this in the current volume. A good overview can be found in Christen (2012a).

1.4   Linkage error

Linkage error occurs when record pairs are misclassified as links or non-links. Errors tend to occur when there is no unique identifier (such as NHS number or National Insurance number) or when available unique identifiers are prone to missing values or errors. This means that linkage relies on partial identifiers such as sex, date of birth or surname (Sariyar, Borg and Pommerening, 2012).

False matches, where records from different individuals link erroneously, occur when different individuals have similar identifiers. These errors occur more often when there is a lack of discriminative identifiers and file sizes are large (e.g. different people sharing the same sex, date of birth and postcode). For records that have more than the expected number of candidate records in the linking file, the candidate(s) with the most agreeing identifiers or with the highest match weight is typically accepted as a link. This may not always be the correct link.

Missed matches, where records from the same individual fail to link, occur where there are errors in identifiers. This could be due to misreporting (e.g. typographical errors), changes over time (e.g. married women's surnames) or missing/invalid data that prevent records from agreeing.

Many linkage studies report the proportion of records that were linked (match rate). Other frequently report measures of linkage quality are sensitivity and specificity (Christen and Goiser, 2005). These measures are directly related to the probability of false matches and missed matches. However, interpretation of these measures is not always straightforward. For example, match rate is only relevant if all records are expected to be matched. Furthermore, such measures of linkage error can be difficult to relate to potential bias in results.

Derivation of measures of linkage error can also be difficult, as estimation requires that either the error rate is known or that the true match status of comparison pairs is known. A common method for measuring linkage error is the use of a gold-standard dataset. Gold-standard data may be an external data source or a subset of data with additional identifiers available (Fonseca et al., 2010; Monga and Patrick, 2001). Many linkage projects create a gold-standard dataset by taking a sample of comparison pairs and submitting the records to manual review (Newgard, 2006; Waien, 1997). The aim of the manual review is to determine the true match status of each pair (Belin and Rubin, 1995; Gill, 1997; Morris et al., 1997; Potz et al., 2010). Once a gold-standard dataset has been obtained, it is used to calculate sensitivity, specificity and other measures of linkage error by comparing the true match status of each comparison pair (in the gold-standard data) with the link status of each pair (Wiklund and Eklund, 1986; Zingmond et al., 2004). These estimates are assumed to apply to the entire linked dataset (the gold-standard data are assumed to be representative). This is a reasonable assumption if the gold-standard data were a random sample; otherwise, potential biases might be introduced.

Manual review is convenient but can take a substantial amount of time, particularly for large files (Qayad and Zhang, 2009; Sauleau, Paumier and Buemi, 2005). It also may not always be completely accurate. If samples are only taken from linked pairs – which is often the case due to the smaller number of links compared to non-links – the rate of missed matches would not be estimated. If the sample of pairs reviewed is not representative, estimates of linkage error may be biased.

1.5   Impact of linkage error on analysis of linked data

Although a large body of literature exists on methods and applications of data linkage, there has been relatively little methodological research into the impact of linkage error on analysis of linked data. The issue is not a new one – Neter, Maynes and Ramanathan (1965) recognised that even relatively small errors could result in substantially biased estimates (Neter, Maynes and Ramanathan, 1965). The lack of comprehensive linkage evaluation seems to be due to a lack of awareness of the implications of linkage error, possibly resulting from a lack of communication between data linkers and data users. However, the relevance and reliability of research based on linked data are called into question in the presence of linkage error (Chambers, 2009).

Data custodians (organisations that hold personally identifiable data that could be used for research) have a responsibility to protect privacy by adhering to legislation and guidelines, avoiding unauthorised copies of data being made and distributed and ensuring data are used only for agreed purposes. For these reasons, data custodians can be unwilling or unable to release identifiable data for linkage. To overcome this issue, many linkage projects adhere to the 'separation principle'. This means that the people performing the linkage (the data linkers – sometimes a trusted third party) do not have access to 'payload' data and people performing the analysis (the data users) do not have access to any personal identifiers. This protects confidentiality and means that linked datasets can be used for a range of purposes (Goeken et al., 2011). Approaches to privacy and security are discussed in detail in Chapter 3.

While the potential knowledge benefits from data linkage can be very great, these have to be balanced against the need to ensure the protection of individuals' personal information. Working with data that is non-personal (i.e. truly anonymous) guarantees such protection but is rarely practicable in a data linkage context. Instead, what is required is the construction of a data linkage environment in which the process of re-identification is made so difficult that the data can be judged as practicably anonymous. This type of environment is created both through the governance processes operating across the environment and the data linkage and analysis models that structure the operational processes. Chapter 3 reviews the main models that are used and their governance processes. Some examples from across the world are presented as case studies.

The separation principle is recognised as good practice but means that researchers often lack the information needed to assess the impact of linkage error on results and are unable to report useful evaluations of linkage (Baldi et al., 2010; Harron et al., 2012; Herman et al., 1997; Kelman, Bass and Holman, 2002). Separation typically means that any uncertainty in linkage is not carried through to analysis. The examples of linkage evaluation that do appear in the literature are often extreme cases of bias due to linkage error. However, as there is a lack of consistent evaluation of linkage, it is difficult to identify the true extent of the problem.

Reported measures of linkage error are important, as they offer a simple representation of linkage quality. However, in isolation, measures of sensitivity and specificity cannot always provide interpretation of the validity of results (Leiss, 2007). Although it is useful to quantify linkage error, it is most important to understand the impact of these errors on results.

The impact of linkage error on analysis of linked data depends on the structure of the data, the distribution of error and the analysis to be performed (Fett, 1984; Krewski et al., 2005). In some studies, it may be important to capture all true matches, and so a more specific approach could be used. For example, if linkage was being used to detect fraud, it may be important that all possible links were captured. In other studies, it might be more important that linked records are true matches, and missed matches are less important. For example, if linked healthcare records were being used to obtain medical history, it might be more important to avoid false matches (German, 2000). For these reasons, it is important that the impact of linkage error is understood for a particular purpose, with linkage criteria ideally tailored to that purpose. Bias due to linkage error is explored in detail in Chapter 4.

1.6   Data linkage: the future

Methods for data linkage have evolved over recent years to address the dynamic, error-prone, anonymised or incomplete nature of administrative data. However, as the size and complexity of these datasets increase, current techniques cannot eliminate linkage error entirely. Manual review is not feasible for the linkage of millions of records at a time. With human involvement in the creation of these data sources, recording errors will always be an issue and lead to uncertainty in linkage. Furthermore, as opportunities for linkage of data between organisations and across sectors arise, new challenges will emerge.

Chapter 9 looks at record linking approaches that are used to support censuses and population registers. There is increasing interest in this with the growing availability of large-scale administrative datasets in health, social care, education, policing, etc. It looks at issues of data security and, like Chapter 3, addresses the balance between individual privacy protection and knowledge and explores technical solutions that can be implemented, especially those that can operate on so-called 'hashed' data or data that is 'pseudonymised at source' where the linker only has access to linking variables where the original information has been transformed (similarly but irreversibly) into non-disclosive pseudonyms.

The second decade of the twenty-first century is an exciting and important era for data linkage, with increasing amounts of resources being applied and a broad range of different disciplinary expertise being applied. Our hope is that the present volume, by setting out some of these developments, will encourage further work and interest.

2

Probabilistic linkage

William E. Winkler

Center for Statistical Research and Methodology, U.S. Bureau of the Census, Suitland, MD, USA

2.1 Introduction

Probabilistic linkage (or record linkage or entity resolution) consists of methods for matching duplicate records within or across files using non-unique identifiers such as first name, last name, date of birth and address, or a national health identification code with typographical error. We refer to fields such as these as *quasi-identifiers*. In combination, quasi-identifiers may uniquely identify an individual.

The term record linkage, introduced by Dunn (1946), refers to linking of medical records associated with individuals. Dunn described an early successful system developed by the Dominion Bureau of Statistics in Canada for which name-related information from microfiche was put on punch cards and then lists were printed for verification and review by different agencies in Canada. The methods were cost-effective at the time because they were far more efficient than purely manual matching and maintenance of paper files.

Modern computerised record linkage began with methods introduced by geneticist Howard Newcombe (Newcombe and Kennedy, 1962; Newcombe et al., 1959) who used odds ratios and value-specific frequencies (common value of last name 'Smith' has less distinguishing power than rare value 'Zabrinsky'). Fellegi and Sunter (1969) gave a mathematical formalisation of Newcombe's ideas. They proved the optimality of the decision (classification) rule of Newcombe and introduced many ideas about estimating 'optimal' parameters (probabilities used in the likelihood ratios) without training data. Training data, which makes suitable parameter estimation much easier, is a set of record pairs for which the true matching status is known, created, for example, through certain iterative review methods in which 'true' matching status is obtained for large subsets of pairs. Fellegi and Sunter's parameter estimates

Methodological Developments in Data Linkage, First Edition. Edited by Katie Harron, Harvey Goldstein and Chris Dibben.
© 2016 John Wiley & Sons, Ltd. Published 2016 by John Wiley & Sons, Ltd.

are not necessarily optimal in a strict mathematical sense but do improve very significantly over parameters obtained by 'guessing' or from training data.

In this chapter, we will give background on the model of Fellegi and Sunter and several of the practical methods that are necessary for dealing with (often exceptionally) messy data. Messy data can have representation differences such as nickname versus legal name, typographical error or differing types of free-form representations of names or addresses. Although the methods rely on statistical models, computer scientists using machine learning or database methods have done most of the development (Winkler, 2006a). Computer scientists refer to record linkage as *entity resolution, object identification* or other terms.

Applications of record linkage are numerous. Early applications of record linkage were almost entirely in health areas involving the updating and maintenance of large national health indexes and death indexes (Gill, 2001). National indexes could be compared against other lists, for example, in epidemiological follow-up studies of infant mortality (Newcombe and Smith, 1975) or in cancer follow-up studies (Newcombe, 1988). The early systems tried to replace many of the clerical review methods with computerised procedures (Newcombe, 1988) that greatly facilitated bringing together pairs using fields such as last name or date of birth.

In other closely related situations, we might use a collection of lists to create a large list (survey frame) or update an existing large list. The updating of lists and list maintenance can assure that we have good coverage of a desired population. The largest applications of record linkage are often during a population census or in updating an administrative list such as a national registry of individuals or households. Large typographical variation or error in fields such as first name, last name and date of birth in a moderate proportion of records can make the updating quite difficult. Historically, some agencies have a full-time staff devoted to cleaning up the largest lists such as population registries (primarily manually). If they did not, then 1–3% error or more might enter the lists every year. Computerised record linkage methods can significantly reduce the need for clerical review and clean-up.

Record linkage can both increase the amount of coverage and reduce the amount of duplication in a survey frame or national registry. Frame errors (duplication or lack of coverage in the lists) can severely bias sampling and estimation. It is nearly impossible to correct errors in estimates that are based on sampling from a frame with moderate error due to duplicates (Deming and Gleser, 1959). After applying sophisticated record linkage, the 1992 US Census of Agriculture (Winkler, 1995) contained 2% duplication, whereas the 1987 Census of Agriculture contained 10% duplication. The duplication rates are based on field validation. Some estimates from the 1987 Census of Agriculture with 10% duplication error may have been substantially biased. The duplication, in particular, can mean that farms in certain areas and their associated crops/livestock are double counted.

Another application of record linkage might be the matching of one list with another list in order to estimate the under-coverage/over-coverage of one of the lists that is believed to be reasonably complete. For the 1990 US Census (Winkler, 1995), a large number of census blocks (contiguous regions of approximately 50 households) were re-enumerated and matched against the main list of individuals. In a re-enumeration, a large number of blocks (and all individuals within their households) are listed and then matched against the main Census using a type of capture–recapture methodology originally developed for estimating wildlife populations. Similar types of coverage procedures are used in the United Kingdom and in Australia.

The computerised procedures for the 1990 US Decennial Census reduced clerical review from an estimated 3000 individuals for 6 months to 200 individuals for 6 weeks. Because of the high quality of the lists and associated skills of individuals, false-match rates of the computerised procedures were approximately 0.2%. More than 85% of matches were found automatically with the remainder of matches easily located among potentially matching individuals in the same household. Because the potentially matching individuals were often missing both first name and age, their records required clerical review using auxiliary information and sometimes field follow-up.

The outline of this chapter is as follows. In the second section following this introduction, we give background on the record linkage model of Fellegi and Sunter (1969), methods of parameter estimation without training data, some brief comments on training data, string comparators for dealing with typographical error and blocking criteria. The examples use US Census Bureau data, but the methods apply to all types of data. The third section provides details of the difficulties with the preparation of data for linkage. Traditionally, file preparation has yielded greater improvements in matching efficacy than any other improvements. We improve matching efficacy by reducing false-match rates or false non-match rates or both (described in the following). In the fourth section, we describe methods for error rate estimation without training data and methods for adjusting statistical analyses of merged files for linkage error. The final section consists of concluding remarks.

2.2   Overview of methods

In this section, we provide summaries of basic ideas of record linkage.

2.2.1   The Fellegi–Sunter model of record linkage

Fellegi and Sunter (1969) provided a formal mathematical model for ideas that had been introduced by Newcombe et al. (1959) and Newcombe and Kennedy (1962). They provided many ways of estimating key parameters. The methods have been rediscovered in the computer science literature (Cooper and Maron, 1978) but without proofs of optimality. To begin, notation is needed. Two files A and B are to be matched. The idea is to classify pairs in a product space $A \times B$ from two files A and B into M, the set of true matches, and U, the set of true non-matches. In comparing information from the two files A and B, we use common information such as names, addresses, date of birth and other fields which we call an agreement pattern and denote by γ. Fellegi and Sunter, making rigorous concepts introduced by Newcombe et al. (1959), considered ratios of probabilities of the form

$$R = \frac{P(\gamma \in \Gamma | M)}{P(\gamma \in \Gamma | U)} \tag{2.1}$$

where γ runs through arbitrary agreement patterns in a comparison space Γ over $A \times B$. For instance, Γ might consist of eight patterns representing simple agreement or not on the largest name component, street name and street number. Alternatively, each $\gamma \in \Gamma$ might additionally account for the relative frequency with which specific values of name components such as 'Smith', 'Zabrinsky', 'AAA' and 'Capitol' occur. Newcombe, a geneticist, looked at odds ratios based on the relative frequencies associated with individual fields that he combined into a total agreement weight associated with each pair in $A \times B$. The ratio R or any mono-tonely increasing function of it such as the natural log is referred to as a *matching weight* (or score). The probability given M in the numerator of (2.1) is called the *m-probability*. The probability given U in the denominator is called the *u-probability*.

The decision rule is given by:

If $R > T_{\mu}$, then designate pair as a match   (2.2a)

If $T_{\lambda} \leq R \leq T_{\mu}$, then designate pair as a possible match and hold for clerical review   (2.2b)

If $R < T_{\lambda}$, then designate pair as a non-match   (2.2c)

The cut-off thresholds T_{μ} and T_{λ} are determined by a priori error bounds on the rates of false matches and false non-matches. False matches are pairs that are designated as matches $\tilde{M}$ that are truly non-matches, false non-matches are pairs that are truly matches that are designated as non-matches, and clerical pairs are pairs that are held for clerical review because there is insufficient or contradictory information for matching. In some situations, resources are available to review pairs clerically. The additive complement of the false-match rate $1 - P(\tilde{M}|U)$ relates closely to precision $P(M|\tilde{M})$.

Rule (2.2) agrees with intuition. If $\gamma \in \Gamma$ consists primarily of agreements, then it is intui-tive that $\gamma \in \Gamma$ would be more likely to occur among matches than non-matches and ratio (2.1) would be large. On the other hand, if $\gamma \in \Gamma$ consists primarily of disagreements, then ratio (2.1) would be small. Rule (2.2) partitions the set $\gamma \in \Gamma$ into three disjoint subregions. The region $T_{\lambda} \leq R > T_{\mu}$ is referred to as the no-decision region or clerical review region. Like Newcombe et al. (1959), Newcombe and Kennedy (1962), Fellegi and Sunter assumed that they knew the underlying truth of whether a given pair was a match or non-match and could estimate directly the probabilities in Equation 2.1. All the authors introduced methods for estimating the unknown probabilities in (2.1) under various simplifying assumptions (Section 2.2.2).

Figure 2.1 provides an illustration of the curves of natural log of frequency versus natural log of the likelihood ratio (Eq. 2.1) for matches and non-matches, respectively. The two verti-cal lines represent the lower and upper cut-off thresholds T_{λ} and T_{μ}, respectively. The x-axis is the log of the likelihood ratio R given by (2.1). The y-axis is the log of the frequency counts of the pairs associated with the given likelihood ratio. The plot uses pairs of records from a contiguous geographic region that was matched in the 1990 US Decennial Census. The cleri-cal review region between the two cut-offs primarily consists of pairs within the same house-hold that are missing both first name and age. Winkler (1989a) observed that the 'optimal' parameters varied substantially in each of approximately 500 regions and allowing this vari-ation significantly reduced the amount of clerical review (Section 2.2.2.3).

Table 2.1 provides examples of pairs of records that might be matched using name, address and age. The pairs give the first indication that matching that might be straightfor-ward for a suitably skilled person might not be easy with naïve rules based on (2.1) and (2.2). If the agreement pattern $\gamma \in \Gamma$ on the pairs is simple agree or disagree on name, address and age, then we see none of the pairs would agree on any of the three fields. In most situations, a suitably skilled person would be able to recognise that the first two pairs may be the same but would be unlikely to put a suitable score (or matching weight) on the first two pairs. The third pair must be taken in context. If the first record in the pair were from a list of indi-viduals in medical school at the University of Michigan 20 years ago and the second record

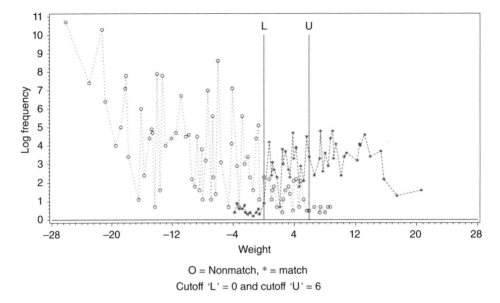

O = Nonmatch, * = match

Cutoff 'L' = 0 and cutoff 'U' = 6

Figure 2.1   Log frequency versus weight, matches and non-matches combined. L, lower; U, upper.

Table 2.1   Elementary examples of matching pairs of records (dependent on context).

Name	Address	Age
John A. Smith	16 Main Street	16
J. H. Smith	16 Main St	17
Javier Martinez	49 E Applecross Road	33
Haveir Marteenez	49 Aplecross Raod	36
Gillian Jones	645 Reading Aev	24
Jilliam Brown	123 Norcross Blvd	43

is from a current list of physicians in Detroit, Michigan, then, after suitable follow-up, we might determine that the third pair is a match.

If we had computerised parsing algorithms (Section 2.3.3) for separating the free-form name field into first name, middle initial and last name and address into house number, street name and other components, then we might have better patterns $\gamma \in \Gamma$ for applying (2.1) and (2.2). If we had suitable algorithms for comparing fields (e.g. Javier vs. Haveir – Section 2.2.3.1) having typographical error, then we might be able to give partial agreement to minor typographical error rather than call a comparison a disagreement. Additionally, we might want standardisation routines that replace commonly occurring words with a common spelling ('Raod' with 'Road' in pair two; 'Aev' with 'Ave' in pair three). There seem to be only a few methods for dealing with typographical error. For example, previously determined typical typographical variations might be placed in lookup tables that could be used for replacing one spelling with another.

2.2.2   Learning parameters

Early record linkage systems were often used for large administrative lists such as a national health index (Newcombe and Kennedy, 1962; Newcombe et al., 1959). The typical fields were name, address, date of birth, city of birth and various fields associated with health information.

In virtually all real-world situations of which we are aware, training data have been unavailable. Practitioners have developed a number of ways for learning 'optimal' record linkage parameters without training data. In all but one of the following subsections, we will describe methods of *unsupervised learning* where training data are unavailable.

2.2.2.1   Ideas of Newcombe

Newcombe's ideas (Newcombe and Kennedy, 1962; Newcombe et al., 1959) are based on odds ratios for individual fields (Eq. 2.4) that are combined into ratios of probabilities (Eq. 2.1) under a simplifying assumption of conditional independence (CI) (Eq. 2.3). One of his breakthroughs was in realising that the parameters needed for the ratio (2.1) could be computed directly from a population register which we denote by E. Both files A and B that were subsequently matched could be assumed to be subsets of E, and the odds ratios computed for individual fields in E could be used for both A and B. The register E had been cleaned up in the sense that duplicates were removed and inconsistent spelling or formatting was eliminated.

Let file $E = (e_{ij})$, $1 \leq i \leq N$, $1 \leq j \leq N_c$ be a file with N records (rows) and N_c fields (columns). Newcombe wished to divide pairs in $E \times E$ into matches M and non-matches U. Although he knew the answer, he wished to be able to match external files A against E (or B) using the odds (conditional probabilities) that he developed from matching E against itself. Let A_i represent agreement on field i, A_i^c represent disagreement on field i, and A_i^x represent agreement or disagreement on field i but not both. Newcombe's first simplifying assumption is the CI assumption that conditional on being in the set of matches M or non-matches U, agreement on field i is independent of agreement on field j:

$$\textbf{(CI)} \qquad P\left(A_i^x \cap A_j^x \mid D\right) = P\left(A_i^x \mid D\right) P\left(A_j^x \mid D\right) \qquad (2.3)$$

where D is either M or U. Under condition (CI), Newcombe then computed the odds associated with each value of a specific field. The intuition is to bring together pairs of common values of individual fields. For instance, with last name, we might consider pairs agreeing on 'Smith' or 'Zabrinsky'. Let (f_{ij}), $1 \leq j \leq I_j$ represent the specific frequencies (number of values) of the ith field. The number of matches is N, and the number of non-matches is $N \times N - N$. Among matches M, there are f_{ij} pairs that agree on the jth value of the ith field. Among non-matches U, there are $f_{ij} \times f_{ij} - f_{ij}$ pairs that agree on the ith value of the jth field. Then the odds ratio of agreement (corresponds to Eq. 2.1) on the ith value of the jth field is

$$R_{ij} = \frac{P\left(\text{agree } j\text{th value of } i\text{th field} \mid M\right)}{P\left(\text{agree } j\text{th value of } i\text{th field} \mid U\right)} \qquad (2.4)$$

$$= \left(\frac{f_{ij}}{N}\right) \bigg/ \left(f_{ij} \times f_{ij} - f_{ij}\right) \bigg/ \left(N \times N - N\right)$$

If pairs are taken from two files (i.e. product space of $A \times B$), then we can use f_{ij} as the frequency in A, g_{ij} as the frequency in B and h_{ij} as the frequency in $A \cap B$ (that is usually approximated with $h_{ij} = \min(f_{ij}, g_{ij})$). There are equivalent random agreement probabilities in the case of $A \times B$.

We notice that the sum of the probabilities of the numerator in Equation 2.4 sums to 1. In practice, we assume that the sum of the probabilities is $1 - \varepsilon$ where $0 < \varepsilon < 0.1$ and multiply all of the numerators in Equation 2.4 by $1 - \varepsilon$. This allows a small probability of disagreement $\varepsilon > 0$ and $P(A_1|M) = 1 - \varepsilon$. The values of the $\varepsilon > 0$ were chosen via experience. In some situations, there was clerical review on a subset of pairs, and the $P(A_1|M)$ were re-estimated. Although the re-estimation (possibly after several iterations) was cumbersome, it did work well in practice.

Newcombe and others had observed the probabilities in the denominator could be approximated by random agreement probabilities

$$P\left(A_i \mid U\right) \approx P\left(A_i\right) = \sum_j \frac{f_{ij} f_{ij}}{N^2} \tag{2.5}$$

Formula (2.5) is a reasonable approximation when the set of matches M is not known. There are equivalent random agreement probabilities in the case of $A \times B$. In the situation of $A \times B$, we replace the second occurrence of f_{ij} with g_{ij} (the corresponding frequency from B) in Equations 2.4 and 2.5 as in Newcombe et al. (1959) or Newcombe and Kennedy (1962).

2.2.2.2   The methods of Fellegi and Sunter

Fellegi and Sunter (1969, Theorem 1) proved the optimality of the classification rule given by (2.2). Their proof is very general in the sense in it holds for any representations $\gamma \in \Gamma$ over the set of pairs in the product space $A \times B$ from two files. As they observed, the quality of the results from classification rule (2.2) were dependent on the accuracy of the estimates of $P(\gamma \in \Gamma|M)$ and $P(\gamma \in \Gamma|U)$.

Fellegi and Sunter (1969) were the first to give very general methods for computing these probabilities in situations that differ from the situations of Newcombe in the previous section. As the methods are useful, we describe what they introduced and then show how the ideas led into more general methods that can be used for *unsupervised learning* (i.e. without training data) in a large number of situations. Fellegi and Sunter observed several things. First,

$$P(S) = P(S|M)P(M) + P(S|U)P(U) \tag{2.6}$$

for any set S of pairs in $A \times B$. The probability on the left can be computed directly from the set of pairs. If sets A^x represent simple agreement/disagreement on a single field, under CI with three fields, we obtain

$$P\left(A_1^x \cap A_2^x \cap A_3^x \mid D\right) = P\left(A_1^x \mid D\right) P\left(A_2^x \mid D\right) P\left(A_3^x \mid D\right) \tag{2.7}$$

then (2.6) and (2.7) provide seven equations and seven unknowns (as x represent agree or disagree) that yield quadratic equations that they solved. Here, D is either M or U. Equation (or set of equations) 2.7 is essentially the same as Equation 2.3 and can be expanded to k fields where $k > 3$. Although there are eight patterns associated with the equations of the form (2.7), we eliminate one because the probabilities must add to one. In general, with more fields but still simple agreement/disagreement between fields, the equations can be solved via the EM algorithm as described in the next section.

Fellegi and Sunter provided more general methods for frequency-based matching (value-specific) matching than those of Newcombe. Specifically, they obtained the general probabilities for simple agree/disagree and then scaled the frequency-based probabilities to the agree/disagree weights. If A_i represents agreement on the ith field and $f_{ij}, 1 \le j \le I_i$ are the frequency values of the ith field, then

$$P(A_i|D) = \sum_j P(A_i \cap f_{ij}|D) \qquad (2.8)$$

where D is either M or U. Typically, $P(A_i|M) < 1$ for the simple agree/disagree weights on field i. This reflects the fact that there is less than 100% agreement for matches on the ith field. Superficially, we can think of the $1 - P(A_i|M)$ as the average error rate in the ith field (usually due to typographical error). To make Equation 2.8 valid under certain restrictions, Fellegi and Sunter assumed that the typographical error rate was constant over all values $f_{ij}, 1 \le j \le I_i$, associated with the ith field. Winkler (1989b) extended the frequency-based ideas of Fellegi and Sunter by showing how to do the computation under significantly weaker form of CI. The details of the computations (which we have greatly simplified) are given in their papers (Fellegi and Sunter, 1969; Winkler, 1989b).

There are a number of implicit assumptions that are often made when matching two files and computing probabilities using (2.6), (2.7) and (2.8). The first is that there is significant overlap between two files A and B. This essentially means that $A \cap B$ is either most of A or most of B. If this assumption is not true, then the probabilities obtained via Newcombe's methods or the Fellegi and Sunter methods may not work well. The second assumption is that neither file A nor B can simultaneously be samples from two larger files A_2 and B_2. Deming and Gleser (1959) provided theory demonstrating the unreliability of determining the sampling overlap (i.e. number of duplicates) from two sample files. As a case in point, if $A_2 = B_2$ each contain 1000 records on which 1% have the last name of 'Smith', among the matches M between A_2 and B_2, there is a 1% probability of being a pair agreeing on 'Smith' actually being a match. If A and B are 10% samples of A_2 and B_2, respectively, then among matches between A and B, there is a 0.1% probability of a pair agreeing on 'Smith' actually being a match. The third assumption is that the typographical error rates are quite low so the frequency-based computations based on the different observed values of the fields are valid. If a relatively rare value of last name such as 'Zabrinsky' has six different spellings in the six records in which it appeared, then it is not possible to compute accurate frequency-based probabilities directly from the file.

2.2.2.3   Expectation–Maximisation algorithm

In this section, we do not go into much detail about the Expectation–Maximisation (EM) algorithm because the basic algorithm is well understood (Dempster et al., 1977). Under CI, EM methods for statistical mixture models (also called latent-class models) are given in Titterington et al. (1988) and for general data and for record linkage in Winkler (1988). If CI does not hold (see, e.g. Bishop, Fienberg and Holland, 1975), then general algorithms are given in Winkler (1993b).

In each of the variants given later, either M and U, C_1 and C_2 or C_1, C_2 and C_3 partition $A \times B$. Smith and Newcombe (1975) were the first to observe that simultaneously accounting for name and address characteristics (three classes: C_1, matches within households; C_2, non-matches within households; and C_3, non-matches outside households partition $A \times B$) yielded substantially better record linkage parameters for certain medical follow-up procedures (see also Gill, 2001). We provide a moderate amount of detail for the record linkage application so that we can describe a number of the limitations of the EM and some of the extensions. The formal extension of the Newcombe–Smith ideas to a three-class EM yielded higher-quality parameters (better separation between matches and non-matches – see Figure 2.1) than the more ad hoc methods of Smith and Newcombe (1975).

For each $\in \Gamma$, we consider

$$P(\gamma) = P(\gamma | M) P(M) + P(\gamma | U) P(U) \tag{2.9a}$$

$$P(\gamma) = P(\gamma | C_1) P(C_1) + P(\gamma | C_2) P(C_2) \tag{2.9b}$$

$$P(\gamma) = P(\gamma | C_1) P(C_1) + P(\gamma | C_2) P(C_2) + P(\gamma | C_3) P(C_3) \tag{2.9c}$$

and note that the proportion of pairs having representation $\gamma \in \Gamma$ (i.e. left-hand side of Eq. 2.8) can be computed directly from available data.

If the number of fields associated with γ is $k > 3$, then we can solve the combination of equations given by (2.9) and (2.7) using the EM algorithm. Although there are alternate methods of solving the equation such as methods of moments and least squares, the EM is greatly preferred because of its numeric stability (Titterington et al., 1988). Under CI (Eq. 2.7), programming is simplified and computation is greatly reduced (from the order of 2^{k+1} to $2k$). If Equation 2.7 is extended to k fields, then there are k parameters for m-probabilities and k parameters for u-probabilities on the right-hand side of the extended (2.7). There are 2×2^k probabilities on the left-hand side of (2.7) when it is extended to interactions between fields.

Caution must be observed when applying the EM algorithm to real data. The EM algorithm that has been applied to record linkage is a *latent-class algorithm* that is intended to divide $A \times B$ into the desired sets of pairs M and U. The probability of a class indicator that determines whether a pair is in M or U is the missing data must be estimated along with the m- and u-probabilities. It may be necessary to apply the EM algorithm to a particular subset S of pairs in $A \times B$ in which most of the matches M are concentrated, for which the fields used for matching clearly can separate M from U and for which suitable initial probabilities can be chosen. Because the EM is a local maximisation algorithm, the starting probabilities may need to be chosen with care based on experience with similar types of files. Because the two-class EM latent-class algorithm is a general clustering algorithm, there is no assurance that the algorithm will divide $A \times B$ into two classes C_1 and C_2 that almost precisely correspond to M and U. Similarly, the three-class EM may not yield three classes C_1, C_2 and C_3 where C_2 are non-matches within the same household, C_3 are non-matches outside the same household and U is given by $U = C_2 \cup C_3$.

Because the EM-based methods of this section serve as a template for other EM-based methods (Section 2.4.1), we provide details of the unsupervised learning methods of Winkler (2006b) that are used for estimating false-match rates. The basic model is that of semi-supervised learning in which we combine a small proportion of labelled (true or pseudo-true matching status) pairs of records with a very large amount of unlabelled data. The CI model corresponds to the naïve Bayesian network formulisation of Nigam et al. (2000). The more general formulisation of Winkler (2000; 2002) allows interactions between agreements (but is not used in here).

Our development is similar theoretically to that of Nigam et al. (2000). The notation differs very slightly because it deals more with the representational framework of record linkage. Let γ_i be the agreement pattern associated with record pair $r_i = (\gamma_{i1}, \ldots, \gamma_{ik})$. Classes C_j are an arbitrary partition of the set of pairs S in $A \times B$. Later, we will assume that some of the C_j will be subsets of M and the remaining C_j are subsets of U. For coherence and clarity Equations 2.10 and 2.11, repeat earlier Equations 2.3 or 2.7 but use a slightly different notation that brings in the parameter Θ that we are estimating and which was implicit in Equations 2.3 and 2.7. The parameter Θ might refer to a specific type of model such as multinomial or Dirichlet multinomial (see, e.g. Agresti, 2007; Bishop, Fienberg and Holland, 1975). Unlike general text classification (Nigam et al., 2000) in which every document may have a unique agreement pattern, in record linkage, some agreement patterns γ_i may have many pairs $p_{i(1)}$ associated with them. Specifically,

$$P(\gamma_i | \Theta) = \sum_i^{|C|} P(\gamma_i | C_j ; \Theta) P(C_j ; \Theta)$$

(2.10)

where i is a specific pair, C_j is a specific class and the sum is over the set of classes. Under the naïve Bayes or CI, we have

$$P(\gamma_i | C_j ; \Theta) = \prod_k P(\gamma_{i,k} | C_j ; \Theta)$$

(2.11)

where the product is over the kth individual field agreement γ_{ik} in pair agreement pattern γ_i. In some situations, we use a Dirichlet prior

$$P(\Theta) = \prod_j (\Theta_{C_j})^{\alpha-1} \prod_k (\Theta_{\gamma_{i,k|C_j}})^{\alpha-1}$$

(2.12)

where the first product is over the classes C_j and the second product is over the fields. With very small values of the Dirichlet prior, we can generally assume that a maximum likelihood estimate exists and estimates of the probabilities associated with each of the cells in the contingency table associated with the γ_{ik} will stay away from zero. We use D_u to denote unlabelled pairs and D_1 to denote labelled pairs. Given the set $D = D_1 \cup D_u$ of all labelled and unlabelled pairs, the complete-data log likelihood is given by

$$L_c(\Theta | D; z) = \log(P(\Theta)) + (1-\lambda) \sum_{i \in D_u} \sum_i z_{ij} \log(P(\gamma_i | C_j ; \Theta) P(C_j ; \Theta))$$

$$+ \lambda \sum_{i \in D_1} \sum_j z_{ij} \log(P(\gamma_i | C_j ; \Theta) P(C_j ; \Theta))$$

(2.13)

where $0 \le \lambda \le 1$ represents the proportional emphasis given to the labelled pairs where we know true matching status. The first sum is over the unlabelled pairs, and the second sum is over the labelled pairs. In the third terms Equation 2.13, we sum over the observed z_{ij}. In the second term, we put in expected values for the z_{ij} based on the initial estimates $P(\gamma_i | C_j ; \Theta)$ and $P(C_j; \Theta)$. After re-estimating the parameters $P(\gamma_i | C_j ; \Theta)$ and $P(C_j; \Theta)$ during the M-step (that is in closed form under condition (CI)), we put in new expected values and repeat the M-step. The computer algorithms are easily monitored by checking that the likelihood increases after each combination of E- and M-steps and by checking that the sum of the probabilities adds to 1.0. We observe that if λ is 1, then we only use training data and our methods correspond to naïve Bayes methods for which training data are available. If λ is 0, then we are in the unsupervised learning situations of Winkler (1993b; 1988). Winkler (2000; 2002) provides more details of the computational algorithms. Because we have never had training data, we delay a discussion of it until Section 2.2.2.4.

More generally, we may wish to account for dependencies (lack of CI) between identifiers directly by using appropriate log-linear models (Bishop, Fienberg and Holland, 1975). Winkler (1993b) provides a general EMH algorithm that accounts for the general interactions between fields and allows convex constraints to predispose certain estimated probabilities into regions based on a priori information used in similar matching projects. The EMH algorithm is a form of Monte Carlo EM (MCEM) algorithm (Meng and Rubin, 1993) that additionally allows convex constraints. The interaction EM can yield parameters that yield slight improvements in matching efficacy (Larsen and Rubin, 2001; Winkler, 2002). The interaction EM is much more difficult to apply because of its sensitivity to moderate changes in the set of interactions and the fact the likelihood surface is quite flat in relation to the CI EM (Professor Donald B. Rubin, personal communication). Winkler (1993b) and Larsen and Rubin (2001) demonstrated that effective sets of interactions can be selected based on experience. The starting point for the interaction EM is the set of parameters from the CI EM.

2.2.2.4   Linkage with and without training data

Representative training data are seldom available for estimating parameters for record linkage classification rules. If training data are available, then it is possible to estimate the parameters by adding appropriate quantities to yield the probabilities in (2.1) and (2.2). In fact, with sufficient training data, it is straightforward to estimate probabilities in (2.1) that account for the dependencies between different matching fields and to estimate error rates.

At the US Census Bureau, we have several high-quality training datasets that were obtained after certain matching operations. All pertinent pairs or a large subset of pairs are reviewed by two individuals. A third individual then arbitrates when there is a discrepancy between the first two individuals. The training (truth) data are used to evaluate the matching operations after the fact and to facilitate of the development of newer methods.

Winkler (1989a) showed that optimal record linkage parameters vary significantly in different geographic regions. For the 1990 US Decennial Census, training data would have been needed for the 457 regions where matching was performed. The amount of time needed to obtain the training data in the 457 regions would have substantially exceeded the 6 weeks that were allotted for the computer matching. In more than 20 years of record linkage at the Census Bureau, there have never been training data. In more than 30 years in maintaining the national health files and performing other large matching projects at Oxford University, Gill (2000, private communication) never had training data.

In the case of no training data, Ravikumar and Cohen (2004) provided EM-based unsupervised learning methods that improved upon the methods of Winkler (1988; 1993b). Bhattacharya and Getoor (2006) provided MCMC methods that improved over previous EM-based methods. The key idea in the unsupervised learning methods was providing more structure (based on prior knowledge such as restrictive distributions in the statistical mixture models.) that forced the parameter estimates into a narrow range of possibilities that were more appropriate for the particular record linkage situation.

Larsen and Rubin (2001) provided MCMC methods of semi-supervised learning where moderate amounts of training data were labelled with true matching status and were combined with unlabelled data. Winkler provided EM-based methods for semi-supervised learning (see Section 2.4.1) that were very slightly worse than the methods of Larsen and Rubin but were between 100 and 1000 times as fast (~10 minutes in each of ~500 regions). The advantage of the semi-supervised learning methods is that if we can take a suitable sample of (say, 100–200) pairs near the upper cut-off T_μ in Equation 2.2 for each of approximately 500 regions, then the amount of clerical review is very significantly reduced and false-match rates can be much more accurately estimated (Section 2.4.1).

2.2.2.5   Alternative machine learning models

The standard model of record linkage is CI (naïve Bayes) that has been extended to general interaction models by Winkler (1989a; 1993b) and Larsen and Rubin (2001). In machine learning, support vector machines (SVMs, Vapnik, 2000) and boosting (Freund and Schapire, 1996; Hastie et al., 2001) typically outperform naïve Bayes classifiers (same as CI) and other well-understood methods such as logistic regression. In this section, we describe the four classifiers in terms of theoretical properties and observed empirical performance. We begin by translating the notation of the four classifiers into a vector space format. If $r_i = (\gamma_{i1}, ..., \gamma_{ik})$ represents an agreement pattern for a record pair r_i of k fields used for comparison and $(\gamma_{i1}, ..., \gamma_{ik})$ are agreement vectors associated with the k fields only taking values 1 or 0 for agree and disagree, respectively, then, in the simplest situations, we are interested in a set of weights $w = (w_1, ..., w_k)$ such that

$$S(r_i) = \sum_{j-1}^{k} w_j \gamma_{ij} > C_H \text{ means the pair } r_i \text{ is a match (in one class),}$$

$$S(r_i) = \sum_{j-1}^{k} w_j \gamma_{ij} \leq C_L \text{ means the pair } r_i \text{ is a non-match (in other class)}$$

and, otherwise, the pair is held for clerical review. In most situations, $C_H = C_L$, and we designate the common value by C. The rule above corresponds to Equation 2.2, but the different methods provide different estimates of the weights w_i that are roughly equivalent to CI. In this section, we assume that representative training data are always available. In logistic regression, we learn the weights w according to the logistic regression paradigm. In SVM, we learn an optimal separating linear hyperplane having weights w that best separate M and U (Vapnik, 2000). With N steps of boosting, we select a set of initial weights w^o and successively train new weights w^i where the record pairs r that are misclassified on the previous step are given a different weighting. The starting weight w^o is usually set to $1/n$ for each record where n is the number of record pairs in the training data. As usual with training data, the number in one class (matches) needs to be approximately equal the number of pairs in the other class (non-matches). Ng and Jordan (2002) and Zhang and Oles (2001) have demonstrated that logistic regression can be considered an approximation of SVMs and that SVMs should, in theory, perform better than logistic regression.

Ng and Jordan (2002) have also demonstrated empirically and theoretically that SVM-like procedures will often outperform naïve Bayes. Various authors have demonstrated that boosting is competitive with SVM. In record linkage under CI, each weight $w_j = P(\gamma_{.j}|M)/P(\gamma_{.j}|U)$ for individual field agreements $\gamma_{.j}$ on the jth field is constant for all records r_j. The weighting of this type of record linkage is a straightforward linear weighting. In theory, SVM and boosting should outperform basic record linkage (possibly not by much) because the weights w are optimal for the type of linear weighting used in the decision rule. One reason that SVM or boosting may not improve much is that record linkage weights that are computed via an EM algorithm also tend to provide better separation than weights computed under a pure CI assumption (Herzog et al., 2010; Larsen, 2005; Winkler, 1990). Additionally, the CI assumption may not be valid. If CI does not hold, then the linear weighting of the scores $S(r)$ is not optimal. Alternate, non-linear methods, such as given by Winkler (1989a; 1993b) or Larsen and Rubin (2001) may be needed.

There are several research issues. The first issue is to determine the situations where SVM or boosting substantially outperforms the Fellegi–Sunter classification rule (2.2). Naïve Bayes is known to be computationally much faster and more straightforward than SVM, boosting or logistic regression. Belin and Rubin (1995) observed that logistic regression classification is not competitive with Fellegi–Sunter classification. The second issue is whether it is possible to develop SVM or boosting methods that work with only unlabelled data (Winkler, 1988; 1993b) or work in a semi-supervised manner as is done in record linkage (Winkler, 2002). Extensions of the standard Fellegi–Sunter methods can inherently deal with interactions between fields (Winkler, 1993b) even in unsupervised learning situations. Determining the interactions can be somewhat straightforward for experienced individuals (Larsen and Rubin, 2001; Winkler, 1993b). SVM can only be extended to interactions via kernels that are often exceedingly difficult to determine effectively even with training data. Fellegi–Sunter methods can deal with nearly automatic methods for estimating error (false-match) rates in semi-supervised situations (Winkler, 2002) or in a narrow range of unsupervised situations (Winkler, 2006b). Accurately estimating error rates is known as the *regression problem* that is very difficult with SVM or boosting even when large amounts of training data are available (Hastie et al., 2001; Vapnik, 2000).

2.2.3   Additional methods for matching

In this section, we describe methods of approximate string comparison that are used to adjust the likelihoods in Equation 2.1 using in the classification rule (2.2) and methods of blocking for only considering greatly reduced subsets of pairs in $A \times B$ without significantly increasing the number of false matches. String comparators and methods for cleaning-up, parsing and standardising names and addresses often yield greater improvements in matching efficacy (reduced false-match and false non-match rates) than improving the parameter-estimation methods given in Section 2.2.2.

2.2.3.1   String comparators

In most matching situations, we will get poor matching performance when we compare two strings exactly (character by character) because of typographical error. Dealing with typographical error via approximate string comparison has been a major research project in computer science (see, e.g. Hall and Dowling, 1980; Navarro, 2001). *Approximate string comparison* refers to comparing two strings containing typographical error such as 'Smith' with 'Smoth'. All string comparators need to deal with the three basic types of typographical error of insertions, deletions and transpositions. In record linkage, we can apply a function that represents approximate agreement, with agreement being represented by 1 and degrees of partial agreement being represented by numbers between 0 and 1. We also need to adjust the probabilities in (2.1) according to the partial agreement values, for example, by multiplying by the partial agreement values. Having such methods is crucial to matching. For instance, in a major census application for measuring under-count, more than 25% of matches would not have been found via exact character-by-character matching (Winkler, 1990). For further developments of the use of string comparators, see Cohen et al. (2003a; 2003b) and Yancey (2005).

Code for the Jaro–Winkler string comparator in C is available at National Institute of Standards and Technology (2005), in C++ at LingPipe (2007) and in Java at StackOverflow (2010). A Google search will yield versions in other languages.

2.2.3.2   Blocking

In practice, it is necessary to perform *blocking* of two files that affects how pairs are brought together. If two files A and B each contain 10000 records, then there are 10^8 pairs in the product $A \times B$. Until very recently, we could not do the computation of 10^8 pairs. In *blocking*, we only consider pairs that agree on certain characteristics. For instance, we may only con-sider pairs that agree on first initial of first name, last name and date of birth. If we believe (possibly based on prior experience) that we are not getting a sufficiently large proportion of matches with a first blocking criteria, we may try a second. For instance, we may only con-sider pairs that agree on first initial of first name, first initial of last name and the ZIP + 4 code (which represents ~50 households). Fellegi and Sunter gave the straightforward theoretical extensions for blocking. In performing computation over pairs P_1 in $A \times B$ obtained via block-ing, there is a fourth implicit assumption: that the pairs in P_1 contain a moderately high proportion of matches (say, $3 + \%$ of P_1 consists of matches). In the next section, we return to the minimal needed proportion of pairs required to be matches in more general situations. The methods of obtaining the probabilities given by (2.6), (2.7) and (2.8) break down when the proportion of matches from M in the set of pairs P_1 is too low. The computations also break down if we do the computation over all 10^8 pairs in $A \times B$. In $A \times B$, at most 0.01% of the pairs are matches.

Bilenko et al. (2006), Michelson and Knoblock (2006) and Kenig and Gal (2013) have done blocking research that relies on training data. The more recent work by Kenig and Gal might be extended to certain unsupervised situations where training data are not available. Ad hoc ideas of blocking based on experience date back to Newcombe and Kennedy (1962), Newcombe (1988) and Winkler (2004). Three individuals at the Census Bureau each indepen-dently developed better blocking criteria than in Winkler (2004) and created the blocking cri-teria used in the production system used in the 2010 Decennial Census (Winkler et al., 2010). The software allowed matching 10^{17} pairs (300×300 million) in 30 hours using 40 CPUs of an SGI Linux machine. Blocking reduced the detailed computation for comparisons to 10^{12} pairs while missing an estimated 1–2% of true matches (based on validations during preliminary testing of methods). BigMatch software (Yancey and Winkler, 2006; 2009) used in the produc-tion matching is 50 times as fast as parallel P-Swoosh experimental matching software (Kawai et al., 2006), 500 times as fast as software tested at the Australia Bureau of Statistics (Wright, 2010) and 10+ times as fast as cloud-based Hadoop technology (Kolb and Rahm, 2013). The timing results are conservative in the sense that the Census Bureau SGI machine used 2006 Itanium chips and all later speed comparisons were done on faster machines.

2.2.4 An empirical example

In the following, we compare different matching procedures on the data where basic matching parameters were determined via an EM algorithm (unsupervised learning). For our production matching in the 1990 Decennial Census, we needed to find automatically 'optimal' parameters without training data and complete matching in less than 6 weeks for approximately 500 regions into which the United States was divided. The 'optimal' parameters reduced clerical review by 2/3. The results we present in the following are slightly worse than the average results over approximately 500 regions. Interestingly, the matching results with the highly structured EM are better than those with a semi-supervised procedure (summarised in the paragraphs immediately below and Table 2.2). The results are based only on pairs that agree on block identification code and first character of the last name. Herzog et al. (2010) provide more details.

The procedures that we use are as follows. The simplest procedure, *crude*, merely uses an ad hoc (but knowledgeable) guess for matching parameters and does not use string comparators. The next, *param*, does not use string comparators but does estimate the *m*- and *u*-probabilities. Such probabilities are estimated through an iterative procedure that involves manual review of matching results and successive reuse of re-estimated parameters. Such iterative-refinement procedures (a type of active or semi-supervised learning) are a feature of Statistics Canada's CANLINK system.

The third type, *param2*, uses the same probabilities as *param* and the basic Jaro string comparator. The fourth type, *em*, uses the EM algorithm for estimating parameters and the Jaro string comparator. The fifth type, *em2*, uses the EM algorithm for estimating parameters and the Winkler variant of the string comparator, which performs an upward adjustment based on the amount of agreement in the first four characters in the string.

In Table 2.2, the cut-off threshold T_μ for designated matches is determined by a 0.002 false-match rate. Each row of Table 2.2 has the same number of total pairs. The designated match pairs correspond to Equation 2.2b. The *crude* and *param* types are allowed to rise slightly above the 0.002 level because they generally have higher error levels. In each pair of columns (designated computer matches and designated clerical pairs), we break out the counts into true matches and true non-matches. In the designated matches, true non-matches are false matches.

By examining the table, we observe that a dramatic improvement in matches can occur when string comparators are first used (from *param* to *param2*). The reason is that disagreements (on a character-by-character basis) are replaced by partial agreements and adjustment of the likelihood ratios (see Winkler, 1990). The improvement due to the Winkler variant of the string comparator (from *em* to *em2*) is quite minor. The *param* method is essentially the same as a traditional method used by Statistics Canada. After a review of nine string comparator

Table 2.2   Matching results via matching strategies (0.2% false matches among designated matches).

	Designated computer match	Designated clerical pair
Truth	Match/non-match	Match/non-match
crude	310/1	9344/794
param	7899/16	1863/198
param2	9276/23	545/191
em	9587/23	271/192
em2	9639/24	215/189

methods (Budzinsky, 1991), Statistics Canada provided options for three string comparators in CANLINK software, with the Jaro–Winkler comparator being the default.

The improvement between *param2* and *em2* is not quite as dramatic because it is much more difficult to show improvements among 'hard-to-match' pairs and because of the differences in the parameter-estimation methods. Iterative refinement is used for *param2* (a standard method in CANLINK software) in which pairs are reviewed, reclassified and parameters re-estimated. This method is a type of (partially) supervised learning and is time-consuming.

The improvement due to the parameters from *em2* can be explained because the parameters are slightly more general than those obtained under CI. If A_i^x represents agreement or disagreement on the ith field, then our CI assumption yields

$$P\left(A_1^x \cap A_2^x \ldots \cap A_k^x \,|\, D\right) = \prod_{i=1}^{k} P\left(A_i^x \,|\, D\right) \tag{2.14}$$

where D is either M or U. Superficially, the EM considers different orderings of the form

$$P\left(A_{\rho,1}^x \cap A_{\rho,2}^x \ldots \cap A_{\rho,k}^x \,|\, D\right) = \prod_{i=1}^{k} P\left(A_{\rho,i}^x \,|\, A_{\rho,i-1}^x, \ldots, A_{\rho,1}^x, D\right) \tag{2.15}$$

where ρ, i represents the ith entry in a permutation ρ of the integers 1 thru k. The greater generality of (2.15) in comparison to (2.14) can yield better fits to the data. We can reasonably assume that the EM algorithm under the CI assumption (as the actual computational methods work) simultaneously chooses the best permutation ρ and the best parameters. Alternate methods for approximating general interaction models (left-hand side of 2.15) called the Generalised Naive Bayes Classifiers were discovered by Kim Larsen (2005). Larsen's extensions use ideas from generalised additive models and should be far slower to compute than the algorithms used by Winkler (1988).

During 1990 production matching, the EM algorithm showed its flexibility. In three regions among a number of regions processed in 1 week, clerical review became much larger with the EM parameters than was expected. Upon quick review, we discovered that two keypunchers had managed to bypass edits on the year of birth. All records from these keypunchers disagreed on the computed age. The clerical review became much larger because first name and the age were the main fields for separating persons within a household.

In this section, we have demonstrated that very dramatic improvement in record linkage efficacy through advancing from seemingly reasonable ad hoc procedures to procedures that use modern computerised record linkage procedures. The issue that affects government agencies and other groups is whether their registers and survey frames are well maintained because of effective procedures.

2.3   Data preparation

In matching projects, putting the data from two files A and B into consistent forms so that the data can be run through record linkage software often requires more work (3–12 months with a moderate or large staff) than the actual matching operations (1–3 weeks with one individual). Inability or lack of time and resources for cleaning up files in preparation for matching are often the main reasons that matching projects fail. We provide details of file acquisition, preparation and standardisation in the next sections.

2.3.1   Description of a matching project

Constructing a frame or administrative list entities for an entire country or a large region of a country involves many steps. The construction methods also hold pairs of lists to help find duplicates within a given list:

1. Identify existing lists that can be used in creating the main list. In this situation, it is important to concentrate on 10 or fewer lists. It is practically infeasible to consider thousands of lists.

2. With each list, obtain an annotated layout. The annotation should include the locations of different fields and the potential values that different fields can assume. For instance, a given list may have several status codes associated with whether the entity is still in business or alive. With lists of businesses, the list may have additional status codes denoting whether the record is associated with another entity as a subsidiary or duplicate. If the annotated layout is not available, then reject the list. If the list is on an incompatible computer system or in an incompatible format such as a typed list or microfiche, then reject the list.

3. Obtain the lists to begin putting them in a standard format that will be used by the duplicate-detection and updating programs. If the list will not pass through name and address standardisation programs (Sections 2.3.3 and 2.3.4), then reject it. If some or many records in the list cannot be standardised, then consider rejecting the list or only use records that can be standardised. The standard format should include a field for the source of a list and the date of the list. If possible, it is a good idea to also have a date for the individual record in the list.

4. If resources permit, greater accuracy may be obtained by matching each potential update source against the main list sequentially. Matching each list in a sequential manner allows more accurate clerical clean-up of duplicates. If the clerical clean-up cannot be done in an efficient manner, then duplicates in the main list will yield more and more additional duplicates as the main list is successively updated. If it appears that an individual list is causing too many duplicates to be erroneously added to the main list, then reject the list as an update source. If a large subset of the update source does not yield a sufficiently large number of new entities in the main list, then it might also be excluded.

5. After the initial matching, additional computerised and clerical procedures should be systematically applied for further identifying duplicates in the main list. A very useful procedure is to assure that the representations of names and addresses associated with an entity are in the most useful form and free of typographical errors. These extra improvement procedures should be used continuously. If updates and clean-ups of lists containing many small businesses are only done annually, then the overall quality of the list can deteriorate in an additive fashion during each subsequent update.

Many matching projects fail because groups cannot even get through the first 1–2 steps above. Maintaining certain types of lists can be difficult because addresses associated with individuals can change frequently. In the United States, the postal change of address files for individuals represent 16% of the population per year. Some individuals may move more than once. With lists of small business (such as petroleum retailers), the change of name or address can exceed 10% per year. In maintaining a large national health file or national death index, 1–3% net error per year can yield substantial error after several years. Certain sources used in updating the national registers can contain typographical error in names or date of birth.

2.3.2   Initial file preparation

In obtaining the files, the first issue is to determine whether the files reside in sequential (standard flat) files, databases or SAS files. As most record linkage software is designed for only sequential files, files in other formats will need to have copies that are in sequential formats. Some groups that do record linkage with many files will have a standard format and procedures so that the files are in the most compatible form for record linkage. An annotated layout will give the descriptions of individual fields that might be compared. For instance, a sex code might be broken out into Sex1 (male=M, female=F, missing=b where b represents blank) or Sex2 (male=1, female=2, missing=0). Simple programs can have tables that are used in converting from one set of codes to another set of codes.

It is very typical for well-maintained files to carry status codes indicating whether an entity is still alive or in business and whether information such as an address or telephone number is current. If a file has status codes indicating that certain records are out of scope, then in most matching applications, the out-of-scope records should be dropped before using the file for updating or merging. In some files, it may be difficult to determine out of scopes. For instance, electric utilities have very good address information that individuals might wish to use in updating a list of residences. Unfortunately, electric utilities typically include small commercial establishments with residential customers because they maintain their lists by flow-rate categories. If the electric utility list is used to update a list of households, many 'out-of-scope' commercial addresses will be added.

It may be necessary to review various fields across two files. For instance, if one file has addresses that are almost entirely of the form house-number-street-name and another file has a substantial portion of the addresses in the form PO box, then it may be difficult to match to two files using name and address information. With lists of businesses, it may be necessary to have auxiliary information that allows separating headquarters from subsidiaries. With many businesses, headquarters fill out survey forms. If a survey form is sent to the subsidiary and returned, then the survey organisation may double count the information from the subsidiary that is also reported in the totals from the headquarters.

In the following, we provide summaries of various procedures that can be used for the preliminary cleaning of files and can often be in straightforward computer routines. In record linkage, a variable (or field) is typically a character string such as a complete name, complete address or a sub-component such as first name or last name. These consistency checks and clean-up procedures prior to running files through a matching program are referred to as *standardisation*:

1. Replacing spelling variants with a common consistent spelling is referred to as *spelling standardisation*:

   (a) Replace 'Doctor' and 'Dr.' with 'Dr'.

   (b) Replace nicknames such as 'Bob' and 'Bill' with 'Robert' and 'William'.

   (c) Replace words such as 'Company', 'Cmpny' and 'Co.' with 'Co'.

Note: The third example is application dependent because 'Co' can refer to county or Colorado.

2. Replacing inconsistent codes is referred to as assuring *code consistency*:

   (a) Replace Sex (male = '1', female = '2', missing = '0') with (male = 'M', female = 'F', missing = ' ').

   (b) Replace 'January 11, 1999' and '11 January, 1999' with MMDDYYYY = '01111999' or YYYMMDD = '19990111'.

Code consistency is sometimes referred to as making the value states of variables (or fields) consistent.

3. Identifying the starting and ending positions of the individual components of a free-form string such as a name or address is referred to as *parsing*:

   (a) Identify locations of first name, middle initial and last name in 'Mr John A Smith Jr' and 'John Alexander Smith'.

   (b) Identify locations of house number and street name in '123 East Main Street' and '123 E. Main St. Apt. 16'.

The idea of parsing is to allow the comparison of fields (variables) that should be consistent and reasonably easy to compare. It is not easy to compare free-form names and addresses except possibly manually. The above three ideas of standardisation are often preliminary to situations when free-form names and addresses are broken (parsed) into components. We cover general name and address standardisation in the next two sections.

2.3.3   Name standardisation and parsing

Standardisation consists of replacing various spellings of words with a single spelling. For instance, different spellings and abbreviations of 'Incorporated' might be replaced with the single standardised spelling 'Inc.' The standardisation component of software might separate a general string such as a complete name or address into words (i.e. sets of characters that are separated by spaces and other delimiters). Each word is then compared to lookup tables to get standard spelling. The first half of Table 2.3 shows various commonly occurring words that are replaced by standardised spellings (given in capital letters). After standardisation, the name string is parsed into components (second half of the following table) that can be compared. The examples are produced by general name standardisation software (Winkler, 1993a) for the US Census of Agriculture matching system. Because the software does well with business lists and person matching, it has been used for additional matching applications at the Census Bureau and other agencies. At present, it is not clear that there is any commercial software for name standardisation. Promising new methods based on hidden Markov models (Borkar et al., 2001; Christen et al., 2002; Churches et al., 2002) may improve over the rule-based name standardisation in Winkler (1993a). Although the methods clearly improve over more conventional address standardisation methods (see following section) for difficult

Table 2.3 Examples of name parsing.

Standardised
1.   DR John J. Smith MD
2.   Smith DRY FRM
3.   Smith & Son ENTP

				Parsed				
	PRE	FIRST	MID	LAST	POST1	POST2	BUS1	BUS2
1.	DR	John	J	Smith	MD			
2.				Smith			DRY	FRM
3.				Smith		Son	ENTP	

situations such as Asian or Indian addresses, they did not perform as well as more conventional methods of name standardisation. Bilmes (1998) provides a tutorial on EM-type algorithms that show that hidden Markov methods are slight generalisations of the simplest EM methods. Among mathematical statisticians, hidden Markov is referred to as the Baum–Welch algorithm.

2.3.4   Address standardisation and parsing

The following table illustrates address standardisation with a proprietary package developed by the Geography Division at the US Census Bureau. In testing in 1994, the software significantly outperformed the best US commercial packages in terms of standardisation rates while producing comparably accurate standardisations. The first half of the Table 2.4 shows a few addresses that have been standardised. In standardisation, commonly occurring words such as 'Street' are replaced by an appropriate abbreviation such as 'St' that can be considered a standard spelling that may account for some spelling errors. The second half of the table represents components of addresses produced by the parsing. The general software produces approximately 50 components. The general name and address standardisation software that we make available with the matching software only outputs the most important components of the addresses.

2.3.5   Summarising comments on preprocessing

Many files cannot be sufficiently preprocessed to clean up much of the data. Examples include legacy files that contain considerable missing data such as blank date of birth and high typographical error rate in other fields. In situations of reasonably high-quality data, preprocessing can yield a greater improvement in matching efficacy than string comparators and 'optimised' parameters. In some situations, 90% of the improvement in matching efficacy may be due to preprocessing. The results of Table 2.2 show that appropriate string comparators can yield greater improvement than better record linkage parameters. Other significant advances in preprocessing to standardise names and addresses using hidden Markov models are due to Christen et al. (2002), Churches et al. (2002), Agichstein and Ganti (2004) and Cohen and Sarawagi (2004).

Table 2.4   Examples of address parsing.

Standardised
1. 16 W Main ST APT 16
2. RR 2 BX 215
3. Fuller BLDG SUITE 405
4. 14588 HWY 16 W

		Parsed							
PRE2	HOUSE NAME	STREET NAME	RR	BOX	POST1	POST2	UNIT1	UNIT2	BUILDING
1. W	16	Main			ST		16		
2.			2	215					
3.								405	Fuller
	14588	HWY	16			W			

2.4   Advanced methods

In this section, we describe more advanced applications of the EM algorithm. We also describe MCMC methods that can often improve the EM algorithm in terms of applications that are presently more advanced and provide more insight than current applications of the EM algorithm. Our initial concern with the EM and the basic MCMC is in providing estimates of false-match rates (closely related to precision) in unsupervised learning situations (no training data) and in semi-supervised learning situations (where modest amounts of training data are combined with readily obtained unlabelled data).

2.4.1   Estimating false-match rates without training data

In this section, we provide a summary of current extensions of the EM procedures for estimating false-match rates. To estimate false-match rates, we need to have reasonably accurate estimates of the right tail of the curve of non-matches and the left tail of the curve of matches such as given in Figure 2.1. Similar methods, but with less data, were given in Belin and Rubin (1995). With any matching project, we are concerned with false-match rates among the set of pairs among designated matches above the cut-off score T_μ in (2.2) and the false non-match rates among designated non-matches below the cut-off score T_λ in (2.2). Very few matching projects estimate these rates although valid estimates are crucial to understanding the usefulness of any files obtained via the record linkage procedures. Sometimes reasonable upper bounds for the estimated error rates can be obtained via experienced practitioners, and the error rates are validated during follow-up studies (Winkler, 1995). If a moderately large amount of training data is available, then it may be possible to get valid estimates of the error rates.

If a small amount of training data is available, then it may be possible to improve record linkage and good estimates of error rates. Larsen and Rubin (2001) combined small amounts of (labelled) training data with large amounts of unlabelled data to estimate error rates using an MCMC procedure. In machine learning (Winkler, 2000), the procedures are referred to as *semi-supervised learning*. In ordinary machine learning, the procedures to estimate parameters are 'supervised' by the training data that is labelled with the true classes into which later records (or pairs) will be classified. Winkler (2002) also used semi-supervised learning with a variant of the general EM algorithm. Both the Larsen and Rubin (2001) and Winkler (2002) methods were effective because they accounted for interactions between the fields and were able to use labelled training data that was concentrated between the lower cut-off T_λ and the upper cut-off T_μ.

Belin and Rubin (1995) were the first to provide an unsupervised method for obtaining estimates of false-match rates. The method proceeded by estimating Box–Cox transforms that would cause a mixture of two transformed normal distributions to closely approximate two well-separated curves such as given in Figure 2.1. They cautioned that their methods might not be robust to matching situations with considerably different types of data. Winkler (1995) observed that their algorithms would typically not work with business lists, agriculture lists and low-quality person lists where the curves of non-matches were not well separated from the curves of matches. Scheuren and Winkler (1993), who had the Belin–Rubin EM-based fitting software, observed that the Belin–Rubin methods did work reasonably well with a number of well-separated person lists.

2.4.1.1   Example: data files

Three pairs of files were used in the analyses. The files are from 1990 Decennial Census matching data in which the entire set of 1–2% of the matching status codes that were believed to have been in error for these analyses have been corrected. The corrections reflect clerical review and field follow-up that were not incorporated in computer files originally available to us.

A summary of the overall characteristics of the empirical data is in Table 2.5. We only consider pairs that agree on census block ID (small geographic area representing ~50 households) and on the first character of surname. Less than 1–2% of the matches are missed using this set of blocking criteria. They are not considered in the analysis of this example.

The matching fields are:

Person characteristics: first name, age, marital status, sex
Household characteristics: last name, house number, street name, phone

Typically, everyone in a household will agree on the household characteristics. Person characteristics such as first name and age help distinguish individuals within household. Some pairs (including true matches) have both missing first name and age.

We also consider partial levels of agreement in which the string comparator values are broken out as [0, 0.66], (0.66, 0.88], (0.88, 0.94] and (0.94, 1.0]. The intervals were based on knowledge of how string comparators were initially modelled (Winkler, 1990) in terms of their effects of likelihood ratios (2.1). The first interval is what we refer to as disagreement. We combine the disagreement with the three partial agreements and blank to get five value states (base 5). The large base analyses consider five states for all characteristics except sex and marital status for which we consider three (agree/blank/disagree). The total number of agreement

Table 2.5   Summary of three pairs of files.

	Files		Files		Files	
	A_1	A_2	B_1	B_2	C_1	C_2
Size	15 048	12 072	4 539	4 851	5 022	5 212
# pairs		116 305		38 795		37 327
# matches		10 096		3 490		3 623

patterns is 140 625. In the earlier work (Winkler, 2002), the five levels of agreement worked consistently better than two levels (agree/disagree) or three levels (agree/blank/disagree).

The pairs naturally divide into three classes: C_1, match within household; C_2, non-match within household; and C_3, non-match outside household. In the earlier work (Winkler, 2002), we considered two dependency models in addition to the CI model. In that work in which small amounts of labelled training data were combined with unlabelled data, the CI model worked well and the dependency models worked slightly better. Dividing the matching and estimation procedures for three classes was first used by Smith and Newcombe (1975) and later by Gill (2001) without the formal likelihood models given by Equations 2.10–2.13.

We create 'pseudo-truth' datasets in which matches are those unlabelled pairs above a certain high cut-off and non-matches are those unlabelled pairs below a certain low cut-off. Figure 2.1 illustrates the situation using actual 1990 Decennial Census data in which we plot log of the probability ratio (2.1) against the log of frequency. With the datasets of this chapter, we choose high and low cut-offs in a similar manner so that we do not include in-between pairs in our designated 'pseudo-truth' datasets. We use these 'designated' pseudo-truth datasets in a semi-supervised learning procedure that is nearly identical to the semi-supervised procedure where we have actual truth data. A key difference from the corresponding procedure with actual truth data is that the sample of labelled pairs is concentrated in the difficult-to-classify in-between region where, in the 'pseudo-truth' situation, we have no way to designate comparable labelled pairs. The sizes of the 'pseudo-truth' data are given in Table 2.6. The errors associated with the artificial 'pseudo-truth' are given in parentheses following the counts. The other class gives counts of the remaining pairs and proportions of true matches that are not included in the 'pseudo-truth' set of pairs of 'matches' and 'non-matches'. In the other class, the proportions of matches vary somewhat and would be difficult to determine without training data.

We determine how accurately we can estimate the lower cumulative distributions of matches and the upper cumulative distribution of non-matches. This corresponds to the overlap region of the curves of matches and non-matches. If we can accurately estimate these two tails of distributions, then we can accurately estimate error rates at differing levels. Our comparisons consist of a set of figures in which we compare a plot of the cumulative distribution of estimates of matches versus the true cumulative distribution with the truth represented by the 45° line. As the plots get closer to the 45° lines, the estimates get closer to the truth. Our plotting is only for the bottom 30% of the curves given in Belin and Rubin (1995; Figures 2, 3). Generally, we are only interested in the bottom 10% of the curves for the purpose of estimating false-match rates. Because of the different representation with the 45% curve, we can much better compare three different methods of estimation for false-match rates.

Our primary results are from using the CI model and 'pseudo-semi-supervised' methods of this section with the CI model and actual semi-supervised methods of Winkler (2002). With our 'pseudo-truth' data, we obtain the best sets of estimates of the bottom 30% tails of the curve of matches with CI and $\lambda = 0.2$ (Eq. 2.13). Figure 2.2a–c illustrates

Table 2.6   'Pseudo-truth' data with actual error rates.

	Matches	Non-matches	Other
A pairs	8817 (0.008)	98 257 (0.001)	9231 (0.136)
B pairs	2674 (0.010)	27 744 (0.0004)	8377 (0.138)
C pairs	2492 (0.010)	31 266 (0.002)	3569 (0.369)

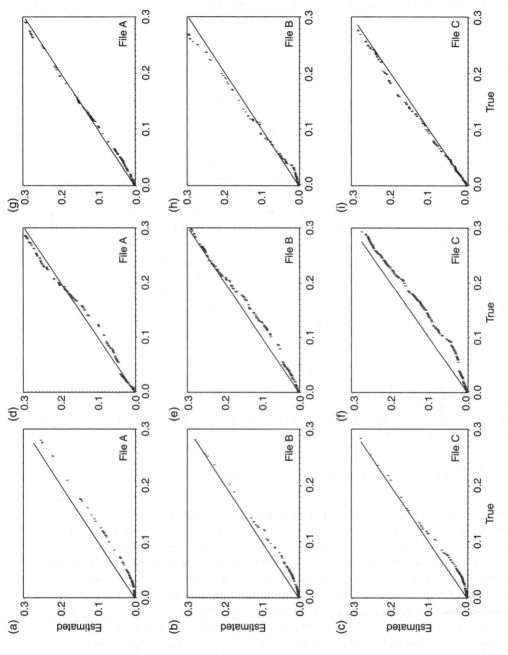

Figure 2.2 Estimates versus truth: (a–c) Cumulative matches (tail of distribution, independent EM, $\lambda = 0.2$); (d–f) Cumulative false-match rates by weight (independent EM, $\lambda = 0.2$); (g–i) Cumulative false matches (independent EM, $\lambda = 0.99$, small sample).

the set of curves that provide quite accurate fits for the estimated values of matches versus the truth. The 45° line represents the truth, whereas the curve represents the cumulative estimates of matches for the right tails of the distribution. The plots are for the estimated false-match probabilities divided by the true false-match probabilities. Although we looked at results for $\lambda = 0.1$, 0.5 and 0.8 and various interaction models, the results under CI were the best with $\lambda = 0.2$ (Eq. 2.13). We also looked at several different ways of constructing the 'pseudo-truth' data. Additionally, we considered other pairs of files in which all of the error rate estimates were better (closer to the 45° line) than those for the pair of files given in Figure 2.2.

Figure 2.2d–f shows the corresponding curves using the methods of Belin and Rubin (1995). The curves are substantially farther from the 45° lines because they are only using the distributions of weights (natural logs of likelihood ratio 2.1). Using the detailed breakout of the string comparator values, the fact that the three-class EM (Winkler, 1993b) provides much better estimates and the breakout available from Equation 2.13, we use more information that allows the estimated curves in Figure 2.2a–c to be closer to the truth than the corresponding curves in Figure 2.2d–f.

The final sets of curves (Figure 2.2g–i) are similar to the semi-supervised learning of Winkler (2002) that achieved results only very slightly worse than Larsen and Rubin (2001) but for which the EM computational speeds (10 minutes in each of ~500 regions) were at least 100 times as fast as the MCMC methods of Larsen and Rubin. It is difficult for the unsupervised methods to perform as well as the semi-supervised methods because the relatively small sample can be concentrated in the clerical review region between the lower cut-off T_λ and the upper cut-off T_μ. Because we had underlying truth data, we knew that in some regions, only 1/40 of the 'truth' sample was truly a match, whereas in other regions, 1/10 of the 'truth' sample was truly a match. In the 1990 Decennial Census, the clerical region consisted almost entirely of individuals within the same household who were missing both first name and age (the only two fields for distinguishing within the household). Because we needed to match all 457 regions of the United States in 3–6 weeks to provide estimates required by law, we could not perform clerical review in each region or use approximations across certain regions because the optimal parameters vary significantly from region to region (Winkler, 1989a).

2.4.2   Adjusting analyses for linkage error

There has been considerable work related to adjusting statistical analyses for linkage error. All the work is theoretically correct given simplifying assumptions and is able to deal with very small problems. The methods do not generally extend to the most realistic record linkage situations and large complex models. In this subsection, we will provide some background on the general problem. We will describe some of the assumptions that are made (either explicitly or implicitly) in the general papers addressing the problem and the commonality of some of the methods across the differing models. With all of the methods, we assumed that the linkage variables are independent of the analysis variables in the statistical models that must be adjusted. In a large exploratory study with more than 100 scenarios, Winkler and Scheuren (1991) had shown that it is often reasonable to assume that the linkage variables are independent of the analysis variables. Goldstein et al. (2012) provide methods for adjusting analyses when linkage variables are not necessarily independent of analysis variables.

2.4.2.1   The general problem

Administrative, survey and other data, when combined in a manner that brings together individuals' data records, have the potential to yield better analyses. Usually, individual files must be data captured in a suitable fashion. Missing/contradictory data must be 'corrected' to remove missing data (e.g. Goldstein et al., 2009) in a manner that assures joint distributions are preserved and edit rules are not violated (Winkler, 2003; 2008). An edit rule might be that a child under 16 cannot have marital status of married. With 'cleaned' files, we assume that there are quasi-identifiers with low or very low error rates for linking records associated with individuals. We initially assume that, if we link two files A and B, then the two files represent approximately the same set of individuals. The high overlap between pairs or sets of files can be relaxed as a number of authors have demonstrated.

There are many potential applications to areas involving health data. One agency might have information about the types and amounts of social benefits received by individuals, a second agency might have information incomes of individuals, and a third agency might have information of use of health services by individuals. Being able to combine the information from a set of files and (partially) correct for linkage errors can yield significantly improved statistical analyses for policy purposes. When there are sets of pairs that do not overlap, then we can impute for missing data using the models developed on the overlapping pairs as in Goldstein et al. (2009; 2012).

Table 2.7 illustrates the general situation of bringing together two files. Scheuren and Winkler (1993) observed that if linkage error is low (3% or even lower at 1%), then it is possible to use statistical modelling methods/software directly without accounting for the linkage error. If linkage error exceeds 1% and the general statistical models are large or complicated, then the linkage error must be accounted for in the modelling. If linkage error is distributed non-randomly in certain groups (subdomains, see Chapter 4), then there are alternative methods (e.g. see Chapter 6).

2.4.2.2   General methods

Under a very simple regression model $Y = \beta X + \varepsilon$ where X is a univariate variable from one file A and Y is a univariate variable from another file B, Scheuren and Winkler (1993) provided a rather crude model for adjusting the statistical analyses for linkage error under various linkage rates. Winkler and Scheuren (1991) also did extensive exploratory and confirmatory work with 100+ data variants and with differing linkage error rates. They concluded three things. Firstly, no adjustment was needed with very low false-match rates (below 3% error). Secondly, the adjustment worked well with false-match rates between 3 and 10% where the probability of match could be computed via a procedure of Belin and Rubin (1995).

Table 2.7   Bringing together two files.

File A	Common	File B
$A_{11}, \ldots, A_{1n}$	Name 1, DOB 1, Address 1	$B_{11}, \ldots, B_{1m}$
$A_{21}, \ldots, A_{2n}$	Name 2, DOB 2, Address 2	$B_{21}, \ldots, B_{2m}$
.	.	.
.	.	.
$A_{N1}, \ldots, A_{nn}$	Name N, DOB N, Address N	$B_{N1}, \ldots, B_{Nm}$

Thirdly, the adjustment would work well for false-match rates between 10 and 20% if the probability of a match could be computed.

The Scheuren–Winkler procedure heavily depended on three things. Firstly, they used very simplistic form of the model. Secondly, they needed good but not totally accurate estimates of the probability of a match for each pair p_{ij} in the set of pairs associated with the analysis. Here, p_{ij} is the probability that the ith record from file A is matched to the jth record from file B. Thirdly, they needed a crude, but appropriate, technique for estimating one term in the estimating equations that suitably counterbalanced the modest bias in their overall procedure. Lahiri and Larsen (2005) greatly extended the Scheuren–Winkler procedure with various multivariate X under the assumption that all match probabilities p_{ij} were available. The Lahiri–Larsen procedure eliminated most of the bias of the Scheuren–Winkler procedure but required all p_{ij} which still today cannot be estimated in the unsupervised situation and cannot be estimated accurately even with large amounts of training data (supervised or semi-supervised learning).

Chambers (2009) (see also Kim and Chambers, 2012a; 2012b) provided the first generalisations of the Lahiri–Larsen procedures under a greatly simplified record linkage model for which all false matches had the same probability. Chambers demonstrated that the estimating-equation approach yielded further reductions to the bias of the Lahiri–Larsen procedure for many statistical analyses. Because of the record linkage model simplification, it was also possible to estimate the match probabilities p_{ij}, but it is not yet clear how well the Chambers procedure would extend to more realistic matching situations. Liseo and Tancredi (2011) used an MCMC approach to provide an adjustment procedure for certain regression analyses.

For a simple undercount procedure, Tancredi and Liseo (2011) provided an MCMC for obtaining estimates for the statistical analyses on discrete data. Tancredi and Liseo applied the 'hit–miss' model described by Copas and Hilton (1990) and first applied by Norén et al. (2005). Other MCMC methods for discrete data are given in Sadinle and Fienberg (2013) and Steorts et al. (2013) and for general data in Goldstein et al. (2012). Gutman et al. (2013) have provided statistical matching methods for determining relationships in logistic regression between variables from two files that might be used to improve some of the previous methods. In general statistical matching, (x, y) pairs from two files where both x and y can be multivariate are brought together according to a weaker criteria such as blocking instead of the stronger procedures of record linkage.

2.4.2.3   A straightforward semi-supervised model for discrete data

In the previous subsection, we primarily considered methods for adjusting a single functional relationship such as ordinary regression or logistic regression of continuous variables. In this section, we consider an adjustment procedure for general contingency tables that might be suitable for several analyses simultaneously (Chipperfield et al., 2011).

The natural way of analysing discrete data is with log-linear models on the pairs of records in $A \times B$. During matching, the ith record in A might be combined with the jth record in B with the true matching status denoted by z_{ij} that would be observed or not. As the methods of Chipperfield et al. (2011) are essentially the same as the semi-supervised methods of Section 2.2.3, we describe the method in terms of Equations 2.10–2.13. Chipperfield needed to begin with a truth sample (in our notation D_l) that would be combined with the unlabelled data (in our notation D_u). The truth sample might need to be enlarged until the EM procedure yields suitably accurate estimates. With larger contingency tables, we might use a suitably chosen very small Dirichlet prior (Eq. 2.12) to assure that the maximum likelihood estimates of the record linkage parameters would almost certainly exist. For each $x \in A$ and $y \in B$, we use p_{xy} to denote the true matching probability in the contingency table where several pairs from $A \times B$ may be mapped to the same cell.

The procedure of Chipperfield et al. (2011) appears to work well in their simple empirical examples that have substantial similarity to Winkler (2002), but the methods of Chipperfield et al. (2011) may be more directly generalised. With their empirical example, the truth sample was large enough to have at least 200 for each cell associated with the p_{xy}. The issue with the semi-supervised learning procedures is whether it is possible to obtain a sufficiently large sample to allow the estimates to converge to plausible values. Without any specific targeting of pairs in the sample that might provide the most improvement in the estimation procedure and best account for the rare patterns with low counts, it seems likely that sample sizes of as much as 25% of the total number of pairs in $A \times B$ may have difficulty providing suitable limiting estimates.

The following example (from Winkler, 2013 without details) illustrates the difficulty of extensions of the Chipperfield et al. (2011). In many situations of matching A with B, it is difficult to get a large subset of pairs in $A \times B$ where the overall false-match rates are below 10% and for which a small but moderate-sized subset of pairs has false-match rates as low as 2–4%. The low false-match rates on a suitable subset of pairs allow creation of an initial model $\hat{p}_{xy}^{(0)}$ as in Scheuren and Winkler (1997) that can gradually be improved. The improved models would help even more with Chipperfield et al. (2011). The issue is the number of values that each multivariate $x \in A$ and each multivariate $y \in B$ can assume. If $x \in A$ takes 600 values and $y \in B$ takes 1000 values, then each false match will bring a $y \in B$ together at random with an $x \in A$. In the situation of Chipperfield et al. (2011), it is difficult to get suitable initial estimates of $\hat{p}_{xy}^{(0)}$ or to get the estimates $\hat{p}_{xy}^{(t)}$ to converge to suitably accurate estimates even with the large sample sizes required in the Chipperfield et al. (2011) procedures. Even with very large truth samples, most cells would have initial values of $\hat{p}_{xy}^{(0)}$ at or near zero and would not move away from their initial values.

2.4.2.4   General models for adjusting statistical analyses

Goldstein et al. (2012) have provided MCMC methods for adjusting statistical analyses for linkage error that build on general imputation methods/software introduced by Goldstein et al. (2009). The methods are suitable for both continuous and discrete data and make use of 'prior-informed imputation' given in Goldstein et al. (2009). For computational efficiency, discrete and general data are converted to multivariate normal where sampling is done and then converted back to discrete and general data. This is discussed in detail in Chapter 6.

2.5   Concluding comments

It is worth mentioning that if extensive 'edit' rules are available from subject matter experts or exceptionally clean auxiliary files are available, then it may be possible to eliminate many false-match pairs in $A \times B$. Such edit rules have been suggested for use in general imputation (Winkler, 2011) and may serve as a starting point as reducing the effects of false matches (Winkler, 2013).

This chapter provides an introductory overview of some well-established methods of record linkage that have been used for different types of lists for more than 40 years. The newer methods deal with adjusting statistical analyses for linkage error and are still subject to considerable research.

3

The data linkage environment

Chris Dibben[1], Mark Elliot[2], Heather Gowans[3], Darren Lightfoot[4] and Data Linkage Centres*

[1] University of Edinburgh, Edinburgh, UK
[2] University of Manchester, Manchester, UK
[3] University of Oxford, Oxford, UK
[4] University of St Andrews, St Andrews, UK

3.1 Introduction

The joining of data records corresponding to the same individual (or sometimes organisations) across multiple datasets is increasingly a required function of research service infrastructures. Through this process, new data structures are built, potentially powerful ones that can facilitate important lines of enquiry within multiple research areas. In many instances, the size of these databases makes it impractical to seek active consent from individuals, and therefore, the data being manipulated in the linkage process is of a special character, where there is an extremely strong need to ensure that there is no disclosure of information to any party about individuals within the datasets. Working with data that is strictly non-personal (i.e. absolutely anonymous) guarantees protection but is rarely achievable in a data linkage context and indeed may actually be impossible with any useful data (Ohm, 2010). Instead, what is required is the construction of a data linkage environment in which the process of re-identification is made so unlikely that the data can be judged as functionally anonymous. This type of environment is formed through the security infrastructure and governance processes that shape the behaviour of those accessing the data and the data linkage and analysis models that structure the operational processes.

---

*The text for the data linkage centre case studies was provided by the Population Data BC (Canada), Centre for Data Linkage (Australia), Secure Anonymised Information Linkage Databank (United Kingdom) and Centre for Health Record Linkage (Australia) and then edited by the authors.

Methodological Developments in Data Linkage, First Edition. Edited by Katie Harron, Harvey Goldstein and Chris Dibben.
© 2016 John Wiley & Sons, Ltd. Published 2016 by John Wiley & Sons, Ltd.

This chapter will introduce the data linkage environment. It will start with an exploration of the law and the linkage of personal data, outlining why a special data linkage environment is a legal necessity. The key elements of the environment that may allow a data stewardship organisation to assert that data are functionally anonymous will then be outlined. The main ways that these elements are organised into models will then be identified, and finally, four case studies from different parts of the world will be discussed.

3.2   The data linkage context

3.2.1   Administrative or routine data

The main driver behind the development of specialist data linkage centres has been the need to provide research access to administrative datasets. The term 'administrative data' refers to information collected primarily for administrative (not research) purposes. This type of information is routinely collected by government departments and other organisations for the purposes of their normal operational activities, such as registration, transaction and record-keeping. Collection usually occurs during the delivery of a service. It has enormous potential to inform social and health research and covers a wide variety of fields.

The owners of these administrative datasets vary between countries, depending largely on their different mix of economies of welfare. Where the state is the provider of a service, government departments are the main (although not exclusive) purveyors of large administrative databases, including welfare, tax, health and educational record systems. In more mixed economies of welfare, administrative datasets will be provided by both the government and the private sector. These datasets have for many years been used to produce official statistics to inform policy making. The potential for these data to be accessed for the purposes of social science and health research is increasingly recognised, although in many counties, it has not been fully exploited.

Administrative datasets are typically very large, covering samples of individuals and time periods not normally financially or logistically achievable through orthodox survey methods. Alongside cost savings, the scope of administrative data is often cited as its main advantage for research purposes. Although the use of administrative data may not be appropriate in every case, the general benefits of using administrative data for research purposes include the following: the data have already been collected for operational purposes and do not therefore incur any costs of collection (other than for extraction and cleaning); the data collection process is not intrusive to the target population; the administrative data are regularly (sometimes continuously) updated; it can provide historical information and allow consistent time series to be built up; it may be collected in a consistent way if it is part of a national system; it is often subject to rigorous quality checks; it often provides near 100% coverage of the population of interest; it is reliable at the small area level; the counterfactuals and controls can be selected post hoc; it captures individuals who may not respond to surveys; and it offers potential for datasets to be linked to produce powerful research resources.

To fully realise the benefits of increased researcher access to administrative data, a variety of modes for data access – including restricted access to confidential data and unrestricted access to appropriately altered public-use data – will need to be used.[1]

---

[1] The trade-off between restricted data and restricted access and the relationship of both with data utility are heavily discussed in the disclosure control literature. See, for example, Doyle et al. (2001), Elliot (2005), Willenborg and De Waal (2001) and Duncan, Elliot and Salazar (2011).

3.2.2   The law and the use of administrative (personal) data for research

The use case for linked administrative data for research is therefore compelling, but of course, any use of administrative data must comply with the law of the country within which the data are collected. The law, as it applies to the use of administrative data and therefore shapes the data linkage environment, is now outlined. A comprehensive exploration of international data protection legislation is beyond the scope of this chapter, but we include here a brief outline of the laws surrounding the use of personal data in several different countries around the world, with a particular focus on the UK, European Union (EU) (which encompasses all the current 28 EU member states) and US data protection and privacy legislation and how it necessitates a particular data linkage environment.

We start with a definition of personal data, a core concept for the data linkage environment. 'Personal data' is defined in the UK Data Protection Act (DPA) as:

> data which relate to a living individual who can be identified:
>
> (a) from those data, or
>
> (b) from those data and other information which is in the possession of, or is likely to come into the possession of, the data controller.

This conceptualisation of personal data (and variations of it in other jurisdictions) frames much of the thinking about how (and whether) linkage can be carried out. If data can be defined as personal data, then particular legal instruments will operate.

The legal protection of an individual's right to privacy in general and the right to privacy over personal data in particular varies around the world. There are comprehensive data protection laws in nearly every country in Europe, as well as in many Latin American, Caribbean, Asian and African countries. By contrast, the United States is notable for not having adopted comprehensive data protection laws. Data linkage programmes that are aimed at linking databases holding information of a personal nature (i.e. not wholly or truly anonymous data) have to take account of any legal constraints surrounding the use of the data in order to lawfully process the information.

The right to data privacy is heavily regulated and actively enforced in Europe. All members of the EU are subject to data protection legislation which stems from the European Data Protection Directive (Directive 95/46/EC on the protection of individuals with regard to the processing of personal data and on the free movement of such data) and which regulates the processing of personal data in the EU.[2] All members of the EU are also signatories of the European Convention on Human Rights which provides for the right to individuals' privacy. The European Data Protection Directive contains eight data protection principles[3] which must be complied with when using or processing personal data.

In the UK, data protection laws require that researchers seeking access to personal data, as well as the data holding organisations providing access to those data, need to consider the implications of sharing data, such as whether the data sharing would breach any common law

---

[2] A European Data Protection Regulation which was drafted in 2012 will supersede the directive in due course.

[3] The eight principles are that the personal data must be (1) fairly and lawfully processed; (2) processed for limited purposes; (3) adequate, relevant and not excessive; (4) kept accurate; (5) kept no longer than necessary; (6) processed in accordance with the data subject's rights; (7) kept secure; and (8) transferred only to countries with adequate protection.

duty of confidentiality,[4] whether there would be any breach of human rights[5] and whether the data sharing would be in accordance with the principles set out in the DPA 1998, of which the most important in this context is that the data are being fairly and lawfully processed. The DPA implemented the European Data Protection Directive in the UK. The main strand of data protection legislation in the United Kingdom is the DPA, which regulates the use of personal data in the United Kingdom. The Act makes a distinction between non-sensitive personal data and sensitive personal data. Sensitive personal data include information about an individual such as their race, political opinion or religion.

The processing of all personal data must be fair and lawful and meet one of the DPA conditions relevant for the purposes of processing any personal data (contained in DPA Schedules 2 and 3). For research purposes, the most relevant conditions for processing non-sensitive data are likely to be either:

- The consent of the data subject or

- The legitimate interests of the data controller

Obtaining consent from an individual is the most straightforward route to allow the processing of their personal data for purposes other than originally collected, but this is frequently practically impossible for many of the use cases for administrative data. Where the data subject has not given consent for the processing, the data processing might be legitimised if the processing is necessary for the 'legitimate interests' pursued by the data controller. The 'legitimate interests' are not defined in the DPA, but the data controller must show that the processing of data is for the legitimate interests being pursued, which requires a balance of the data controller's legitimate interests against the interests of the data subject (who must come first), and the data controller must also show that there are no unjustified adverse effects on the data subjects. Where the requirements of the 'legitimate interests' condition can be satisfied, it may be possible to rely on this condition to use non-sensitive personal data for research purposes without consent from the data subject but only where there has been a consideration of a balance between the legitimate interests of those to whom the data would be disclosed and between any prejudice to the rights, freedoms and legitimate interests of

---

[4] The common law tort of breach of confidence offers protection to individuals' private interests and their confidential information by dealing with the unauthorised use or disclosure of certain types of confidential information. It may protect such information on the basis of actual or deemed agreement to keep such information private. A breach of confidence will only occur where the disclosure of information is considered to be an abuse or unconscionable to a reasonable man. In certain circumstances, the law relating to contracts may apply, so, for example, where an explicit statement has been made by a data controller relating to the confidentiality of an individual's personal information, that statement may constitute a written or verbal contract.

[5] The Human Rights Act 1998 allows an individual to assert the rights of the European Convention on Human Rights (ECHR) against public bodies in UK courts and tribunals. Personal data (particularly medical data) is therefore protected by Article 8 of the ECHR as part of an individual's right to respect for a private life. The Human Rights Act is intended to prevent any communication or disclosure of personal data as may be inconsistent with the provisions of Article 8 of the ECHR. Article 8 of the ECHR provides for the right to respect for private life, family life and one's home and correspondence and that there shall be no interference by a public authority with the exercise of this right, except if it is in accordance with the law, for a legitimate social purpose or for the protection of the rights and freedoms of others. In order to justify an infringement of Article 8 of the ECHR and therefore any infringement of privacy under the Human Rights Act, a public authority must be able to show that any interference is in accordance with the law or for a legitimate aim, necessary in a democratic society (this would require a court judgement as to whether the sharing of data was necessary, whether there were sufficient safeguards in place and whether the aims were legitimate and sufficiently defined) and proportionate. Data holding organisations need to address such issues prior to releasing of any personal data.

data subjects. It is therefore within this subtle, nuanced and subjective deliberation that the legality of administrative data linkage within a specialist 'data linkage environment' is made.[6]

It is worth noting, however, that UK and European data protection legislation is in a state of flux. In January 2012, the European Commission issued a draft Data Protection Regulation to replace the existing Data Protection Directive 95/46/EC and the legislation required to implement it in each EU member state. The main purpose of the original proposed draft of the regulation is to strengthen individuals' rights, but it also contains several changes that will have an impact on research and is likely to force changes in practice, including implementing a 'right to be forgotten or have information erased' and the removal of certain exemptions that currently exist for research. It also embodies a much greater emphasis on the right to have the 'specific, informed and explicit' consent before processing (i.e. linkage) is allowed. It is probable that, without research exemptions, within this new legislation, many of the data linkage environments outlined in this chapter will be illegal.

In contrast to data protection legislation in the UK and other European countries, the United States has adopted limited data protection legislation, based on Fair Information Practices, rather than having adopted comprehensive data protection laws. The basic principles of data protection in the United States are not too dissimilar to European data protection principles[7]; however, Fair Information Principles are only recommendations, and they are not enforceable by law. Data privacy is not as highly legislated or regulated in the United States as it is in EU countries. There is some partial regulation surrounding the access of personal data, but unlike the UK and other European legislation, there is no all-encompassing law regulating the acquisition, storage or use of personal data in the United States. In general, there tends to be legal provision in the United States which favours the flow of information and permits personal data to be used and stored by data processors, irrespective of whether the data was collected without the data subject's permission.[8] Very few US states recognise individuals' rights to privacy, a notable exception being California.

Unlike the US approach to privacy protection, which relies on industry-specific legislation and regulation, the EU relies on comprehensive data protection legislation. Following the introduction of the European Data Protection Directive in 1995 (which required implementation in

[6] If the processing of personal data is fair and lawful and meets one of the conditions outlined above, Section 33 of the DPA also provides a 'research exemption' aimed at facilitating the researchers' use of personal data in respect of the processing (or further processing) of personal data for research purposes (which, although not specifically defined in the DPA, includes statistical or historical purposes). Section 33 provides exemptions to some of the eight data protection principles contained in the DPA, but it is quite narrow. Provided that the data are not processed to support measures or decisions in relation to particular individuals and provided that the data are not processed in such a way that substantial damage or distress is, or is likely to be, caused to any data subject, the exemption permits personal data to be used for purposes other than they were originally collected for; personal data to be kept indefinitely, if the conditions under which the data were obtained allow and personal data are exempt from the subject access rights if the results of the work are not made available in a form which identifies any data subject(s). These provisions do not remove the duty to comply with the remainder of the DPA – the processing of personal data must still comply with the other data protection principles which apply to personal data provided and/or used for research purposes.

[7] US Fair Information Principles are that there should be a stated purpose for all data collected; information collected by one individual cannot be disclosed to other organisations or individuals unless the individual concerned has given consent, or it is authorised by law; records kept on an individual should be accurate and up to date; there should be mechanisms for individuals to review data about them to ensure accuracy; data should be deleted when it is no longer required for the stated purpose; it is prohibited to transmit personal information to locations where 'equivalent' personal data protection cannot be assured; and some data are deemed too sensitive to be collected, unless there are extreme circumstances (e.g. sexual orientation, religion).

[8] For example, the Health Insurance Portability and Accountability Act of 1996 (HIPAA), the Children's Online Privacy Protection Act of 1998 (COPPA) and the Fair and Accurate Credit Transactions Act of 2003 (FACTA) are all US federal laws with provisions favouring information flow and operational profits over the rights of individuals to control their own personal data.

EU member states by 1998), the US Department of Commerce in consultation with the European Commission developed 'Safe Harbor Privacy Principles' in order to provide a means for US companies to comply with the European directive.[9] The 'Safe Harbor' framework was approved as providing adequate protection for personal data for the purposes of the directive in July 2000.[10] The debate in this area in the United States remains focused on privacy, whereas the debate in the EU is on data protection.

The introduction and implementation of privacy and data protection laws in any legal juris-diction aim to ensure that a series of safeguards are in place to limit the risk of personal data being processed in such a way as to cause any distress or harmful consequences related to the rights and freedoms of individuals around the world. However, changes and developments in technology and the mere size of many new data structures have highlighted the insufficiencies in the protection that individuals can expect to be offered by data protection legislation. There is therefore the question of whether many of the data protection laws currently embedded in differ-ent jurisdictions are capable of being sufficiently resilient to answer the new technological chal-lenges.[11] The EU viewpoint on the implications of this is that '[t]he protection of fundamental human rights such as privacy and data protection stands side-by-side with public safety and security. This situation is not static. It changes, and both values are able to progress in step with technological advances. But it also means that there must be lines which cannot be crossed, to protect people's privacy'.[12] This point of view rests upon an approach which depends on the need to ensure total anonymity as much as possible, rather than adopting a more risk-based approach to anonymity. The risk-based approach to anonymity (which is reflected in the US approach to data privacy, discussed in the next section, rather more than is the case in the highly regulated EU countries) does have support and seems to be accepted in some societies, but there remains a dilemma as to how to bridge the gap between the two different approaches. Data protection laws around the world recognise the need for some form of protection of individuals' privacy, but there remains a divergence between the degree of regulation required, which in turn is responsi-ble for a recurring tension regarding the scope of legally enforced personal data protection.

One approach to determining the extent to which anonymity must be protected is to consider whether disclosure of any personal data without the consent of the data subject can be justified in any circumstances as being within the public interest or the public good (bearing in mind that what is of interest to the public is not necessarily in the public interest). This requires an exacting and rigorous balancing of factors, such as whether it would be in the interests of society as a whole; whether it would promote openness and transparency by public bodies, while also protecting individuals' personal data; and the extent to which it would cause any substantial damage or distress to any individual. The 'greater good' argument may ultimately not be sufficient to justify the dis-closure of any personal data without consent, where there is any concern that it would cause any adverse effects (which may be particularly relevant to particular datasets, such as medical- or insurance-related datasets); and anonymity will be considered paramount.

---

[9] The directive requires that personal data may only be transferred from countries within the European Economic Area to countries which provide adequate data protection (Chapter IV, Article 25).

[10] It is regarded by some critics as an imperfect solution because it is not legally imposed on all US organisations and it does not adequately address data protection compliance with onward transfer obligations, where data originating in the EU is transferred to the US Safe Harbor and then onto a third country.

[11] For examples of legal implications of forensic profiling, see http://www.fidis.net/resources/fidis-deliverables/forensic-implications/d67c-forensic-profiling/doc/17/.

[12] European Commissioner Franco Frattini responsible for Justice, Freedom and Security: Conference on Public Security, Privacy and Technology, Brussels, 20 November 2007.

3.2.3   The identifiability problem in data linkage

In many countries, therefore, the legal justification for having access to administrative data – in the absence of consent – rests on an argument that it is non-personal or not identifiable. This of course presents a problem: without some sort of unique identifier, accurate linkage is effectively impossible. In practice, a pragmatic approach to anonymisation – which is about minimising risk rather than providing absolute guarantees – is necessary for any secondary data usage to take place. Mackey and Elliot (2013) describe how such risk is crucially moderated by the data environment – the total context in which the processing of data takes place. This approach applies to linkage just as much as to analysis; and so the identifiability problem is solvable through conceptualising the re-identification risk of a data linkage process as not simply lying with the data but also with the data environment within which it is processed. If all components that make up this environment (people, data, space, technologies, etc.) in concert ensure that the re-identification risk is sufficiently small, the data are seen to be in a state where they are functionally anonymous.

At first, this may appear to be a sleight of hand, but the approach is supported in the UK by the Information Commissioner's 2012 code of practice on anonymisation. It is really just an embodiment of the decision-making processes that underpin all human activity, from the design of safety features in transport systems to the setting of government budgets. We accept that there are individual-scale risks accompanying these collective-scale decisions, so why would we expect zero risk in the realm of data?

Of course, that does not mean that the data controller, the linker and the researcher can all relax into laissez-faire. Rather, they must proceed with extreme caution, taking care to minimise the re-identification risk while producing data resources that maximise the wider social benefit. Duncan, Elliot and Salazar (2011) call this data stewardship, a concept which neatly conveys both the wider social responsibility and the duty of care to individuals. In the UK, the notion is even embodied in the role of the Information Commissioner, who is responsible for both data protection and freedom of information. Similarly, the Office for National Statistics has the twin responsibilities of protecting the confidentiality of individuals and disseminating useful data about those individuals.

So, if we accept that in order to reap the benefits of the reuse and linkage of administrative data, we must accept that it carries some individual-scale risk of re-identification; and if we accept the dual responsibilities of data stewardship, then we are necessarily working with an optimisation problem rather than an absolute anonymisation problem. This still is no trivial task, and in the next section, we discuss the mechanisms that have been developed for tackling it – all of which involve in some way control of elements of the data environment.

Data linkage centres, often independent secure environments set up for the sole purpose of joining two or more datasets together to form a single dataset for research purposes, are often used for this purpose.

3.3   The tools used in the production of functional anonymity through a data linkage environment

Data linkage centres have developed methods of operating that aim to minimise, in all parts, the risk of re-identification of individuals in datasets. Taken in concert, it is argued that these measures lead to the overall risk of any disclosure of information on individuals being acceptably small, thus making the data within this system functionally anonymous. The methods that, together, result in this situation of functional anonymity are typically diverse but aim to impact all parts of the data linkage process and subsequently the research activity that then follows.

3.3.1 Governance, rules and the researcher

Governance procedures that direct a researcher applying for and accessing data will form part of the data linkage environment. The tighter and more regulated these procedures are, the more likely that an individual will not be able to accidentally achieve or maliciously attempt re-identification. There are a variety of multiple and common approaches used by data controllers to govern researchers when using their identifiable data. These are now summarised.

3.3.2 Application process, ethics scrutiny and peer review

Formal requests to access data are usually made through an application. Details collected generally include information about the applicant(s) (perhaps checked through law enforcement agencies) and institution, details of the data required, aims of the project, audience, possible outputs and impacts of research. In some cases, for access to more sensitive data, a detailed business case justifying the need for such data will be required. Some organisations may require more in-depth information covering areas such as research methodology, details of external datasets that may be linked and security plans for the protection of data against misuse, loss or unauthorised access.

Where access to data is granted for research purposes, it typically requires a panel of people to consider whether it is legal to disclose the data. The panel may also consider whether the research is in the public interest, a common argument used for relaxing data protection principles for research reuse of data. Public interest could rarely be served by poorly designed research, and therefore, a common basis for panel decision-making on a particular project is whether it is 'good' research. This of course will not always be uncontroversial.

Researchers putting forward proposals for a piece of research are usually guided by their institution or a data linkage centre to seek ethical scrutiny of their research endeavour. Typically, health data holding organisations (such as the Health and Social Care Information Centre and NHS Scotland in the UK) will have their own dedicated ethics committee for reviewing applications for patient identifiable data. The committee will take into account the benefits of the research as well as its potential harms and the credentials of the researchers and organisation before approving any access.

The end product of these processes is typically some form of licence or contract allowing access to the dataset and including a set of instructions on how the researchers must behave within the data linkage environment.

3.3.3 Shaping 'safe' behaviour: training, sanctions, contracts and licences

Any breaches of licence agreements could cause reputational and political damage to the original supplier of the data and more generally would undermine the argument that the data are functionally anonymous. Therefore, sanctions are often put into licence agreements to act as a deterrent to such behaviour. Dependent on the type of breach, sanctions can include legal proceedings which could lead to imprisonment, a suspension (either temporary or permanent) for the researcher and/or their institution from using the data in the future or access denial to any linked funding sources.

So, for example, in the UK, provisions under the DPA allow data controllers to be penalised up to £500 000 for serious breaches of the Act. The way in which a researcher handles personal data may make them a data controller and therefore liable to be served with a monetary penalty if any data protection principles are breached. It is common for data controllers who provide access to personal data to insist that researchers have received some form of information governance training prior to any access. Courses may be particular to a data holding organisation (e.g. government department) or provided by a third-party organisation (e.g. national statistical agency or university).

If an application is successful, a contract or licence may be issued to a researcher which sets out the terms and conditions that a researcher must adhere to when using their data. Typically, this will cover who can use it, where it can be used, what it can be used for and for how long it can be kept. There is also likely to be a data destruction policy, details on output clearance, sanctions for breach of procedures and procedures for data publication.

3.3.4   'Safe' data analysis environments

3.3.4.1   Safe setting

The setting where a researcher can access and analyse data forms a crucial part of the data linkage environment. Both the physical and psychological attributes of a safe setting will affect the behaviour and attitude of the researcher towards the data once they enter into it. A safe setting (also known as a safe haven) is a secure physical location where data are accessed for analysis purposes. The data may also be located in this environment or held elsewhere and accessed through a secure network link. There are various considerations that need to be taken into account when designing a secure safe setting, such as its physical security, hardware security, data handling practices, who can access the room, and how to ensure appropriate behaviour in the setting (i.e. behaviour that meets the governance standards). Safe settings are generally not designed to a common standard or specification and instead are usually designed around the sensitivity of the data that is to be held or accessed from the safe setting.

However, safe settings are likely to have several of the following features:

- Access controlled in and around the setting (e.g. 'onion-skin' levels of security, alarms, etc.).

- Designed so that only authorised personnel can enter the safe setting location (e.g. dual lock, swipe card access).

- All other points of access are strong against attack (e.g. if there are accessible windows, they are secured).

- Any stand-alone PCs or thin clients are chained down and not connected to the Internet. Password systems are also likely to be in operation to boot the PC. External drives and USB ports are likely to be disabled.

- Only essential software is installed on the machine. Antivirus and malware software are installed and kept up to date.

- CCTV and other monitoring technologies are fitted in order to monitor the behaviour of the individual while in the room.

Safe settings typically have strict access arrangements in place to ensure that only authorised personnel can have access. Other issues to be considered include key holder responsibilities (such as changing pin codes regularly), procedures for when safe setting support staff leave the organisation and how access to the safe setting is logged. A comprehensive procedural document would normally be in place to cover these issues.

How data are transferred to the safe setting is of equal importance and will depend on an assessment of the sensitivity of the data. Such an assessment would take into account the detail and type of identifiable variables in the dataset, together with a risk assessment and impact that the loss or control of the data could make. Data being transferred is nearly always encrypted using dedicated software. Transfer to the safe setting is most commonly done over a network but can also be physically couriered. Once at its destination, consideration will then be given to an assessment of its secure storage.

A safe setting can be costly to set up, as it involves the allocation, building or modification of a room. In some cases, safe settings can also be resource intensive to manage. These factors can then be prohibitive to the number and geographical location of safe settings within which a data controller or research institution may wish to provide access to data. A new concept which overcomes some of these barriers is to develop a prefabricated secure room (PSR) which can provide for a fully controlled and consistent environment for data analysis without the need for a room conversion. A PSR shares similar features to a traditional safe setting and would allow researchers to access data over a secure network with the following advantages:

- The PSR sits within an existing room.

- The design of a PSR can be standardised and therefore easy to reproduce. This allows data controllers to be confident that the same standards apply in multiple locations.

- A PSR can be manufactured to be moved and rebuilt in a new location if needed.

- A PSR is suitable for organisations where there are space constraints.

- The build of a PSR can incorporate strong psychological cues (i.e. that this is an environment that requires a different form of behaviour).

- The individual and their behaviour can easily be monitored in a PSR. The design can also be easily modified to help control behaviour.

- A PSR can be customisable to provide a pleasant working environment.

A suggestive set of features for a PSR might include the following:

- The PSR should be small (perhaps 2 m width × 2 m depth × 2 m height) to provide a comfortable space for a single researcher to work in. This will reduce the chance that multiple users of a workspace will lead to an unauthorised person viewing the data. This will also provide enough space for wheelchair access to the room.

- An Internet protocol CCTV camera can be installed to allow authorised personnel to monitor the behaviour of the researcher from outside the PSR.

- The PSR could incorporate a conductive RF-shielding layer, something which would be difficult to achieve in a room converted to a safe setting.

- Door entry should be secured multiple entry control, for example, a traditional mortice lock and pin entry.

- Adequate and adjustable lighting should be provided in the PSR for the comfort of the researcher. Flexible ventilation solutions can be added to the PSR, dependent on the environment within which the room is to be placed.

- Intruder and emergency alarms should be fitted.

An ideal location for the room would be within a building that has its own security and access controls, with staff available to support the running of the room and with extended opening hours to assist researchers to use the room for long periods of time as needed. The hosting organisation would need to abide by standard PSR security, access, monitoring and auditing procedures. Any connection from a PSR to a server for remote access to data would need to be secured. There are many solutions available which involve the use of virtual private networks (VPN) to securely send and receive data across the Internet using Transport Layer Security (TLS) protocol and Secure Sockets Layer (SSL) protocol. A penetration test should be used to evaluate the security of the network by simulating an attack and outlining any possible measures to reduce risks.

One final consideration to take into account when establishing a safe setting would be the potential vulnerability to the monitoring of any computer equipment signals (i.e. compromising emanations). This would be dependent on a number of factors such as the existing shielding of the computer, the build materials and how close an attacker could get to the safe setting. To manage protection, the safe setting electrical equipment would need to contain additional conductive shielding, shielded external cables and the provision of additional filters in interfaces and power supply lines to help comply with emission limits. The NATO 'TEMPEST' specification describes emission test requirements for three different security levels based on how close the attacker can get to their targeted equipment. Any decision to provide additional shielding in the safe setting should balance such cost with a realistic assessment of an attack and the implications of a loss of data. For further information on electromagnetic emanations, see Kuhn and Anderson (1998).

3.3.4.2   The problem of output and statistical disclosure control

After data analysis, the researcher will naturally want to take output from the safe setting. By definition, the output will be moving outside governance processes and security infrastructure that maintain functional anonymity of the data that have been linked and analysed (and indeed may be published) and are therefore de facto open. Functionally, the output is a representation of the data which is moving from one (safeguarded) data environment to another (with effectively no safeguards).

The data controller will therefore either stipulate that outputs are checked by them prior to any publication or ensure and have confidence in such procedures at the processing institution (details of which are normally collected through the application form). This is essentially a reassessment of the risk of re-identification, given the change in the environment compensated for by the much reduced information content of the output compared to the original data.

The checking process is essentially one of statistical disclosure control (SDC). SDC is a complex and highly technical field with its own journals, conferences and research teams which we will not be attempting to describe herein its entirety; the interested reader should refer to Duncan, Elliot and Salazar (2011) or Hundepool et al. (2012) for extensive reviews of the field. In essence, SDC is the mechanism by which two processes, identification and attribution, are (severely) limited. Duncan, Elliot and Salazar (2011) describe attribution as 'the association of information in a data set with a particular population unit' and identification as 'the association of a particular population unit whose identity is known with a particular data unit'. A unit is often an individual but can also be an organisation such as a school or business. In lay terms, identification is finding somebody, and attribution is finding out something about somebody.[13] The SDC process is first to assess the risk and then (if necessary) to mitigate that risk.

There is no single comprehensive method of assessing risk in output, simply because it comes in many forms. Nevertheless, high-risk features include low or zero counts[14] in aggregate outputs, unusual or unique combinations of characteristics, overlapping outputs (where one may be subtracted from the other to produce small subpopulations), linkable outputs and output that allows reconstruction of the original data (typically models and residual information). Actions to mitigate those risks include refusing release of the output, suppressing some part of it, giving similar output with less detail or perturbing some part of the output.

3.3.5   Fragmentation: separation of linkage process and temporary linked data

Trusted third parties (TTP) are a widely used mechanism for the indexing and enhancement of datasets across the world while also minimising the amount of information any one group holds and therefore reducing the risk of disclosure and maintaining functional anonymity. The involvement of a TTP is necessary for research where, even though the end product of the process is not sensitive, the process of carrying out the linkage carries data security and/or privacy risks. The TTP mechanism allows a reduction in risk by separating functions or processes and therefore

---

[13] It may not be immediately obvious, but these two processes can occur independently of one another. See Elliot (2005) for an explanation of this.

[14] This is another point which may not be immediately obvious. As a general principle with tables of counts without zeros (raw or derivable), no disclosure can take place. For example, if the counts of Y conditional on $X=x$ are $\{100,0,0,0\}$, then if I know $X=x$ for a given person, then I know their value of Y. On the other hand, if the values of Y conditional on $X=x$ are $\{100,1,1,1\}$, then I cannot be certain of the value of Y. See Smith and Elliot (2008) for a full treatment of this.

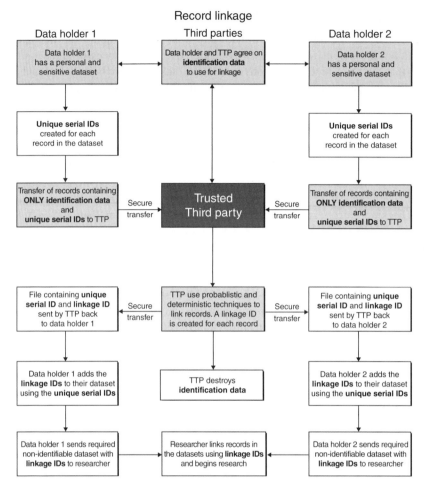

Figure 3.1   Record linkage within a trusted third-party mechanism.

allowing each stage of the research dataset construction process to be carried out using a very minimum amount of data (see Figure 3.1). This is very important during the indexing process, where, although identifiers are necessary, no ancillary (payload) information is required.

The data necessary for indexing (the linkage variables), although individually identifying, hold no information on the individual beyond their presence in a dataset; and this in itself could be hidden by not alerting the TTP to the data owners involved in the indexing process or by supplementing the 'genuine names' with other names – perhaps all names that could possibly be in the dataset. However, this could still be seen as disclosive. One solution is to encrypt the identifiable data at source, so that this encrypted data can then be shared and linked without revealing the identity of the individual, known as privacy-preserving record linkage or 'pseudonymisation' where a cryptographic hash of the linkage variables is made (see Chapter 9). For this to work, the encrypted identifier must be non-reversible, or near impossible to reverse, and it must also be recorded without error (i.e. identical between sources). This is because a good cryptographic hash of two slightly differently spelt words will be massively different by design. Therefore, no similarity algorithms will be able to identify the similarity of the original two words.

Schnell, Bachteler and Reiher (2009) proposed a method for hashing the information used in linkage that still allows similarity of two encrypted strings to be calculated. This method, in combination with other aspects of the data managing model, can be used to remove the need to transfer any identifying data and therefore significantly decrease the risk of any disclosure. It also allows the argument that any processing (sharing) does not involve personal data. This of course is a fairly new technique but one that has been tested fairly extensively by the research team which developed it and now by other research groups. It, however, has one significant drawback, namely, that it does not easily allow manual matching as the final step of the linkage process (see Chapter 9).

Whether a linked administrative dataset is produced for a short period of time for a specific research project or is more permanently established as a 'study' dataset, serving a wider set of research projects, is an important aspect of existing and future programmes. There are strengths and weaknesses associated with both, in most cases the weaknesses in one being the strength in the other. On the whole, the benefits of temporary linkage are largely accrued as privacy/control enhancements, with the benefits of more permanent linkage being to research utility.

Strengths of temporary linkages

- Privacy – The linkage is more clearly associated with a single project and a set of users. It is therefore possible to state why and for what purpose the use of personal data was sanctioned.

- Flexibility – Where data are drawn from live databases, the latest version of the dataset is used. The data are therefore more likely to be up to date.

- Control – Data owners may have a stronger sense of control over the data they manage.

Strengths of maintaining a 'study'

- Quality – A permanent 'study' allows incremental improvement in dataset quality (e.g. dealing with missing data, biases, etc.). This can take many years and there is no 'loss' of this work at the end of each temporary project/linkage.

- Efficiency – Requires linkage, cleaning, etc. to be carried out once rather than multiple times or by multiple data owners. Repeating this process, as particular sets of linked datasets become more popular, will become increasingly costly.

- Archiving – Where data are being drawn from live databases overwriting older information, important information that would otherwise be lost is archived.

- Longitudinal studies – May be the only way of effectively producing a longitudinal study unless all data holders are archiving regular 'cuts' of their data.

- Replicating research – A study makes the replication of studies quicker and efficient and therefore more likely.

3.4   Models for data access and data linkage

Looking across existing centres around the world, a number of the 'archetypal' models can be identified. These are now outlined. All of these models would include the characteristics of the data linkage environment outlined in Section 3.3.

3.4.1   Single centre

The single-centre model is the simplest of the structures described in this section (Figure 3.2). It involves the transfer of multiple datasets to a trusted research centre. The centre then constructs a research dataset by linking data from different organisations and makes the resulting data available within a safe setting to authorised researchers. The data made available to researchers will almost always be reduced in content to ensure that within the controlled environment of the safe setting, the data are non-identifiable. Part of the control operated through the safe setting is over the level of information that can be taken out of the research centre. This will typically only be information that is entirely non-disclosive (i.e. where re-identification is set at a suitable level of risk). The data transferred will need to involve sufficient information to allow linkage (i.e. either an individual reference or uniquely identifying characteristic of the individual). This model is therefore highly likely to involve the transfer of identifiable data and therefore will represent a sharing (processing) of personal data.

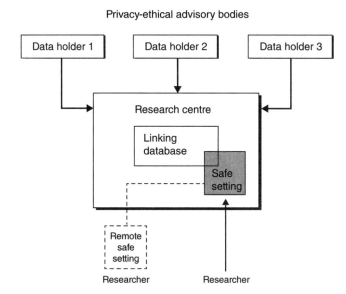

Figure 3.2   Single-centre model – solid (heavy) weighted arrow shows movement of data, and the dashed line indicates a remote 'view' of the data but no transfer of actual data.

3.4.2   Separation of functions: firewalls within single centre

The second model is a modification of the single centre with a privacy enhancement structural change (Figure 3.3). It requires a physical separation of functions during the dataset linkage process within the single centre. Here, the process of creating a link between records for the same individual and then the linking of the full research dataset are separated. In the first instance, the data holders send a limited amount of information to an area of the research centre to enable matching between the different datasets. This would be limited to only the data necessary to achieve a satisfactory level of matching – the linking variables. This would typically include name or parts of, date of birth, address information and an identifier unique and interpretable only by the data holder. The indexer within the research centre then either deterministically or probabilistically matches records, giving ones believed to be for the same person a unique study identifier. The study identifier and the relevant data holder identifiers are then passed back to the data holders, together with any additional information – in the case of probabilistic linking, information about the probability of a match being correct (see Chapter 6). Each data holder then adds the study identifier to their datasets, removes any other identifier information and sends the research relevant data to a separate area of the

---

Strengths: Single centre model

- The single centre minimises the number of data transfer stages, and this therefore reduces the inherent danger of loss of data in transit.

- Involves only one organisation which makes scrutiny by overseeing bodies easier (i.e. they can simply visit one site to audit security).

- Linkage will be more efficient and easier to organise because it involves one organisation.

- Because the linkage is carried out by a single entity, it will be easier for the one centre to know the biases within the dataset because it has been involved in all stages.

- The research centre over time can collect and organise metadata, collect programming algorithms and foster a deep understanding of administrative datasets because it is involved in all stages of the data processing.

Weaknesses: Single centre model

- From the outside, there are no 'visible' barriers to dishonest behaviour. The public has to trust that the data centre will not attempt to identify individuals and link information to them.

- There are no structural aids (e.g. separation of functions) to support an argument that the processing is of non-personal data – that is, that individuals cannot be identified.

- On the whole, it therefore relies on the research centre being entirely honest, because the centre will actually hold all the information necessary to identify and learn things about individuals.

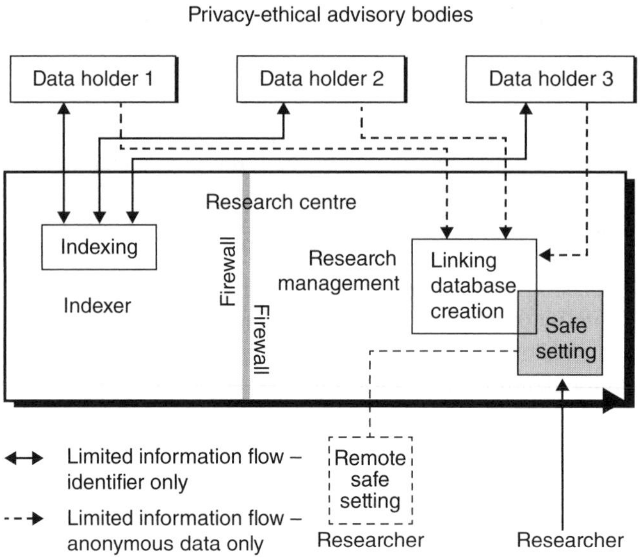

Privacy-ethical advisory bodies

Figure 3.3   Functions separated within a single research centre through the use of firewalls.

research centre. In the meantime, the linkage data would be destroyed by the research centre. The research management part of the research centre then links the various datasets using the study identifier and makes it available to researchers under the single centre model conditions. There is, as a result, a clear separation of function that acts to ensure that the identifier information cannot be used in conjunction with the research dataset to reattached identifiers.

Strengths: Firewall model

• This model offers a structural barrier to dishonest behaviour. It would be difficult, and involve deliberately 'illegal' behaviour, for a research centre worker to bring together identifier and payload information on an individual.

• It has the same strengths (2–5) as the single centre model.

Weaknesses: Firewall model

• Unlike the single centre model, it does offer a structural/temporal barrier to dishonest behaviour. However, this is not particularly visible to the public, and it may simply appear that identifier and payload information on individuals are being held by the same centre.

• The privacy enhancement of the firewall separation of functions relies on the research centre behaving honestly, adhering strictly to the firewall.

• There is more transfer of data in this model, and this increases the inherent danger of loss in transit.

3.4.3 Separation of functions: TTP linkage

The third model is a slight but important refinement of the firewall model. Instead of the indexing process taking place in a firewall separated part of the same organisation, it takes place in an entirely separate organisation. Importantly, the TTP that will carry out the indexing does not transfer any data to the research centre. Indeed, any form of direct communication between the indexer and the research centre can be limited. This then means that the research centre does not need to hold identifier information (i.e. names, addresses, etc.). Indeed, it is possible that the research centre only needs to receive data that – through SDC processes – may also be non-identifiable (particularly within the context of a controlled environment) and therefore is, arguably, not personal data (Figure 3.4).

3.4.4 Secure multiparty computation

This model is an entirely different approach. Here, there is no research centre, but instead, the researcher makes an approach to a set of data holders requesting that they set about a process of 'secure multiparty computation', at the end of which the relevant summary statistics are generated for the researcher. These summary statistics can be controlled so that they cannot be disclosive. The data holders do need to have a common identifier among them, and so a TTP may have to be used if an existing linking index does not already exist (i.e. a national identity number).

Secure multiparty computation involves the transfer of quantities of data[15] that allow the computation of the necessary statistics without revealing the values of the underlying data. For example, in the case of secure least squares regression, in the context of a simple vertically partitioned dataset, each data holder holds different sets of records on all of the individuals in

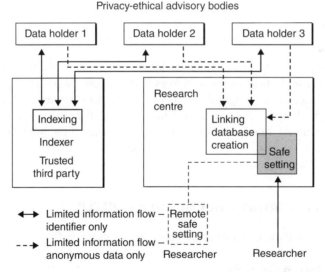

Figure 3.4 Functions separated spatially and organisationally.

[15] Although the idea of secure multiparty computation dates back to a paper by Yao (1982), the huge communication cost means that only very recently have we had sufficient bandwidth to allow its use in dealing with real-world problems. The most notable recent example was the development of a system in the prevention of collisions between satellites owned by different countries who wish to reveal no information about their satellites to others: http://mpclounge.wordpress.com/2013/04/09/using-secure-computation-to-avoid-satellite-collisions/ (accessed 21 July 2015).

Strengths: TTP model

- This model offers a visible structural barrier to dishonest behaviour. It will be extremely difficult, even if a research centre worker is intent on 'illegal' actions, for them to link identifier information to payload data on an individual.

- The separation of functions offers structural aids to support an argument that the processing is of non-personal data and therefore lies outside the scope of data protection law.

- It has the same 5th strength as the single centre model but has lost the strengths outlined in 2–4.

Weaknesses: TTP model

- Because there are now a greater number of organisations involved, auditing the entire process becomes harder. There may be an increased cost in auditing, and this may lead to a reduction in levels of scrutiny.

- The greater number of organisations involved will almost always lead to a loss in efficiency. The need for different organisations to act in concert in a timely manner means that the time taken to process is likely to increase.

- The calculation of linkage quality and the inclusion of this assessment into analysis are likely to be harder.

- It has the same third weakness as the firewall model.

---

any of the other datasets, that is, each data holder has access to all the variables that the data analyst wishes to use. Data agencies need to exchange a privacy-preserving matrix that will allow the calculation of off-diagonal elements of a relevant 'sufficient statistic' such as a covariance matrix, but that does not reveal the values of the underlying data (Karr et al., 2009). This then allows, through a chain process, the construction, over all agencies, of the required statistical information, such as the full variance–covariance matrix across all the variables in the analysis (Figure 3.5).

3.5   Four case study data linkage centres

We now outline how these broad principles have been enacted in four case study centres.

3.5.1   Population Data BC

Population Data BC (PopData) facilitates research access to individual-level, de-identified longitudinal data on British Columbia's (BC) four and a half million residents. These data are linkable to each other and to external datasets, where approved by the data provider (public body).

Under BC's Freedom of Information and Protection of Privacy Act, PopData is permitted to enter into data sharing agreements to receive data collected by public bodies for research

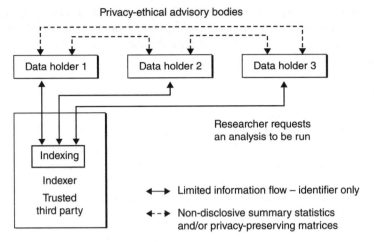

Figure 3.5   Secure multiparty computation.

Strengths: Multiparty model

- This method has the benefit of offering a visible structural barrier to dishonest behaviour by researchers because they have no access to individual-level data. It also requires no sharing of individual information between data holding organisations.

- Arguably, there is no transfer of personal data, and therefore, the system, if combined with privacy-preserving record linkage, is outside the scope of data protection legislation.

Weaknesses: Multiparty model

- This is a developing area of computer/statistical science, and only a limited set of analysis is currently possible, and certain kinds of data modelling, for example, Bayesian methods, are not available.

- The method involves a high degree of participation among multiple data holders in every analysis – automation is possible, but may not be desirable.

- It requires the data holders to provide research ready data (e.g. clean, robust, accurate, etc.). Researchers by design can have no access to the datasets.

- It typically involves very large amounts of data transfer; however, this will be in a privacy-preserving form – loss/interception should not therefore lead to disclosure.

---

purposes. PopData is also authorised to make the data it controls available to eligible research-ers for approved research projects. To access the data, eligible researchers are required to submit a research application to the public body responsible for the data. The public body approves the research application if legislative conditions are met for data release including the benefits of data linkage, contribution to public interest and data security and privacy considerations. Given all necessary approvals are in place, PopData facilitates the release of the approved data to the researcher and oversees the data access process through to data destruction.

3.5.1.1   Operational model

PopData currently holds over 3.2 billion health records from a variety of data providers including the BC Ministry of Health (hospitalisations, physician visits, continuing care, mental health, registration and billing), the BC Vital Statistics Agency (births, deaths, marriages and stillbirths), the BC Cancer Agency (cancer registry, cancer treatment), the WorkSafeBC (claims, firm level data and exposure data) and child development data from the Human Early Learning Partnership. The sources of data continue to expand, with additional sources being added at an increasing rate.

3.5.1.2   Data linkage

With no research programme of their own, PopData acts as a TTP for linkage in addition to being a data repository. In order to achieve this, they follow strict technical and operational guidelines within a high-security environment.

A number of precautions are taken to maximise security and privacy. In no particular order, these are as follows:

- Data are delivered to PopData only through a secure mechanism – typically through a secure upload site. The data files themselves are encrypted with 256-bit AES encryption. They are then uploaded to a secure upload site (transfer and identity of the site are protected by SSL encryption). The uploader separately communicates the encryption key to PopData. Data are moved into the Red Zone (moated network), and the key is communicated to the systems and security manager who decrypts the file.

- Data are characterised as 'content data' (eligible for research use) and 'identifiers' (used for linkage). Identifiers are removed from the content data at the earliest possible time following intake of new data. Identifiers are securely stored separately from content data.

- Linkage (using identifiers only) happens proactively on intake rather than on a per-project basis, to minimise their use.

- Data are handled only by specially trained programmers who have signed confidentiality agreements.

- Following linkage, meaningless but unique internal IDs (identification numbers) – PopData IDs – are applied to the content data.

- As soon as linkage is resolved and a new content data collection is completed, the raw data are sent to an encrypted archive on an unmounted drive.

- All work on raw, content or identifiers is performed in the 'Red Zone' – a highly secure space accessible only to select personnel.

- Programmers work on 'Red Zone' terminals which have no direct connection to the outside world. This space is separated and secured both physically and electronically.

- When content data are released to researchers for approved research projects, the PopData ID is replaced with a study ID – a person-specific number which is unique to each research extract. In this way, records for one research project cannot trivially be linked to records for the same individual from another research project.

- Data minimisation is applied, and researcher access is limited to the subset of files and fields required; records are limited to the study population.

- Released geographic variables are typically limited to larger regions unless otherwise approved.

- Demographic variables like date of birth are commonly limited in their granularity unless otherwise approved.

- Other IDs (facility, group, practitioner) provided on a record are commonly transformed to a study-specific ID unless otherwise approved.

- Researchers must send research materials to the public body in advance of public dissemination.

- Researchers must successfully complete a privacy training programme and test before they are given access to the data extract.

- Staff are required to take annual privacy training.

PopData performs proactive linkage on intake of a new dataset from a data provider. New datasets are received from data providers throughout the year and incorporated into PopData's holdings on an ongoing basis.

PopData uses any personal identifiers available, in unencrypted format, to perform linkage (e.g. name, date of birth, address, personal health number, personal education number, gender). Linkage is done using both probabilistic and deterministic techniques, employing purpose-built software developed in-house and refined over the last 25 years. Linkage enables PopData to identify records that belong to the same individual across files and over time.

Anonymisation typically takes place in terms of (i) data minimisation (only data needed for the study is released), (ii) suppression of identifiers and (iii) limitation of geographic granularity. Approaches to this vary by the specific needs of the project. PopData does not make guarantees of anonymity of the data. Access to identifiable information for research purposes is permitted under legislation, but practice is to limit the potential for identifiability as far as possible without hindering the research objectives. PopData also adds many other layers of privacy protection (e.g. privacy training for researchers, access through the Secure Research Environment (SRE) only, agreements signed by researchers).

3.5.1.3   Ethics

PopData's operations are guided by a governance and oversight committee comprising representatives from BC's research institutions and representatives from the research community. An advisory board provides direction and guidance to PopData's executive director. Lastly, a data stewards working group, comprised of one representative from each public body whose data are accessible through PopData, advises and supports the development of common standards and processes that relate to data access and legislation.

3.5.1.4 Data access

Researchers access their data extract via the SRE. The SRE is a central server accessible only via an encrypted VPN through a firewall and use of a YubiKey for two-factor authentication. The SRE provides secure storage and backup, a centralised location for access and processing of research data, a range of software for use and security standards that meet data provider requirements. Researchers are *not* permitted to download research extracts (raw data) or identifiable information from their study-specific space on the SRE to any local drive. Researchers are *not* allowed to upload data not specified in the data access request. Information that is to be transferred out of the SRE is dropped into a special 'yellow folder'. This triggers a transfer programme, which logs the data and transfers it to a location that is accessible from the outside.

This process allows PopData to keep an audit trail for transfers, and the explicit action required by the researcher will minimise accidental releases of data. The log information is regularly reviewed by PopData and upon request by the applicable data provider(s).

3.5.2 The Secure Anonymised Information Linkage Databank, United Kingdom

The Secure Anonymised Information Linkage (SAIL) Databank links together a wide range of person-based data using robust anonymisation techniques for health-related research (Ford et al., 2009; Lyons et al., 2009; Rodgers et al., 2009; 2011). It represents collaboration between academia, government and the NHS in Wales and is operated by the Health Information Research Unit (HIRU) based at Swansea University. A consumer panel guides the work carried out by HIRU, and lay members are included on the steering committees of virtually all projects.

3.5.2.1 Operational model

The Databank holds over 500 million records and continual growth is in progress. Datasets held at the SAIL Databank include anonymised versions of the All Wales Injury Surveillance System, NHS hospital inpatient and outpatient statistics, Welsh Demographic Service, disease registries, data from about a third of GPs, some laboratory data, Office for National Statistics births and deaths, educational attainment and housing.

3.5.2.2 Data linkage

SAIL operates a combination of privacy-protecting methodologies including TTP, safe haven, multiple encryption, safe setting and safe researcher approaches. A split-file approach to anonymisation is used to overcome the confidentiality and disclosure issues in health-related data warehousing. Through this method, datasets being provided to the SAIL Databank are split at the source organisation into demographic data and clinical data. A system linking field is used to ensure the data can be rejoined later. Clinical data are transferred directly to the HIRU. The demographic data are transferred to NHS Wales Informatics Service (NWIS) for first-stage pseudonymisation and the allocation of an anonymous linking field (ALF) to each record in place of the demographic data. An ALF takes the form of a unique 10-digit number assigned to each individual in a dataset. This product is transferred to the HIRU where it is joined to the clinical data via the system linking field and encrypted a second time before being stored in the SAIL Databank. The SAIL Databank does not hold any personally identifiable data. The identities of small area geographies and service provider codes are also encrypted before being made available for analysis.

3.5.2.3   Ethics

All proposals to use SAIL datasets must comply with HIRU's Information Governance policy. To apply to use SAIL data, individuals must contact the HIRU before being sent a Data Access Agreement and Enquiry form. The forms are modelled on the Secure Data Service's 'approved academic researchers' system and carry the same sanctions for researchers and universities. Once the forms are received back, the research proposal will be considered for approval by the independent Information Governance Review Panel (IGRP) which includes members from different backgrounds: lay people, Caldicott guardian, NWIS Information Governance, NRES and chair of the British Medical Association Ethics Committee. This process usually takes around 1–2 months.

3.5.2.4   Data access

The data held in the SAIL Databank can be accessed remotely through the development of a secure remote access system which is known as the SAIL Gateway. The SAIL Gateway has a number of key features, and these ensure its safe and effective operation. Data are encrypted a third time before being made available for approved projects. It has a secure firewalled network to safeguard the data; and data users are only able to access the data via remote desktops, running Windows in a virtualised environment (VPN). These machines operate the full remote desktop protocol with all desktop and server group policies applied. This ensures that data users cannot copy or transfer files out of the gateway. All requests to export files are reviewed by a data guardian who scrutinises the files before release, an approach modelled on that used in the Office for National Statistics Virtual Microdata Laboratory.

3.5.3   Centre for Data Linkage (Population Health Research Network), Australia

The Centre for Data Linkage (CDL) is an Australian government initiative established in 2009 and funded under the Population Health Research Network (PHRN).[16] The PHRN was established to provide Australian researchers with access to linked de-identified data from a diverse and rich range of health datasets, across jurisdictions and sectors. This supports nationally and internationally significant population-based research to improve health and enhance the delivery of healthcare services in Australia. The CDL is the national linkage component of the PHRN (Boyd et al., 2012).

3.5.3.1   Operational model

CDL's operational model incorporates a separated and layered linkage approach where state/ territory linkages are conducted by individual state-based or 'jurisdictional' linkage units, while cross-jurisdictional or 'national' linkages are conducted by the CDL (O'Keefe, Ferrante and Boyd, 2010a). This layered model builds on the success of well-established linkage units in several Australian states.

---

[16] NCRIS: Funding Agreement for the National Collaborative Research Infrastructure Strategy's Research Capability known as 'Population Health Research Network'. Canberra: Commonwealth Department of Education Science and Training; 2009.

This model does not involve a central data repository, which means that custodians only release data on a project-by-project basis. The CDL does not hold clinical or content data, but links the demographic data that has been separated from the remainder of each dataset to create 'linkage keys'. Clinical or service information is not needed by the CDL and is not provided to it, and the researcher receives only that part of the record that they have approval to see (without any demographic or identifying information).

3.5.3.2   Data linkage

Linkage is carried out using probabilistic methods, without the use of any linkage 'spine' or relatively complete list of individuals.

Data flows for cross-jurisdictional linkage comprise three distinct phases:

1. *Flow of data for linkage*

   The data used for cross-jurisdictional linkage involve only a limited set of variables, typically demographic data (e.g. name, date of birth, address, date of event). The CDL uses this information to link data across multiple jurisdictions.

2. *Provision of project-specific linkage keys*

   The provision of project-specific linkage keys from the CDL enables research datasets to be extracted and merged. For each cross-jurisdictional project, the CDL returns a file with a unique set of project-specific linkage keys (O'Keefe, Ferrante and Boyd, 2010b).

3. *Extraction of research data*

   For each cross-jurisdictional research project, content data are extracted by the data custodian. These data consist of project-specific linkage keys and only those variables which the researcher has been authorised to access. The dataset does not contain any identifying data items (e.g. name). The linkage keys in the dataset are project specific so that researchers cannot collude and bring together data from different projects. Once the researcher is provided with data from all relevant data custodians, records can be merged using the project-specific linkage key and then used in analyses.

This protocol provides an approach suitable for most projects that draw large volumes of information from multiple sources, especially when this includes organisations in different jurisdictions.

3.5.3.3   Ethics

A major challenge for all members of the PHRN has been to ensure that the collection, use and disclosure of personal information comply with applicable information privacy legislation (Boyd et al., 2012).

Among the governance structures instituted by the PHRN is a Management Council overseeing the implementation of the national data linkage programme, with subcommittees which provide advice and direction to Management Council members. These subcommittees include the Ethics, Privacy and Consumer Engagement Advisory Group; an Operations Committee (providing technical advice); an Access Committee (providing advice on access, accreditation and eligibility); a Data Transfer Working Group; and Proof of Concept Reference Group.

Additional governance features of the PHRN include a strict reporting regime, a privacy framework, an Information Governance framework, rigorous approval processes for each research project and binding agreements related to data release, date confidentiality and security and network-wide policies and guidelines.

3.5.4   The Centre for Health Record Linkage, Australia

The Centre for Health Record Linkage (CHeReL) was established in 2006 to provide a mechanism for researchers, health planners and policymakers to access linked data from the health and human service sectors in New South Wales and the Australian Capital Territory. The functions of the CHeReL include (i) advising potential users on design, process, feasibility and cost of linkage studies; (ii) building data linkage infrastructure to deliver timely, cost-effective access to high-quality linked data; (iii) providing tailored linkage services for research and evaluation; and (iv) making the use and outputs of linked data transparent.

3.5.4.1   Operational model

As of 2013, the CHeReL's core linkage system contained more than 70 million records relating to 9.8 million people from 17 different health and related datasets. The records within this linkage system are regularly updated, and the range of datasets is being expanded over time. This comprehensive system of enduring links between personal identifiers enables timely and cost-effective access to linked population-based data. The current range of data collections includes hospital admissions, emergency presentations, perinatal and mental health ambulatory data, cancer and infectious disease notifications, early child development and birth and death registrations. This system has been used in more than 250 projects since 2006. The CHeReL infrastructure has supported projects that have attracted research income from competitive grant funding in excess of $38 million and has delivered services to over 1000 researchers, evaluators and policymakers. In addition, the CHeReL has linked 85 external datasets to parts of the core system on request, subject to data custodian and ethics approval. Examples include public laboratory, toxicology and screening data, administrative data from other sectors (including transport, education, justice and community services) and primary research data collections of cohort or trial participants.

3.5.4.2   Data linkage

The CHeReL carries out record linkage using best practice privacy-preserving procedures (Kelman, Bass and Holman, 2002). These ensure that the process of record linkage, which requires access to personal identifiers, is completely separated from the data analysis, which does not require personal information.

The CHeReL holds only the personal information such as name, date of birth, gender and address required for record linkage and uses this to create a linkage key (or unique number) that points to where records for the same person can be found in different databases (e.g. hospitalisation, cancer registry, birth and death databases). For each research project, the CHeReL provides project-specific keys back to the relevant data custodians, who provide the approved health information to the researchers with a project-specific person number. This enables researchers to create linked files without accessing or using personal information. A comprehensive suite of information security controls is in place in accordance with NSW government policy. The CHeReL does not mandate the use of secure remote access facilities. Arrangements for use and storage of linked data files must comply with the policies and conditions imposed by relevant ethics committees and the agencies that have disclosed the data.

Record linkage methods used by the CHeReL include both deterministic and probabilistic approaches. The CHeReL currently uses ChoiceMaker™ software for probabilistic linkage (Goldberg and Borthwick, 2004), a system originally developed to assist the New York City Department of Health in de-duplicating its child immunisation register. ChoiceMaker provides for standardisation and parsing; and it differs from traditional approaches primarily in the use of an automated blocking algorithm and machine learning technique for 'scoring' or assigning weights. A group matching process follows the pairwise matching and identifies cohesive clusters from the analysis of transitivities. Clerical reviews are performed on a small percentage of linked record groups to assess the accuracy of the linkage and correct any incorrect links that are identified. Researchers are provided with a document that describes the linkage methods and error rates for their project.

3.5.4.3   Ethics

The CHeReL is managed by the NSW Ministry of Health. Other organisations may become members of the CHeReL and participate in a Data Linkage Advisory Committee. The Data Linkage Advisory Committee plays a key role in providing advice to the NSW Ministry of Health on the CHeReL's strategic plan, the development of record linkage infrastructure and services and the use of linked data to enhance policy-relevant research and inform policy and practice. A Community Advisory Committee for the CHeReL has been functioning since 2007, providing advice on issues of community interest regarding data linkage.

3.5.4.4   Data access

A dedicated research liaison officer provides individual guidance and advice to interested individuals and organisations wishing to access data. Contact details and detailed information on the application and linkage process can be found on the website (www.cherel.org.au).

3.6   Conclusion

The advantages of sharing and linking data through well-organised, secure data linkage environments are numerous and include the following: the level of access permitted to potentially disclosive data increases, while the risk of disclosing personal information without consent or approval decreases; safe settings represent a model with standardised procedures for academic researchers to securely access administrative data, which in turn can provide a consistent approach to certain limited circumstances in which personal data can be shared without the data subject's knowledge or consent; there is likely to be less risk of the occurrence of complaints and disputes about the way in which personal data are shared if a rigorous procedure has been followed during the application stage for access to personal data; there is consequently less risk of reputational damage for data holding organisations caused by inappropriate or insecure sharing of data; the more secure the environment in which a researcher is accessing confidential information, the more relaxed a data holding organisation is likely to be in permitting access to sensitive information; the probability of breaching the confidentiality of the data reduces as the security increases; and safe settings consequently minimise the risk of security breaches and any resulting enforcement action by regulators.

4

Bias in data linkage studies

Megan Bohensky

Department of Medicine, Melbourne EpiCentre, University of Melbourne, Parkville, Victoria, Australia

4.1 Background

Given the widespread use of data linkage and the likelihood of its applications growing further in the future, consideration must be given to some of the potential methodological limitations of the uses of linked data for scientific studies. As various new data linkage centres and methods for data linkage have emerged over recent years, there may be a lack of consistency among the choice of software, techniques being used and quality of the linkage processes between linkage operators and centres. Furthermore, linkage methods and quality are not always clearly described in the published literature, making it difficult to assess the validity and generalisability of research findings.

As described in previous chapters, data linkage involves one or more existing data sources and a number of different methods that can be applied to facilitate the linkage. Error can be introduced to the data linkage process if there are records that belong to a person or entity that fail to be matched (missed matches) or if there are cases not belonging to the same person or entity that are erroneously matched (false matches) (Figure 4.1). Factors such as missing data, incomplete participant inclusion or recruitment, duplicate records and inaccuracies in the data such as transpositions or misspellings can all contribute to missing or inaccurate data leading to error in research findings. All of these data quality issues have been identified in administrative databases (Chattopadhyay and Bindman, 2005; Iezzoni, 1997a; Westaby et al., 2007) and clinical registries (Aylin et al., 2007; Wang et al., 2005), both of which are commonly used for data linkage.

While the data linkage process attempts to minimise these issues, the availability and accuracy of data does influence the quality of this process. Pinto da Silveira and Artmann conducted a systematic review of the peer-reviewed literature (up to 2007) to examine probabilistic

Methodological Developments in Data Linkage, First Edition. Edited by Katie Harron, Harvey Goldstein and Chris Dibben.
© 2016 John Wiley & Sons, Ltd. Published 2016 by John Wiley & Sons, Ltd.

		True match status		
		Matches	Non-matches	
Link status (as determined by data linkage process)	Identified links	True links or true positives (TP)	False matches or false positives (FP)	Total links*
	Identified non-links	Missed matches or false negatives (FN)	True non-links or true negatives (TN)	Total non-links**
		Total matches	Total non-matches	Total record pairs

Figure 4.1 Classification of missed and false matches; *positive predictive value = true positives/total links; **negative predictive value = true negatives/total non-links.

data linkage accuracy (Pinto da Silveira and Artmann, 2009). They identified six studies that had complete data on summary measures of linkage quality and found that the sensitivity of the linkage process, or the number of correct matches identified, ranged from 74 to 98%, while the specificity, or the proportion of true negatives detected, ranged from 99 to 100%. The authors suggested that the strongest predictor of high linkage accuracy was the number and quality of linkage variables with high rates of missing data being one of the biggest factors to compromise linkage results. For example, one of the studies with the lowest linkage sensitivity discussed in the review linked a cohort of 250 hospital records to death records. Despite the small number of records in the study and the use of manual review, a relatively low matching rate (86%) was achieved due to the high proportion of records with missing names. Linkage analysts were unable to determine if a number of records contained homonymous demographic information or were true matches.

It is important to consider the limitations of data linkage in balance with its benefits, to make an accurate assessment of its validity and utility when choosing these methods for research or to answer policy questions. 'Selection bias' is a term used in epidemiology, which means that a systematic error has been introduced into the process of selecting individuals or groups to participate in a research study (Rothman, 2002). In data linkage studies, selection bias can occur if the records of certain subgroups of individuals have different linkage rates to other groups. These differences in the accuracy of linkage ('linkage errors') may impact the assessment of study outcomes if people from certain groups are more or less likely to have the risk factors or outcomes of interest ('selection bias'). Bias will produce estimates that are either diluted (bias towards the null) or overly exaggerated (bias away from the null); however, this will be dependent on the source of error and how it creates bias.

Given these considerations, this chapter will explore some of the common issues affecting quality in the data linkage process. The second part of the chapter will go on to present a narrative review of the literature describing how the limitations of data linkage can impact the quality of research findings. Lastly, it will provide some recommendations for practice to improve the linkage process and the interpretation of results based on linked data.

4.2   Description of types of linkage error

4.2.1   Missed matches from missing linkage variables

Missed matches are perhaps the most challenging issue in data linkage, as they lead to issues of missing data in the final linked dataset. Missed matches can be missing completely at random (MCAR), missing at random (MAR) or missing not at random (MNAR), and this will play a role in how they can influence study results. The following example illustrates how each of these three types of missingness can occur.

A study is being undertaken which will involve linkage of an infectious disease registry dataset to a cancer registry to examine the number of people with hepatitis B (Y) who go on to develop liver cancer in the next year (X). The linkage variables to be used include patient names and dates of birth, and some of these variables may be missing or incorrectly recorded in each dataset. There are three possible scenarios by which linkage errors can occur:

1. There may be no pattern to patients' names and dates of birth being missing or incorrectly recorded. Therefore, the proportion of linkage errors is similar for all types of patients, and the chance that people with hepatitis B (Y) have missing or incorrectly linked records bears no relationship to X or Y. In this scenario, the data are MCAR.

2. Patients belonging to one ethnic group may be more likely to have errors in their names or dates of birth. The proportion of unlinked cancer registry records in this group will be higher, but they are no more or less likely to have hepatitis B. Therefore, the probability that Y is missing is proportional to the value of X. These data are MAR.

3. Patients belonging to one ethnic group may be more likely to have missing values or errors in their names and dates of birth and have unlinked cancer registry records, and they are also more likely to have hepatitis B. Hence, the probability that Y is missing depends on the unobserved value of Y in the linked dataset. In this scenario, data are MNAR.

Methods are available for dealing with data that are MCAR or MAR, but data that are MNAR can render errors in estimates through systematic bias. Therefore, it is important to understand why linkage errors have occurred, how these are distributed across different participant groups and how this may impact the assessment of outcomes.

Issues of missing data and linkages are harder to detect and quantify than false matches, as most manual case review processes typically only consider a selection of probable links. When a number of key linkage variables contain missing data, it is a challenge to assess whether paired records are true matches. In a review of 105 multicentre clinical databases across the United Kingdom, undertaken in 2003, Black and colleagues surveyed data custodians about the completeness of their data sources. They found that less than half (40%, 42 of 105 databases) said that most (>90%) or almost all (>97%) variables had small amounts of missing data (5% or less cases). Notably, over 40% of data custodians did not know the completeness of their data (Black, Barker and Payne, 2004). In Australia, Evans et al. assessed

28 registries in 2006–2007 and found that 6 (21%) registries did not assess variable completeness, or had less than 80% of variables, with less than 5% missing data (Evans et al., 2011). In administrative data sources, the completeness of coding may be lower than clinical registries, as data are typically drawn from medical records and coded into a finite number of coding slots (Iezzoni, 1997b). A recent study in the United States looked at data linkage of 381 719 injured patient records in seven regions. They found that sites with data missing for key variables had the lowest rate of matched records, with the lowest site having less than 20% of records match. It was also noted that the cases that did match appeared to be unrepresentative, as they possessed less common values (e.g. unusual zip codes, older or younger ages) (Newgard et al., 2012).

4.2.2   Missed matches from inconsistent case ascertainment

The choice of inclusion criteria or participant recruitment method can affect the population coverage of registries and databases, impacting the validity and generalisability of research findings. Kho et al. conducted a systematic review of the literature and identified 17 studies reporting bias in registry recruitment (Kho et al., 2009). The authors reported registry participation rates ranging from 36.3 to 92.9% and identified biases in age, sex, race, education, income and health status. Despite these individual differences in participation rates, no consistent trends in the magnitude of effects were identified across all studies, and reasons for non-participation were unclear. Black and colleagues, in their aforementioned review of 105 UK clinical registries, found that 45 (43%) of registries either did not know the completeness of their recruitment processes or recruited less than 90% of the eligible population. In their review of 28 Australian clinical registries, Evans et al. also found that 13 registries (46%) did not assess or recruited less than 80% of the eligible population (Evans et al., 2011). As cancer notifications are mandated by governments to estimate the population burden of cancer in many countries, it is generally expected that they have a high degree of accuracy in their case-finding procedures. However, various estimations undertaken have demonstrated that some registries may miss up to 10% of cases for certain types of cancer (Brenner, Stegmaier and Ziegler, 1995; Dickinson et al., 2001; Stefoski Mikeljevic et al., 2003).

4.2.3   False matches: Description of cases incorrectly matched

False matches, or two cases belonging to different people being mistakenly matched, can also impact the quality of the linkage process. Matches that are near the threshold cut-off value, or have 'close agreement' in a probabilistic linkage process (e.g. a name that is similar in spelling), may be reviewed by clerical checking, and the match will be determined by human judgement or face validity (e.g. 'it looks correct'). However, these manual methods of reviewing close matches can introduce a degree of subjective judgement into the process (Newcombe, 1984). The impact of technical experience and inter-operator reliability of data-matching accuracy are not well documented. As the data linkage process is often outsourced to data custodians or linkage centres who may not be familiar with each dataset or the research questions, there is a risk that matching criteria could be inappropriate. Brenner et al. simulated the effects of different threshold values on follow-up studies using linkage to a death registry (Brenner, Schmidtmann and Stegmaier, 1997). They found that using a lax definition for a match, or a lower threshold value without clerical review, overestimated the death rate by 115.6%. At the optimal rate, where false negative and false positives were in the same order of magnitude, there was an underestimation of deaths by 3.3%. While this had a small net effect on the outcome, the individual rate of false negative and false positive links was noted to be large (5% and 8%, respectively).

Additionally, there are various types of linkage methods and software available, and many of the latter can be readily accessed by researchers at low cost with little training. The degree of control a user has over the data preparation phases and linking process may vary, and it is often unclear how the accuracy and reliability of new software are validated. One study compared linkage results of two different linkage technologies (The Link King and Link Plus) using a blinded clerical review of a subsample of the records as the 'gold standard' for determining correct matches. Link King generated 229 189 linked records, while Link Plus matched 225 170 records, corresponding to a sensitivity of 96.7% compared to 94.1% and a positive predictive value of 96.1% compared to 94.8% (Campbell, Deck and Krupski, 2008). While the absolute differences between software performances may not seem large, if the error in the linkage process is not randomly distributed, these differences can introduce bias into the final results.

More recently, the Centre for Data Linkage in Western Australia undertook an evaluation of 10 data linkage software packages (Bigmatch, dfPower Studio, FEBRL, FRIL, HDI, LinkageWiz, LINKS, QualityStage, The Link King and a program developed in-house based on the Scottish Record Linkage System) (Ferrante and Boyd, 2012). The authors reviewed the quality of linkage, including both a de-duplication and file-to-file linkage process, for a synthetic population of 4 million people. Linkage quality was based on matching sensitivity (proportion of true matches), positive predictive value (number of true matches divided by the total number of cases considered to be matches) and the F-measure, which assesses the balance between sensitivity and positive predictive value. For the de-duplication linkage, the authors ranked only 3 of the 10 software packages as producing 'good' quality linkage, with the remaining being ranked as fair (sensitivity ranged from 96 to 84%). For the file-to-file linkage, one package was ranked 'very good', four were ranked 'good', and the remaining five were ranked 'fair' (sensitivity ranged from 97 to 91%). Thus, the choice of technologies used for linkage and the operator's experience and knowledge of the software may affect the derived data, and depending on the research questions, incorrectly linked cases may bias the final results.

The choice of probabilistic versus deterministic linkage will also have an impact upon study results. A number of studies have compared the use of deterministic linkage strategies with probabilistic strategies to ascertain the number of false positives and negatives (Campbell, 2009; Gomatam et al., 2002; Grannis et al., 2003; Jamieson, Roberts and Browne, 1995; Roos and Wajda, 1991; Tromp et al., 2011). Most of these studies have demonstrated the superiority of probabilistic linkage methods. Gomatam et al. compared deterministic and probabilistic linkage methods without clerical review in a cohort of paediatric intensive care patients (Gomatam et al., 2002). It was shown that deterministic links that match accurately had a higher degree of certainty and that links were valid (higher positive predictive value), but there was a lower degree of sensitivity in achieving correct matches, where there may be inaccuracies in the data. Given the effects of these methodological differences, the authors suggested that the choice of the linkage method largely be determined by the availability and quality of identifying variables held within the datasets, resources available and the level of precision required for the specific research questions. Tromp et al. found that their full deterministic linkage approach produced 330 false negatives in a simulation study, while the probabilistic strategy outperformed the deterministic strategy on all linkage scenarios. They suggested that deterministic strategies could be tailored to have similar performance to probabilistic strategies, but linkage analysts required a priori knowledge about the data, and which disagreements would be acceptable (Tromp et al., 2011).

The sources of error and reasons for incorrect linkages may not be known in certain studies. If a linked record implies an outcome (e.g. linkage to a mortality registry indicates a death), a false negative link will be assumed to imply a negative outcome (e.g. survival) and the effects on the derived data are difficult to estimate without clerical review. Similarly, if the linkage has a one-to-many relationship (e.g. a number of birth records per mother), it can also be difficult to identify where records have not linked accurately, without another data source to verify the true number of links to be achieved.

4.3   How linkage error impacts research findings

The review in this section aims to provide a summary of identified quality issues with data linkage and how these may introduce selection bias into research results. To gain an understanding of the extent of these issues with data linkage, we conducted a structured qualitative synthesis of the literature (Medline, EMBASE and CINAHL databases) to identify studies that described patient or population characteristics that may be associated with lower linkage rates or changes in the sensitivity or specificity of data linkage, thereby introducing bias into reported outcomes. This review is an update to our previous review (Bohensky et al., 2010), utilising similar methods, and includes literature from 2007–2013. To be included in the review, the article had to empirically evaluate methodological issues relating to data linkage, report on patient characteristics in matched versus unmatched records or report how differing linkage strategies impacted study outcomes. Articles were excluded if they did not involve data linkage, such as a discussion of another form of health information technology; if they did not include an evaluation of data (e.g. a commentary, letter or discussion of data linkage methodology without an empirical evaluation); or if they presented a linkage project without comparing characteristics in matched and unmatched records. We also restricted our search to studies reported in the English language and to human studies.

For each study, data were extracted and entered into an evidence table. Items included the author, year, country, a brief description of the type of data sources that were used in the linkage, participant inclusion criteria, total number of participants, the linkage methods (e.g. probabilistic, deterministic), variables on which the linkage process was based, linkage rates (overall and for specific subgroups, if applicable) and a brief summary of any linkage bias in outcomes that was identified. The data in the review were synthesised with descriptive statistics and qualitatively. There were not a sufficient number of studies with similar outcomes or similar measures to consider extensive quantitative analysis (meta-analysis or statistical pooling) of data.

4.3.1   Results

There were 4158 potentially relevant reports identified, of which 4094 were excluded based on their titles and abstracts. The complete texts of the remaining 31 studies were retrieved and screened against the inclusion criteria. This detailed screening of the full reports led to the exclusion of 18 reports, leaving 13 studies over the time period which met the inclusion criteria (Figure 4.2).

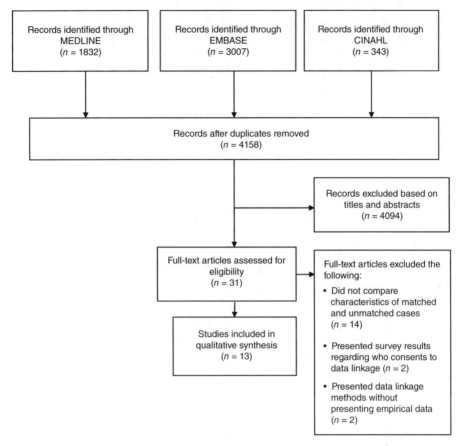

Figure 4.2   Flowchart of study inclusion criteria.

4.3.1.1   Excluded studies

The majority of the 18 excluded articles (78%) presented a linkage study with rates of unlinked records, but did not compare characteristics of matched and unmatched cases. Two studies presented survey results regarding who consents to data linkage, and two studies presented data linkage methods without presenting actual data.

4.3.1.2   Included studies

The 13 included studies (Table 4.1) utilised 28 different datasets from six countries (six studies from Australia, three from the United States, one from France, one from the UK, one from Switzerland and one from the Netherlands). The clinical focus of the studies included perinatal outcomes (four studies), cancer research (two studies), intensive care (one study), cardiovascular disease (one study), drug rehabilitation outcomes (one study), surgical outcomes (one study), hospitalisation of people in aged care (one study), minority health service utilisation (one study) and respiratory disease in children (one study). All studies were cohort designs. The key characteristics that were examined among the included studies in relation to data linkage quality and potential biases are reported herein.

Table 4.1 Summary of included studies.

First author, year, country	Data source types	Inclusion criteria	Number of participants	Linkage method/ variables	Linkage rate(s)	Bias outcomes
1. Bentley, 2012, Australia	1. Statutory birth records 2. Hospital records: birth records linked to both mother and infant hospital birth admission records	All mothers who gave birth, and their infants, in NSW, Australia, from 1 January 2001 to 31 December 2008	706 685 deliveries	Probabilistic linkage (ChoiceMaker). Based on first name, last name, address, sex, date of birth and country of birth. Hospital admission details, birth plurality and birth order used where available	96% at 37 weeks' gestation <90% at 30 weeks gestation <70% at 25 weeks gestation	The unlinked birth records had higher proportions of nulliparous, Australian-born women, aged 35 and over, births in private hospitals, by caesarean section and the lowest levels of social disadvantage
2. Bohensky, 2011b, Australia	1. Critical care registry data 2. Hospital records	All patients ≥16 years with an intensive care unit (ICU) admission at one of the study hospitals in VIC, Australia, from 1 January 2001 to 31 December 2006	20 907 patients	A backward stepwise deterministic linkage method using indirect identifiers (SAS). Based on hospital of the patient's ICU admission, patient's age at admission, hospital admission date, hospital discharge date, length of hospital stay and number of days in the ICU	92.3% (95% CI 91.9–92.6%)	The factors most strongly associated with unsuccessful linkage were patients at hospital C, admissions in years 2002 and 2003, transferred patients, non-Australian-born patients and patients with a hospital length of stay of 20 days or more

Study	Data sources	Population	Sample size	Linkage method	Result	Findings
3. Bopp, 2010, Switzerland	1. Linked census and mortality records 2. Cardiovascular cohort study (MONICA study)	All participants enrolled in the 1984–1986, 1988–1989 and 1992–1993 waves of the cohort study	15 893 individuals	Multi-step linkage process. Based on sex, exact date of birth and place of residence. If available, nationality, marital status, educational category and profession were used	97.8% of MONICA participants could be linked to a census or mortality record	The proportions of unlinked individuals were negligible (2.2%), and socio-demographic characteristics did not substantially differ from successfully linked individuals
4. Campbell, 2009, United States	1. Administrative dataset for state alcohol and substance abuse services 2. State police records 3. Death records	All clients receiving alcohol and substance abuse services in 2005	15 562–16 044 admissions (depending on de-duplication strategy)	Three linkage methods were used: exact match, deterministic linkage and probabilistic linkage (The Link King). Based on first name, last name, middle name, birth date and SSN	Not reported	The probabilistic linkage strategy produced the highest estimates of performance indicators. A disproportionate number of links missed by the exact and deterministic linkage strategies (but captured by the probabilistic algorithm) were female or belonged to a minority racial/ethnic group
5. Duvall, 2010, United States	1. Inpatient and outpatient medical records 2. Family history and vital records	All patients with inpatient and outpatient medical records since the database inception (in 1993)	1 850 683 demographic records	Probabilistic record linkage. Based on first, middle, last name, addresses, phone numbers and names of next of kin	74.3% with 11.3% linked to multiple records (duplicate linkages)	Many of the names over-represented in the duplicate set were traditionally Hispanic. Common Vietnamese, Korean, Chinese, Navajo and Arabic names exhibited the same over-representation in the duplicate set

(Continued)

Table 4.1 (*Continued*)

First author, year, country	Data source types	Inclusion criteria	Number of participants	Linkage method/variables	Linkage rate(s)	Bias outcomes
6. Fournel, 2009, France	1. Hospital data 2. Mortality data	All patients hospitalised for the first time between 1998 and 2000 at one hospital with a malignant tumour or a tumour suspected to be malignant were included	10089 patients	Probabilistic linkage with manual validation. Based on last name, first given name, date of birth and code of place of birth. Other variables (marital name, second and third given names) were used for validation	98.4% patients were properly classified 93.7% of patients born abroad were properly classified	The linkage method was less efficient for patients born abroad and the place of birth was more efficient for men than for women
7. Huntington, 2012, United Kingdom	1. HIV cohort data 2. National surveillance data	All women in the HIV cohort receiving HIV clinical care in 1996–2009 who were found to have a pregnancy	8 286 women	Deterministic decision criteria (SAS). Based on DOB, CD4 date, drug start/stop dates, HIV diagnosis date and ART profile	24.9% had a record in the national surveillance data	Timing of HIV diagnosis, repeat pregnancies, attendance at clinics in London, age, and ethnicity varied between matched and unmatched records
8. Karmel, 2008, Australia	1. Hospital data 2. Residential aged care data	All permanent and respite admissions and hospital and social leave events for 2000–2001 for people aged >65 years	19636 admissions	Probabilistic matching. Person-based matching on surname, given names, sex, date of birth and address. Event-based matching (WebSphere software) on hospital separation date and residential care admission date and other discharge information	Event-based linkage had a positive predictive value of 97% and sensitivity of 80.7%	The event-based linkage strategies underestimated movement between hospital and residential aged care, with permanent residential aged care admissions being particularly affected

Study	Data sources	Population	Sample size	Linkage method	Result	Conclusion
9. Lain, 2009, Australia	1. Midwives dataset 2. Hospital records 3. Pathology dataset	Randomly selected women who were expected to deliver before 31 December 2006 with pathology tests between 1 January and 30 June 2006	1 882 women	Probabilistic matching. Based on full name, date of birth, sex, address, hospital code and hospital record number	89.3% of pathology records had an established linkage to a pregnancy outcome	There was no evidence that the unlinked pregnancies were different in regard to their pathology results (PAPP-A and free β-hCG), days of gestation, maternal age or maternal weight
10. Lawson, 2013, Australia	1. Surgical registry 2. Hospital claims	All surgical inpatients at participating hospitals aged <65 years from 2005 to 2008	150454 records	Deterministic linkage algorithm (SAS). Based on hospital, age, sex, diagnosis, procedure category and dates of admission, discharge and procedure	80.5% surgical registry records matched to a hospital claims record	Linkage rates varied significantly by surgical procedure type, age group, year of procedure and geographic region
11. McCusker, 2012, United States	1. Cancer registry 2. Biorepository data	All patients in California diagnosed with cancer during 2005–2009	1 040 records	Probabilistic data linkage. Based on name, gender, date of birth, race, medical record number, tumour site, tumour behaviour, date of diagnosis, pathology report number and site of care	81.2% of records were matched	The number of records that matched between the two databases varied by year and cancer site

(Continued)

Table 4.1 (*Continued*)

First author, year, country	Data source types	Inclusion criteria	Number of participants	Linkage method/ variables	Linkage rate(s)	Bias outcomes
12. Moore, 2012, Australia	1. Hospital records 2. Laboratory data	All hospital admissions for acute lower respiratory illness between January 2000 and December 2005	8 980 hospital admissions	Probabilistic data linkage. Based on a unique child identifier key (developed by data linkage service), specimen dates and hospital admission dates	45.2% admissions were linked with laboratory records	Predictors of non-linkage included birth region, private hospital type, aboriginal status, age group and year of hospital admission
13. Tromp, 2008, Netherlands	1. Newborn registry 2. ICU	All admission records from 5 neonatology wards and all 10 neonatal intensive care units (NICUs)	30 082 admission records	Deterministic and probabilistic internal linkage. Based on date of child's birth (blocking variable), date of mother's birth, postal code, gestational age, gender, birth weight and APGAR scores	The sensitivity of links where the status was uncertain was 73% and the specificity was 64%	There were a substantial number of errors in the linkage of readmissions of twin brothers or twin sisters

4.3.1.3 Description of data sources

Of the 28 datasets utilised in the study reports, 29% were hospital admission data, 18% were clinical registry data (intensive care, newborn registry, cancer registry, surgical registry), 14% were mortality data, 7% were laboratory or pathology data, 7% were cohort study data (cardiovascular disease cohort, HIV cohort), and the remaining 21% were other sources of administrative data (residential aged care, police records, birth records, substance abuse treatment records, HIV surveillance data). Given the range of datasets, it was expected that the data would vary in terms of quality and completeness. However, this was not always discernible, based on reports. Nearly all reports (92%) contained the dataset inclusion criteria, 11 (85%) reports discussed some potential sources of bias and inaccuracies at the data collection phase, 7 (54%) studies reported the data collection methods (who collects the data and how data are obtained), 7 (54%) discussed coding methods used (e.g. international classification of diseases coding), 7 (54%) reported the total number of records held in each dataset, 5 (38%) reports included the total duration of the data source (i.e. for how many years it has been established), and 4 reports (31%) gave some indication of the amount of missing data.

Similarly, the descriptions of the linkage process and results were variable in reports. All studies reported the number of linked records; however, some did this via flowchart, while others reported numbers or proportions. All studies presented the type of linkage that was undertaken, with 7 (54%) using probabilistic methods, 4 (31%) using deterministic methods, 2 (15%) using a combination of these at different stages in the linkage process and nearly half (46%) outsourcing the linkage process to a linkage group or data custodian. The majority of studies (92%) reported a linkage rate or sensitivity and listed which linkage variables were used. Fewer studies reported the specificity (31%), positive predictive value (15%) or negative predictive value (15%) of the linkage process. There were 8 (62%) studies that described the linkage process in further detail, including threshold values, or steps in the deterministic processes, such that the linkage methods could potentially be replicated based on the information provided.

4.3.2 Assessment of linkage bias

There were 11 studies (85%) that identified some type of bias in the linkage results. Linkage bias was assessed in a number of ways. Most commonly, authors compared characteristics of linked and unlinked records on key factors in their clinical areas of research (reported in more detail in the next section). However, three of these studies presented the linkage rates only, without statistical tests for significance. Other studies used regression methods to assess factors that were predictive of linkage or non-linkage. The study by Duvall et al. assessed the frequency of ethnic names on duplicate records (Duvall et al., 2010). The authors assumed that the duplicate records would occur at random and that each name should have an equal probability of being duplicated. Tromp et al. validated matches that were thought to be probable links via each person's admission history and then examined characteristics of those records that were inaccurately linked (Tromp et al., 2008). While this is the most accurate form of validation, the time and resourcing required only permitted the authors to validate 200 records. Karmel and Rosman (2008), Bopp et al. (2010) and Campbell (2009) all examined the impact of their linkage results on the analysis of key study outcomes.

Common factors where bias was identified among study participants included health status or condition type, age group, geographical location, ethnicity, gender, year and socio-economic status. The reasons for the inaccuracies and bias in the linkage results varied depending on the datasets, their inclusion criteria and the linkage criteria. These are each described further herein by the category of bias.

4.3.2.1   Health status/condition type

A total of seven studies examined results by the participant's health status or condition type. Lain et al. linked pathology results to hospital admission and midwives datasets, using probabilistic matching on mother's full name, sex and date of birth, and found no statistically significant differences in pathology test results (maternal serum levels of PAPP-A or free β-hCG) for the records of linked and unlinked pregnancies, based on a linkage rate of 89.3% (Lain et al., 2009). The remaining six studies all identified differences, generally showing that people with more severe conditions were less likely to have matched records. In the study by Bohensky et al., the authors linked intensive care registry data with hospital admission records, using a combination of deterministic and probabilistic linkage methods, and achieved a linkage rate of 92.3% (95% CI 91.9–92.6%) (Bohensky et al., 2011b). As the linkage process relied partially on admission and separation dates, they found that participants with longer lengths of stay (>20 days), who would also be the most severe cases, were less likely to have linked records, due to less accurate dates being recorded in their admission and intensive care unit records.

4.3.2.2   Age

Five studies (Bentley et al., 2012; Huntington et al., 2012; Lain et al., 2009; Lawson et al., 2013; Moore et al., 2012) examined whether the linked and unlinked results had differences by age of participants. Again, Lain et al. found no statistically significant differences in maternal ages or days gestation for the records of linked and unlinked pregnancies. The remaining four studies all found a bias in the age of participants. Probabilistic linkage was conducted in two of these studies (Bentley et al., 2012; Moore et al., 2012), and deterministic linkage was undertaken in the other two (Huntington et al., 2012; Lawson et al., 2013), with linkage rates ranging from 24 to 80.5%. Bentley et al. matched birth records with hospital admission records for mothers and infant birth admissions. They used probabilistic linkage methods based on name, date of birth, country of birth and hospital admission details. Unlinked records for births were more common for older women (aged >35 years) and may have been the result of a greater number of these births occurring in private hospitals, where information capture is not as complete. Conversely, unlinked records for mothers were more common among women aged less than 25 years. This group were also more likely to have risk factors and adverse pregnancy outcomes. As more of these pregnancies resulted in stillbirths, the authors suggested that this may partly explain why they were not able to be linked to birth records, which are more likely to capture live births only (Bentley et al., 2012).

4.3.2.3   Geographical location

Four studies identified differences in the geographical location of participants, with linked records compared to unlinked records (Bohensky et al., 2011b; Huntington et al., 2012; Lawson et al., 2013; Moore et al., 2012). Huntington and colleagues (2012) matched HIV cohort data to national HIV surveillance records in the UK, using a deterministic decision criterion, where they achieved a 25% linkage rate. They found that participants attending clinics in London were more likely to be included in the cohort data, which has a greater number of sites in the London area. In the study by Moore et al., researchers matched hospital records to laboratory samples taken from children with asthma, using a probabilistic linkage method. Less than half (45.2%) of all hospital admissions were linked to a laboratory record, with admissions to public and metropolitan hospitals more likely to link (Moore et al., 2012). Data from rural hospitals were more likely to be missing, as these sites maintained separate data systems, which needed to be combined with metropolitan systems in a separate process. Also, the authors suggested that there may be limited resourcing in regional hospitals for routinely collecting pathology samples from all children.

4.3.2.4   Ethnicity

Differential rates of linkage by participant ethnicity was considered and identified in four studies (Bohensky et al., 2011b; Campbell, 2009; Duvall et al., 2010; Fournel et al., 2009). Duvall et al. matched vital records with inpatient and outpatient medical records using probabilistic matching on participant names. They found that Hispanic, Vietnamese, Korean, Chinese, Navajo and Arabic names were more likely to be false positives in their analyses of duplicate records. The authors suggested that it was likely that ethnic names, unfamiliar to registration clerks and other hospital staff, would have increased occurrences of misspellings. Also, the fields for each person's name consisted of a first name, a middle name and a last name, which might not be suitable in many cultures. Hispanic names often include more than one first or middle name, and it may be appropriate to use different last names in different situations. Many Asian names also have the last or family name presented before the first or given name (Duvall et al., 2010). Similarly, Fournel et al. found that their linkage method, which used place of birth as a linkage variable, was less efficient for patients born abroad, as the place of birth coding for patients born abroad was not as precise as the place of birth for patients born in France (where the study was undertaken) (Fournel et al., 2009).

4.3.2.5   Gender

Linkage rates by gender were considered in two studies (Campbell, 2009; Fournel et al., 2009). The previously described study by Fournel et al., which used the participants' full name as a linkage variable, found that linkage performance was better for men than for women, as the maiden name was not always recorded in databases or was entered as a compound name with the marital name. Campbell compared three linkage strategies and found that two of the methods, which were both deterministic in nature, had lower linkage rates for women. He also suggested that this may be related to a last name mismatch, with female names changing over the life course more commonly than male names. Of all three linkage strategies, the probabilistic linkage method seemed to be the best in accounting for the name differences, although the linkage algorithm and weights were not specified in the report.

4.3.2.6   Year

Two studies identified differences in linkage rate by year (Bohensky et al., 2011b; McCusker et al., 2012). Both McCusker et al. and Bohensky et al. found lower linkage rates in the earlier years of their respective studies, as datasets were still in the development, and implementation phases and data were not collected as robustly as they were in later years.

4.3.2.7   Socio-economic status

Lastly, two studies examined bias relating to the socio-economic status of participants (Bentley et al., 2012; Bopp et al., 2010). Bopp et al. identified no differences, while Bentley et al. found that mothers in the most socially disadvantaged groups were less likely to have records that linked to infant hospital records. The authors suggested that lower matching rates with the infant records could be related to an association between missing information, social disadvantage and adverse outcomes. It was also suggested that severely ill infants, with prolonged hospitalisations, may not be coded as birth admissions in hospital data.

4.4   Discussion

Overall, the results of the review suggest that bias was common in studies involving linked data, with the overwhelming majority of studies (85%) identifying bias based on the characteristics examined. The findings in the review are consistent with the findings of our previous review, based on studies published up to 2007, which also found that linkage error can impact key participant characteristics and that these factors were not consistently evaluated or reported (Bohensky et al., 2010).

Of the 11 studies that identified potential bias in results, factors such as missing data (MAR/MNAR), inaccurate data and incomplete participant recruitment all contributed to sources of bias in research findings based on linked data. The method of linkage, such as a deterministic or probabilistic strategy, may also impact the completeness and accuracy of results, as demonstrated in the report by Campbell (2009). The impact of technical experience and inter-operator reliability of data matching may also have influenced the results, although this was not examined in the included studies. Interestingly, nearly half of the studies (46%) outsourced their linkage processes to data linkage groups. While linkage groups are likely to have more technical experience and data linkage knowledge than researchers, outsourcing may also make researchers less aware of quality issues impacting the linked data that they use for their studies. This can have implications for the interpretation and generalisability of research findings.

There were two studies that did not identify any sources of bias in the factors that were considered in their linkage results. There are several potential reasons why these two studies did not identify any bias. The study by Bopp et al. had a high linkage rate at 97.8%, which may have been due to a number of high-quality demographic variables available from the cohort study, which were collected through participant interview and self-administered questionnaire data (Bopp et al., 2010). The study by Lain et al. had a linkage rate of 89.3% and a smaller number of cases ($n = 1882$) (Lain et al., 2009). The linkage process in this study was outsourced to a data linkage centre, which may have utilised more extensive clerical review processes, especially given the relatively small number of cases. Both studies also involved data sources with high rates of completeness, as three were administrative data sources developed for legislative or funding purposes and one was a high-quality cohort study. It may also be that sources of bias did exist in other participant characteristics that were not assessed by the authors.

Our initial database search identified 4158 studies, with the keywords of 'data linkage' or 'medical record linkage'. Of these, only 13 studies were identified, examining potential sources of bias within the data linkage process. The authors of the included studies used various linkage methods and measures of bias, linkage quality and reporting of characteristics within studies, so findings were heterogeneous. Not all factors that were of interest were reported consistently in publications. A number of studies only compared linked and non-linked cases on a select few number of characteristics. Hence, there may have been other biases that were overlooked.

The methods for assessing the completeness of linkage were also inconsistent. Some studies compared proportions of different patient characteristics among matched and unmatched records, others examined the odds of a successful match using regression analysis, while Duvall et al. examined overall trends in duplicate records. Karmel et al. and Campbell both quantified the impact of linkage bias on results. Examining linkage quality in this way provides a useful insight, as data analysts can determine when suboptimal linkage quality may be acceptable for their research purposes. For example, the study by Karmel et al. examined trends in residential aged care transitions to hospital. They found that the patterns of use identified, and the characteristics of people making particular types of transitions for both linkage methods, led to very similar conclusions. Given the lower effort associated with their event-based linkage method, this may be the most cost-effective choice in a given scenario, despite its slightly lower linkage rate. Bopp et al. assessed the quality of their linkage results by comparing survival rates of their linked data to population-based life table estimates to determine if their results departed from population norms. This method allowed for an assessment of the generalisability of their linked data results, which was vulnerable to systematic bias at both the data collection and linkage phases.

4.4.1   Potential biases in the review process

This review focused on studies which examined observed differences between linked and unlinked cases through the data linkage process. However, the overall impact of these differences on measures of risk and outcomes assessment was only tested in three studies. As such, the impact of selection bias on the study overall results can be variable and difficult to quantify without prior knowledge of the relationship between covariates and a study outcome (Ellenberg, 1994). While most studies (85%) considered potential sources of bias at the data collection phase, this was not evaluated quantitatively in any of the reports. As seven studies involved registries ($n=5$) or cohort studies ($n=2$) which are not likely to be population-based data sources, there is potential for additional bias during recruitment to the registry or cohort study (Rochon et al., 2005). The review relied only on published academic literature. As many linked data projects have been undertaken by government agencies and may not be publicly accessible, it is possible that we have overlooked these. It is also possible that this review suffered from publication bias, so readers should consider the possibility that it may overestimate the impact of linkage error.

4.4.2   Recommendations and implications for practice

There has been an increasing use of studies reliant on existing data sources and linked data, as data linkage studies are more cost-effective than randomised control trials (RCTs) or prospective cohort studies. Given the huge expense inherent in these large-scale prospective studies, it has been proposed that researchers focus on clinical registries and leverage RCTs off these to save on costs (Lauer and D'Agostino, 2013). However, where data linkage is used in existing data sources, issues of bias need to be carefully assessed. While perfect data collection and linkage processes are likely to be too expensive and impractical to achieve, those involved in data linkage studies must consider the available resources and whether these are likely to achieve an acceptable level of study quality and selection bias for the intended study outcomes.

The following recommendations for practice have been proposed to ensure that a high-quality linkage standard can be achieved:

- For countries that do not already have them, direct, unique identifiers, such as national health identifiers, should be developed and included within datasets. These will assist in having higher-quality linkage, as bias from incorrectly coded or missing demographic variables may otherwise be introduced. This issue of bias was clearly illustrated in the previous example describing the use of female and ethnic surnames, which, in the case of females, may change across the lifespan or, in the case of certain ethnicities, be partitioned differently to Anglo-Saxon surnames, leading to lower rates of linkage. National health identifiers, which are in standard formats and routinely included within datasets, could help to address many of these issues of differential coding. As discussed in Chapter 3, various mechanisms exist for managing privacy issues around the use of such identifiers.

- Increasing the use of routine data linkage between disparate datasets should be encouraged. As data linkage can be used to assess aspects of data quality, including accuracy, completeness, consistency and currency, linkage will help to identify errors and enhance data quality. Teppo et al. describe how record linkage has been used between the Finnish cancer registry and hospital admission data to identify incorrectly coded cancers in the hospital data, missing cases in the cancer registry and misclassified benign tumours within the hospital data (Teppo, Pukkala and Lehtonen, 1994). Similarly, Roos et al. describe how linked data in Canada have been used to compare agreement on mortality information, procedures, diagnostic information, double counting of hospital procedures and the accuracy of case ascertainment (Roos et al., 2005).

- Systematic, high-quality methods should be used for data linkage. Some of these are described in other sections of this book. Furthermore, quality indicators for describing the linkage accuracy and bias should be estimated and provided to data users. These may include quantitative metrics or a qualitative assessment of the final linked cohort. Various quantitative measures for assessing linkage error have been described previously, and a summary of these is presented in Table 4.2 (Christen and Goiser, 2007; Leiss, 2007; Sariyar, Borg and Pommerening, 2011). Ideally, several of these measures would be presented in combination to provide a justification for the chosen linkage threshold and an understanding of its accuracy and precision. Equally, qualitative descriptions of data, linkage quality and potential linkage bias may also be presented to data users to ensure they understand the limitations of the linked data to be used for their analyses.

- Ensure criteria for the integrity and completeness of datasets are met before including them in linkage processes. Part of this process may include quality control procedures (e.g. business rules at the point of data entry and quality assurance activities) and financial incentives to improve data quality with data custodians and ensure data quality from different sites is comparable. Nationally (if not internationally) consistent coding systems and definitions should be used whenever possible. International disease and health coding standards have been developed by the World Health Organization (2001; 2008), with some nations making local clinical modifications to these. National initiatives, such as the National Health Data Dictionary in Australia, the NHS Data Model and Dictionary Service in the UK and the 3M Healthcare Data Dictionary in the United States, have also been developed to encourage greater consistency in health information across national datasets (3M Health Information Systems, 2013; National Health Service, 2013). Reporting guidelines and frameworks for evaluating secondary data sources have also been developed (Langan et al., 2013; Sorensen, Sabroe and Olsen, 1996). These can also be utilised by linkage analysts to better understand the integrity of the data being used for linkage.

Table 4.2   Quantitative measures for assessing linkage quality.

Measure name	Description	Method of calculation
Sensitivity	This is often referred to as the 'matching rate' and is commonly reported in data linkage studies	True positives/(true positives + false negatives)
Specificity	This measure is also known as the 'true negative rate'. It refers to the proportion of non-matches which have been correctly identified	True negatives/(true negatives + false positives)
Positive predictive value	This is often known as the 'precision rate' and presents the proportion of matches that are true links	True positives/(true positives + false positives)
Negative predictive value	This measure presents the proportion of non-matches that are not true links	True negatives/(true negatives + false negatives)
F-measure	This measure will have a high value only when sensitivity and positive predictive value have high values. It allows for an assessment of the balance between both measures	This is the harmonic mean of the positive predictive value and sensitivity
False match rate	Also known as the 'false positive rate', this measure reports the proportion of total matches that are false matches	False positives/(true negatives + false positives) This measure can be estimated through various modelling techniques (Christen and Goiser, 2007; Sariyar, Borg and Pommerening, 2011)
Missed match rate	This measure presents the proportion of total links which are missed matches	Fellegi and Sunter (1969) have reported methods for calculating this metric, which requires obtaining the probabilities of having a false link and missed link for each linkage variable (Fellegi and Sunter, 1969)
Duplicate link rate	A duplicate link occurs when a record from one file is linked to more than one record on the other file (where a 1:1 match is expected). The duplicate link rate can be used to assist in the construction of appropriate cut-off weights	The number of duplicate links can be evaluated at different values of record comparison weights to determine where the optimal linkage threshold lies (Bishop and Khoo, 2007)

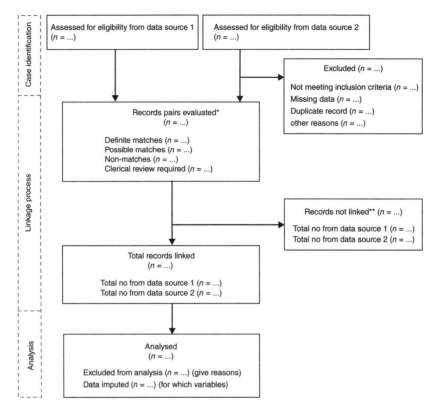

*Match classification categories may differ depending on the linkage methods used.
**The number of unlinked records may not always imply a missed match or false negative. However, if a one-to-one match between datasets was expected then any characteristics of unlinked records which are significantly different to linked records should also be reported.

Figure 4.3   Hypothetical data linkage inclusion flowchart for cross-sectional data linkage.

- Similar to the CONSORT statement which is used for reporting RCTs, it is necessary to report information from data linkage studies in a clear and systematic manner (Moher et al., 2010). Reporting should include the number of participants at several stages during the linkage study process, from the initial cohort of subjects included from each original data source to the cohort which is utilised in the data linkage study (see Figure 4.3 for a hypothetical example of a data linkage inclusion flowchart for a cross-sectional data linkage. This can be modified for other types of linkage processes, such as de-duplications). Similarly, linkage methods should be documented, or a link to such documentation provided, in such a manner that they are repeatable at a later stage. The potential for linkage bias needs to be routinely considered within the limitations of linked data studies (Bohensky et al., 2011a).

- There is a need for more validation studies by linkage centres and researchers to understand which populations are most vulnerable to selection bias and which methods are most likely to bring about bias. Validation will enable linkage analysts to focus on vulnerable record pairs and help to decrease sources of bias in data collection processes and during the linkage process.

5

Secondary analysis of linked data

Raymond Chambers and Gunky Kim

National Institute for Applied Statistics Research Australia (NIASRA),
School of Mathematics and Applied Statistics, University of Wollongong,
Wollongong, New South Wales, Australia

5.1   Introduction

Record matching, or data linking, is now firmly established as an important research tool. Separate datasets that individually contain the values of study variables can be used to investigate their marginal behaviour, but a linked dataset is necessary for investigation of relationships between them. A common type of linked data analysis is regression analysis, where the underlying relationship between a response variable and a set of explanatory variables is explored by fitting a regression model to linked data. When we do so, we implicitly assume that the linked dataset is made of correctly matched records. Without unique identifiers, however, perfectly correct linkage is usually not possible. In such cases, the linked dataset is typically created via some form of probabilistic record matching, where linkage errors are almost certain. That is, some of the records on the linked dataset will actually be made up of values taken from two, or sometimes more, distinct individuals or population units. Standard regression modelling using such linked data is then biased, with relationships between the study variable and the explanatory variables typically attenuated.

There are essentially two options available in this situation. The first is to improve the record matching algorithm in order to minimise, or at least reduce, the incorrect linkage rate (i.e. the proportion of linked records that contain data from distinct individuals). This has been the focus of much of the research in data linkage over the last quarter century, starting with the pioneering work of Fellegi and Sunter (1969). The other approach is to model the bias due to incorrect linkage and then develop methods of correcting it. Somewhat surprisingly, this avenue of research has received comparatively little attention over the same time period.

Methodological Developments in Data Linkage, First Edition. Edited by Katie Harron, Harvey Goldstein and Chris Dibben.
© 2016 John Wiley & Sons, Ltd. Published 2016 by John Wiley & Sons, Ltd.

In most cases, an analyst using a linked dataset will not have been involved in its creation. In particular, such a 'secondary' analyst will not have access to information from the record matching process and so will be severely restricted as far as modelling the probabilities underpinning the linkage outcome are concerned. Occasionally, partial information about the matching process may be available, depending on privacy protection regulations governing it, but this is rare. This access to complete matching process information is implicit in the inferential methods for linked data developed in Scheuren and Winkler (1993; 1997), Lahiri and Larsen (2005) and, more recently Goldstein, Harron and Wade (2012).

On the other hand, the bias correction ideas explored in Chambers (2009) and Kim and Chambers (2012a; 2012b) are motivated by secondary analysis, in that these authors assume a model for linkage errors that only requires non-sensitive summary information about the performance of the data linkage method. This chapter will take the same approach, using linear regression analysis to illustrate the basic ideas. That is, we shall typically assume that the aim is to use the linked dataset to fit a linear regression model linking a target variable Y and a vector of covariates X of the form

$$\mathbf{y} = \mathbf{X}\beta + \varepsilon, \tag{5.1}$$

where $\mathbf{y}$ is the vector of population values y_i of Y, $\mathbf{X}$ is the matrix whose rows correspond to the population values $\mathbf{x}_i$ of X and β is the target of inference, and we make the usual assumption that the components of ϵ are independently and identically distribution with zero mean and finite variance σ^2. Note that (5.1) implicitly assumes that the same rows of $\mathbf{y}$ and $\mathbf{X}$ correspond to values from the same individual in the population. Also, since most of the subsequent development casts the estimation problem as the solution of an estimating equation, extensions of the methods we describe to more complex models are usually straightforward.

5.2   Measurement error issues arising from linkage

The impact of linkage errors on regression analysis is not dissimilar to the impact of measurement errors in regression model covariates, in the sense that both sources of error lead to attenuation of estimated regression coefficients. However, models for linkage error are quite different from the additive models often used to characterise measurement errors in covariates. Consequently, we now discuss the different types of outcomes that result following a linking procedure.

5.2.1   Correct links, incorrect links and non-links

Most linked datasets are not perfect, even though most of records they contain will be correctly linked. Studies investigating the rate of correct linkage have been carried out, and by and large, these indicate that the linkage error rate, though small, is not negligible. For example, the Australian Bureau of Statistics (ABS), as a part of its Census Data Enhancement project, investigated linkage error rates under a number of different record matching scenarios (see Bishop and Khoo (2007)). In this study, records from a sample of individuals were linked back to their census records. When name and address were used as linking fields, 87% of linked records were correctly linked. This figure is consistent with other linking studies in

Australia, with Holman et al. (1999) stating that the correct linkage rate in linked datasets created by the Western Australian Data Linkage Unit during 1996–1997 was 87% and that correct linkage rates for linked hospital morbidity data in Victoria over 1993–1994 were in the range 78–86%. Note that these rates are for situations where names and addresses are used as linking fields. However, many linking exercises do not have access to this type of information, reflecting confidentiality concerns. When name and address are removed from the set of linking fields, Bishop and Khoo (2007) report that the correct linkage rate drops sharply to 68%.

In reality, many records cannot be linked with certainty because the linking fields are ambiguous. This ambiguity is usually quantified by a score that characterises the likelihood that the records contributing to a potential link or 'match' are actually from the same individual. Many linkage operations only 'declare' a link when this score is above a pre-specified threshold. In this case, all record pairs on the datasets contributing to the linkage operation with a score below this threshold can never be linked. As a consequence, there will be records on these datasets that are not linked. Clearly, the person or organisation carrying out the linking could potentially increase the rate of correct linkage by lowering the threshold and thus reducing this non-linkage rate. However, this might also increase the incorrect linkage rate. That is, the choice of the threshold is a compromise between the incorrect linkage rate and the non-linkage rate. Increasing the threshold reduces the incorrect linkage rate but increases the non-linkage rate. Decreasing the threshold has the opposite effect. The optimal choice is one that maximises the correct linkage rate while simultaneously minimising these two sources of error. Any statistical inference using linked data must therefore take account of both these sources of error. In what follows, we develop models for both linkage error and incomplete linkage that only require marginal information about the performance of the linking procedure. This information is essentially the minimal information that linker could supply along with the linked dataset, which then could be used by a secondary analyst to control for biases arising from linkage errors as well as non-linking errors associated with the final linked dataset.

5.2.2   Characterising linkage errors

We start by restricting development to linkage error models where the only linkage error is in the vector $\mathbf{y}$ in (5.1). In particular, we assume that the records defining $\mathbf{y}$ and $\mathbf{X}$ in (5.1) are stored on two separate registers. Ideally, the linkage procedure ensures that each record in the $\mathbf{y}$ register is correctly matched with its corresponding record in the $\mathbf{X}$ register. However, under probabilistic linkage, this is unlikely. Instead of identifying each true $(y_i, \mathbf{x}_i)$ pair, this process will produce a set of matched $\left(y_i^*, \mathbf{x}_i\right)$ pairs, where y_i^* denotes the record in the $\mathbf{y}$ register that is matched to the record $\mathbf{x}_i$ in the $\mathbf{X}$ register. Let $\mathbf{y}^*$ denote the vector of matched values assumed to correspond to $\mathbf{y}$. Most components of these two vectors will be identical. However, there will also be a small number of cases where y_i and y_i^* correspond to values from different individuals. A secondary analyst interested in fitting the linear regression model (5.1) to the population defining the two registers will only have access to the linked data $(\mathbf{y}^*, \mathbf{X})$. If this analyst is unaware of potential linkage errors and assumes $\mathbf{y}$ and $\mathbf{y}^*$ are identical, then he or she will be effectively fitting the linked data model

$$\mathbf{y}^* = \mathbf{X}\boldsymbol{\beta}^* + \boldsymbol{\varepsilon}^*,$$

where $\beta^* \neq \beta$ if the linkage error rate is not negligible. That is, using $(\mathbf{y}^*, \mathbf{X})$ to estimate β in (5.1) under the assumption that $\mathbf{y}^*$ is identical to $\mathbf{y}$ will lead to biased inference, with the extent of the bias depending on the linkage error rate.

5.2.3   Characterising errors from non-linkage

As noted in Subsection 5.2.1, there will typically be records in both the $\mathbf{y}$ and $\mathbf{X}$ registers that remain unlinked following the linkage process. These non-linked records can be thought of as similar to non-response. The crucial issue then is whether non-linked records represent a 'special' subset of the population. The simplest case is where it is reasonable to assume that the non-linked records on the $\mathbf{X}$ register can be treated as a random sample from this register. In this case, it is clear that beyond the loss of efficiency because of the reduced number of linked records available for analysis, this non-linkage is ignorable. However, such cases are rare. In most cases, because of the nature of the linkage process, the probability that records in either the $\mathbf{y}$ or the $\mathbf{X}$ registers remain unlinked is related to their values y_i and $\mathbf{x}_i$, respectively (see Chapter 4). The former case is essentially the same as non-response that is missing at random (MAR) given $\mathbf{x}_i$ and can be handled by either judicious imputation or weighting. The latter case is equivalent to non-response that is not missing at random (NMAR) and provides the same level of difficulty as NMAR in allowing for its impact on inference. In what follows, we will either assume ignorable non-linkage or, if this is not the case, assume access to appropriate weights (akin to propensity weights) that can be used to correct for non-linkage bias in inference. We will also investigate how access to population summaries from the $\mathbf{y}$ and $\mathbf{X}$ registers can be used as auxiliary information in order to reduce biased inference based on linked incomplete data from these registers.

5.3   Models for different types of linking errors

We assume throughout that all links are *one to one* (i.e. we do not allow the same record in one register to be linked to multiple records in other registers) and start by considering the simplest type of linking, which is *binary linking*. Here, every record in the $\mathbf{y}$ register is linked to a different record in the $\mathbf{X}$ register, and we propose a simple model that can be used to characterise linkage errors for this situation. We then extend this model to the *multi-linking* case, where $\mathbf{X}$ itself is also created via linking, thus allowing for more than two files to be linked, and finally to the *sample to register linking* case, where only a selected sample of records from the $\mathbf{X}$ register is linked to records in the $\mathbf{y}$ register. This last case allows us to examine methods for dealing with non-linking in our inference.

5.3.1   Linkage errors under binary linking

Under binary linking, two datasets are linked to form a new dataset. This is the simplest linking case and has been the focus of much of the research on the analysis of linked data. Clearly, if the linking is precise (e.g. via a unique identifier), then the resulting linked dataset can provide a rich source of relational information, something that was not available before record linking. However, precise linking is typically impossible, and so some sort of probabilistic linking process may be used. By its very nature, there will then be some (hopefully not many) records in the linked dataset that are incorrectly linked. Furthermore, depending on the type of linking algorithm used, there will be some records in the original datasets that remain unlinked at the conclusion of the linking process. We focus initially on the incorrect linking issue.

Following the notation introduced earlier, we suppose that there are two separate registers, say, $\mathbf{X}$ and $\mathbf{y}$, that contain the values of variables X and Y, respectively. Following the record matching process, we will have a linked dataset of the form $\left(\mathbf{y}^{*}, \mathbf{X}\right)$ where $\mathbf{y}^{*} \neq \mathbf{y}$ due to possible linkage errors. Under one-to-one linking, $\mathbf{y}^{*}$ can be regarded as a permutation of the records in $\mathbf{y}$, such that

$$\mathbf{y}^{*} = \mathbf{A}\mathbf{y} \tag{5.2}$$

where $\mathbf{A}$ is an unknown permutation matrix. That is, $\mathbf{A}$ is made up of ones and zeros, with a value of one occurring just once in any row and column. Under probability linking, $\mathbf{A}$ is a random variable, with linkage errors defined by the off-diagonal values of one in this matrix. A standard assumption then is that the distribution of $\mathbf{A}$ does not depend on the distribution of the regression errors in (5.1). That is, linkage errors are *non-informative* about $\mathbf{y}$ given $\mathbf{X}$. This allows us to write

$$E\left(\mathbf{y}^{*} \mid \mathbf{X}\right) = E\left(\mathbf{A} \mid \mathbf{X}\right) E\left(\mathbf{y} \mid \mathbf{X}\right).$$

The expression for $E\left(\mathbf{y} \mid \mathbf{X}\right)$ above depends on the regression model assumed to underpin the correctly linked data, for example, (5.1) implies $E\left(\mathbf{y} \mid \mathbf{X}\right) = \mathbf{X}\beta$. In contrast, the value of $E\left(\mathbf{A} \mid \mathbf{X}\right)$ depends on the type of probabilistic linkage scheme used to create the linked dataset. As a consequence, the information available to a secondary analyst for modelling $E\left(\mathbf{A} \mid \mathbf{X}\right)$ is typically very limited. We put

$$E\left(\mathbf{A} \mid \mathbf{X}\right) = \mathbf{T}_{A} \tag{5.3}$$

for the time being and explore models for this quantity that require minimal information about the linking process in later subsections. Let $E\left(\mathbf{y} \mid \mathbf{X}\right) = \mathbf{f}\left(\mathbf{X};\beta\right)$ denote the population vector of values of the regression function of interest. Then

$$E\left(\mathbf{y}^{*} \mid \mathbf{X}\right) = E\left(\mathbf{A} \mid \mathbf{X}\right)\mathbf{f}\left(\mathbf{X};\beta\right) = \mathbf{T}_{A}\mathbf{f}\left(\mathbf{X};\beta\right). \tag{5.4}$$

Note that in the linear regression case (5.1)

$$E\left(\mathbf{y}^{*} \mid \mathbf{X}\right) = \mathbf{T}_{A}\mathbf{X}\beta. \tag{5.5}$$

which implies that it is the regression of $\mathbf{y}^{*}$ on the product $\mathbf{T}_{A}\mathbf{X}$, rather than on $\mathbf{X}$, that is linear.

Before we move on, we need to point out that the assumption of non-informative linking is a strong one. In reality, one would expect that the capacity to correctly link the $\mathbf{y}$ and $\mathbf{X}$ registers will depend on the values in both. When an analyst has access to the complete linkage process (i.e. a primary analyst), this dependence can be allowed for when modelling $\mathbf{T}_{A}$. For example, Lahiri and Larsen (2005) equate $\mathbf{T}_{A}$ to the matrix of matching probabilities used in creating the observed links, while Chipperfield and Chambers (2015) use bootstrap replication of the linkage process to estimate $\mathbf{T}_A$. Here, however, we put ourselves in the position of a secondary analyst, without access to the precise details of how the linkage was carried out. In this situation, a non-informative linking assumption represents an obvious first step in trying to model the distribution of $\mathbf{y}^*$ given $\mathbf{X}$.

5.3.2   Linkage errors under multi-linking

In many cases, a linked dataset will be the outcome of a number of separate linking processes. We illustrate this multi-linking by considering the situation where the values in the linked dataset are obtained from three distinct registers, $\mathbf{y}$, $\mathbf{X}_1$ and $\mathbf{X}_2$. Here, the final linked data can be considered to be the result of two distinct binary linking operations: $\mathbf{y}$ is linked to $\mathbf{X}_1$ to create $\mathbf{y}^*$ and $\mathbf{X}_2$ is linked to $\mathbf{X}_1$ to create $\mathbf{X}_2^*$, so that the linked matrix of regression covariates corresponding to $\mathbf{X}$ in (5.1) is $\mathbf{X}^* = \begin{bmatrix} \mathbf{X}_1 & \mathbf{X}_2^* \end{bmatrix}$. As a consequence, we can model the resulting linkage errors as functions of two potentially correlated random permutation matrices $\mathbf{A}$ and $\mathbf{B}$ such that

$$\mathbf{y}^* = \mathbf{A}\mathbf{y} \quad \text{and} \quad \mathbf{X}_2^* = \mathbf{B}\mathbf{X}_2. \tag{5.6}$$

Note that this model includes the case where $\mathbf{y}$ and $\mathbf{X}_2$ are actually drawn from the same register, since then $\mathbf{A} = \mathbf{B}$.

5.3.3   Incomplete linking

Linking two (or more) population registers can be extremely expensive. In such cases, a common strategy is sample to register linking, where a sample from one register, say, $\mathbf{X}$, is linked to the other register $\mathbf{y}$. For example, the Census Data Enhancement project of the ABS aims to link a sample of records from the 2011 Australian Census with corresponding records in subsequent censuses. We use a subscript of s to denote the set of sampled records in such a situation. Since most linkage errors will now involve incorrectly matching a sampled record to a non-sampled record, we can no longer treat the linked sample records as a permutation of the records defining s, and so we need to modify the linkage error models developed in the preceding two subsections. In doing so, we will assume that a set of sample weights $\mathbf{w}_s$ exists (or can be calculated) such that weighted averages of correctly linked sample quantities are valid estimates of the corresponding population quantities.

Unsampled records in $\mathbf{y}$ represent one way in which non-links occur. However, a more pernicious problem is where there are records in the selected sample from $\mathbf{X}$ that cannot be matched with records from $\mathbf{y}$. An obvious example is when the number of records in these registers is not the same, for example, the population numbers in different censuses differ because of death, births and migration during the intercensal period. More generally, non-linked records can arise in probabilistic linking because of the tension between linkage accuracy and the number of records linked, with some sampled records in $\mathbf{X}$ deliberately excluded from linkage because of low match probabilities. Compared to non-links due to sampling, non-links due to non-availability of suitable matches or due to matching restrictions can be considered as similar to non-contacts due to coverage errors and non-response due to refusals, respectively, and analogously to weighting for sampling prior to linking, we can think of weighting after linking to correct for these types of non-linkage errors.

Like the non-informative linking assumption discussed earlier, there are two further assumptions that we make in order to be able to deal with the different types of errors associated with non-links. The first is relatively uncontroversial and corresponds to assuming that the sampling process is non-informative given $\mathbf{X}$ (e.g. some form of probability sampling is used) and is independent of the linkage process. The second, however, is more controversial, but practically necessary, in a secondary analysis situation. This is to assume that the sampling weights can be modified so that these weights continue to be valid in the presence of non-linked sample records. This is a controversial assumption since it is essentially the same as assuming that non-response is MAR given response-adjusted weights in sample data analysis. However, without this assumption, it is hard to see how one can allow for non-linking in secondary analysis of linked data.

Finally, we note that weighting is not the only way non-linking can be accommodated in secondary inference of linked data. Depending on the amount of available information about the non-linked records, we can adapt the methods for sample-based inference given summary population information described in Chambers et al. (2012) to linked data inference. However, exploration of this approach is outside the scope of this chapter.

5.3.4   Modelling the linkage error

It is clear from (5.4) that if we wish to use the linked data to fit the regression of $\mathbf{y}$ on $\mathbf{X}$, then we need to model $\mathbf{T}_A$ (as well as $\mathbf{T}_B$ in a multi-linking situation). Since $\mathbf{A}$ is unobservable, modelling it requires more information than that contained in the observed linked data $(\mathbf{y}^*, \mathbf{X})$. For the primary analyst (i.e. the linker), information for modelling $\mathbf{T}_A$ can be obtained from the record matching procedure. To illustrate, suppose that the linking procedure is based on a priori matching probabilities:

$$\Pr\left(y_i^* = y_j\right) = p_{ij}$$

with $\sum_j p_{ij} = 1$. Then one could define an estimator of $\mathbf{T}_A$ of the form

$$\hat{\mathbf{T}}_A = \left[p_{ij}\right].$$

This idea has been developed by Scheuren and Winkler (1993) and has been used in Lahiri and Larsen (2005) to adjust for bias due to linkage errors under (5.1). In particular, Lahiri and Larsen (2005) use the linear regression identity (5.5) to suggest an estimator of β of the form

$$\hat{\beta} = \left[\left(\hat{\mathbf{T}}_A \mathbf{X}\right)^T \hat{\mathbf{T}}_A \mathbf{X}\right]^{-1} \left(\hat{\mathbf{T}}_A \mathbf{X}\right)^T \mathbf{y}^*. \tag{5.7}$$

In contrast, Chipperfield and Chambers (2015) describe how $\mathbf{T}_A$ can be estimated by parametrically bootstrapping the linking process and demonstrate that (5.7) can be biased if in fact the matching probabilities p_{ij} used in linking do not correspond to achieved correct linkage probabilities.

However, our focus is on secondary analysis, and in this context, we note that, by definition, secondary analysts do not have the same amount of information about the operation of the linking procedure as do primary analysts. To illustrate this information 'gap', Kelman,

Bass and Holman (2002) describe how technicians involved in record linking carried out using the Western Australian Data Linkage system cannot take part in the analysis of the linked datasets that they create. This provides protection against loss of data confidentiality by ensuring that researchers only have access to the linked datasets required for their specific projects. As a result, the bias correction techniques developed by Scheuren and Winkler (1993), Lahiri and Larsen (2005) and Chipperfield and Chambers (2015) cannot be used.

In contrast, there is no loss of confidentiality (though perhaps some credibility) if linking agencies were to release summary statistics about correct linkage rates at the same time as they release linked datasets for secondary analysis. At its most basic, this information could literally be just the linking agency's estimate of the proportion of correct links in the linked dataset. In particular, let M denote the number of records in $\mathbf{y}^*$ and put λ equal to the estimated correct record linkage rate and $\gamma = 1 - \lambda/M - 1$. Then, following ideas first set out in Neter, Maynes and Ramanathan (1965), we could consider the following model for $\mathbf{T}_A$:

$$\mathbf{T}_A = \left(\lambda - \gamma\right)\mathbf{I}_M + \gamma \mathbf{1}_M \mathbf{1}_M^T = \begin{pmatrix} \lambda & \gamma & \gamma & \cdots & \gamma & \gamma \\ \gamma & \lambda & \gamma & \cdots & \gamma & \gamma \\ \vdots & \vdots & \vdots & \vdots & \vdots & \vdots \\ \gamma & \gamma & \gamma & \cdots & \gamma & \lambda \end{pmatrix}, \tag{5.8}$$

where $\mathbf{I}_M$ is the identity matrix of order M and $\mathbf{1}_M$ is the vector of ones of size M. Chambers (2009) refers to (5.8) as the *exchangeable linkage error* or ELE model, because it assumes that probability of successful linkage (λ) is the same for all records and the probability of incorrect linkage (γ) is the same for all record pairs. It has been criticised by Scheuren and Winkler (1993) as being too simplistic. This criticism is valid from the viewpoint of a primary analyst since the matching probabilities used in the linking process are typically unequal. However, as it stands, (5.8) represents a first-order approximation to $\mathbf{T}_A$ based on the common sense realisation that if the linking is properly carried out, then correct linking is much more likely than incorrect linking. Furthermore, it can easily be made more realistic by partitioning the population into groups of records within which (5.8) provides a better approximation to linking reality. Of course, such a partitioning then requires that the linking agency be willing (and able) to release estimates of correct linkage rates for each of the resulting groups. In what follows, we shall assume that a version of (5.8) holds at some level of publicly available data about the estimated distribution of correct linkage error probabilities in the linked dataset.

5.4   Regression analysis using complete binary-linked data

This is the simplest case. It allows us to develop key concepts in an accessible fashion and hence lays the groundwork for more complex situations considered later. We assume that both $\mathbf{y}$ and $\mathbf{X}$ contain M records. We also assume that the record matching procedure is one–one and complete, that is, all records in both registers are linked. We focus on fitting a regression relationship to $\mathbf{y}$ and $\mathbf{X}$ of the form $E\left(\mathbf{y} \mid \mathbf{X}\right) = f\left(\mathbf{X};\beta\right) = \mathbf{f}$ where f is a known function, while β is unknown and has to be estimated. Following on from the discussion in the preceding paragraph, we also assume that the linked records can be partitioned into Q distinct and non-overlapping groups indexed by q in what follows such that linkage errors only occur within these groups. These groups are referred to as *match*-blocks or *m*-blocks in what follows, with restriction to *m*-block q indicated by a subscript of q.

Note that the *m*-block concept is not the same as the *blocking* concept used in data linking theory. In the latter case, linking is carried out in stages, with each stage in the linkage process corresponding to attempted matching of so far unmatched records within groups defined by the same value of a categorical variable that is usually referred to as a blocking variable. The definition of this blocking variable changes from stage to stage. That is, a block in data linkage corresponds to a stage in the data linkage process. In contrast, an *m*-block represents a group of linked records which contains all realistic alternative links for those records. In effect, the categorical variable with values equal to the values taken by the *m*-block index q defines a stratification of the population such that records in different *m*-blocks can never be from the same population unit, while records in the same *m*-block represent potential alternative links, that is, linkage errors are confined to *m*-blocks. There can never be linkage errors involving two or more *m*-blocks.

5.4.1   Linear regression

We consider fitting the linear model (5.1) given the probabilistically linked dataset $(\mathbf{y}^*, \mathbf{X})$. To start, we note that the usual ordinary least squares (OLS) estimator $\hat{\beta}_{\text{OLS}}$ of the regression parameter β given these data is

$$\hat{\beta}_{\text{OLS}} = \left[\sum_q \left(\mathbf{X}_q^T \mathbf{X}_q \right) \right]^{-1} \left[\sum_q \left(\mathbf{X}_q^T \mathbf{y}_q^* \right) \right] = \left[\sum_q \left(\mathbf{X}_q^T \mathbf{X}_q \right) \right]^{-1} \left[\sum_q \left(\mathbf{X}_q^T \mathbf{A}_q \mathbf{y}_q \right) \right].$$

Hence,

$$E\left(\hat{\beta}_{\text{OLS}} \mid \mathbf{X} \right) = \left[\sum_q \left(\mathbf{X}_q^T \mathbf{X}_q \right) \right]^{-1} \left[\sum_q \left(\mathbf{X}_q^T \mathbf{T}_{Aq} \mathbf{X}_q \right) \right] \beta = \mathbf{D}\beta.$$

Unless $\mathbf{D}$ is close to the identity matrix, $\hat{\beta}_{\text{OLS}}$ is biased. Chambers (2009) uses this bias expression to motivate a ratio-type bias-corrected estimator:

$$\hat{\beta}_{\text{R}} = \mathbf{D}^{-1} \hat{\beta}^* = \left[\sum_q \left(\mathbf{X}_q^T \mathbf{T}_{Aq} \mathbf{X}_q \right) \right]^{-1} \left[\sum_q \left(\mathbf{X}_q^T \mathbf{y}_q^* \right) \right].$$

Alternatively, we can substitute $\mathbf{T}_A$ defined by (5.8) in the bias-corrected estimator (5.7) suggested by Lahiri and Larsen (2005):

$$\hat{\beta}_{\text{LL}} = \left[\sum_q \left(\left(\mathbf{T}_{Aq} \mathbf{X}_q \right)^T \mathbf{T}_{Aq} \mathbf{X}_q \right) \right]^{-1} \left[\sum_q \left(\left(\mathbf{T}_{Aq} \mathbf{X}_q \right)^T \mathbf{y}_q^* \right) \right].$$

A more efficient approach to fitting a regression function based on an estimating equation framework is described in Chambers (2009). When there are no linkage errors, an efficient estimator of the regression parameter β can be defined by solving the unbiased estimating equation

$$\mathbf{H}(\beta) = \sum_q \mathbf{G}_q \left(\mathbf{y}_q - \mathbf{f}_q \right) = 0,$$

where $\mathbf{G}_q$ is a suitably chosen weight. With linked data, the corresponding unbiased estimating equation is

$$\mathbf{H}^* (\beta) = \sum_q \mathbf{G}_q^* \left(\mathbf{y}_q^* - \mathbf{T}_{Aq} \mathbf{f}_q \right) = 0, \tag{5.9}$$

where $\mathbf{G}_q^*$ is an appropriately modified version of $\mathbf{G}_q$. Under the linear model (5.1), it is straightforward to see that the solution to (5.9) is

$$\hat{\beta}^* = \sum_q \left(\mathbf{G}_q^* \mathbf{T}_{Aq} \mathbf{X}_q \right)^{-1} \mathbf{G}_q^* \mathbf{y}_q^*. \tag{5.10}$$

Note that the estimators $\hat{\beta}_R$ and $\hat{\beta}_{LL}$ derived earlier are special cases of (5.10), defined by $\mathbf{G}_q^* = \mathbf{X}_q^T$ and $\mathbf{G}_q^* = \left(\mathbf{T}_{Aq} \mathbf{X}_q \right)^T$, respectively. The efficient estimator of β is defined by the optimal weights

$$\mathbf{G}_q^* = \left[\frac{\partial E \left(\mathbf{y}_q^* | \mathbf{X}_q \right)}{\partial \beta} \right]^T \left[\mathrm{var} \left(\mathbf{y}_q^* | \mathbf{X}_q \right) \right]^{-1} = \left(\mathbf{T}_{Aq} \mathbf{X}_q \right)^T \left[\mathrm{var} \left(\mathbf{y}_q^* | \mathbf{X}_q \right) \right]^{-1}. \tag{5.11}$$

When $\mathbf{T}_{Aq}$ is the identity matrix (i.e. there are no linkage errors), substitution of (5.11) into (5.10) defines the *best linear unbiased estimator* (BLUE) of β. We therefore denote the value of (5.10) corresponding to (5.11) by $\hat{\beta}_{BL}$ in what follows.

The asymptotic variance of (5.10) can be obtained using Taylor series approximation, treating $\mathbf{G}_q^*$ as fixed, and is given by

$$\mathrm{var} \left(\hat{\beta}^* | \mathbf{X} \right) \approx \left[\frac{\partial \mathbf{H}^* (\beta)}{\partial \beta} \right]_{\beta = \beta_0}^{-1} \mathrm{var} \left(\mathbf{H}^* (\beta_0) | \mathbf{X} \right) \left(\left[\frac{\partial \mathbf{H}^* (\beta)}{\partial \beta} \right]_{\beta = \beta_0}^{-1} \right)^T \tag{5.12}$$

where β_0 is the true value of β. Here,

$$\frac{\partial \mathbf{H}^* (\beta)}{\partial \beta} = \sum_q \mathbf{G}_q^* \mathbf{T}_{Aq} \frac{\partial \mathbf{f}_q}{\partial \beta}$$

and

$$\mathrm{var} \left(\mathbf{H}^* (\beta_0) | \mathbf{X} \right) = \sum_q \mathbf{G}_q^* \mathrm{var} \left(\mathbf{y}_q^* | \mathbf{X}_q \right).$$

The asymptotic variance (5.12) can be estimated by replacing β_0 with $\hat{\beta}^*$. Furthermore, under non-informative linkage,

$$\text{var}\left(\mathbf{y}_q^*\right) = \text{var}\left(\mathbf{y}_q\right) + \text{var}\left(\mathbf{A}_q\mathbf{f}_q\big|\mathbf{X}_q\right) = \sigma^2\mathbf{I}_q + \text{var}\left(\mathbf{A}_q\mathbf{f}_q\big|\mathbf{X}_q\right). \tag{5.13}$$

Chambers (2009) shows that

$$\hat{\sigma}^2 = N^{-1}\left(\sum_q\left(\mathbf{y}_q^* - \mathbf{f}_q\right)^T\left(\mathbf{y}_q^* - \mathbf{f}_q\right) - 2\sum_q\mathbf{f}_q^T\left(\mathbf{I}_q - \mathbf{T}_{Aq}\right)\mathbf{f}_q\right)$$

is an unbiased estimator of σ^2, while

$$\text{var}\left(\mathbf{A}_q\mathbf{f}_q\big|\mathbf{X}_q\right) \approx \text{diag}\left[\left(1 - \lambda_q\right)\left\{\lambda_q\left(f_i - \overline{f}_q\right)^2 + \overline{f}_q^{(2)} - \left(\overline{f}_q\right)^2\right\}\right],$$

where $\mathbf{f}_q = \left(f_i\right)$ and $\overline{f}_q$ and $\overline{f}_q^{(2)}$ denote the mean and the mean of the squares of the components of $\mathbf{f}_q$, respectively. Substituting $\hat{\beta}^*$ for β in these two expressions then back substituting into (5.13) allows iterative calculation of the optimal weights (5.11) as well as estimation of $\text{var}\left(\hat{\beta}^*\right)$ via the asymptotic variance approximation (5.12).

The aforementioned development assumes that the correct linkage rate λ_q in each m-block is known. In practice, it will be estimated by $\hat{\lambda}_q$. This does not change the estimation of β, but it does change how we estimate the variance of $\hat{\beta}^*$ since we now need to include the variability due to estimation of these correct linkage rates. Let $\hat{\lambda}$ denote the vector of estimated correct linkage rates. Extending the Taylor series approximation to this case, Chambers (2009) shows that under the assumption that $\mathbf{y}^*$ and $\hat{\lambda}_q$ are mutually uncorrelated, the asymptotic variance of $\hat{\beta}^*$ can be approximated by

$$\text{var}\left(\hat{\beta}^*\big|\mathbf{X}\right) \approx \left(\frac{\partial\mathbf{H}_0^*}{\partial\beta}\right)^{-1}\left[\text{var}\left(\mathbf{H}_0^*\big|\mathbf{X}\right) + \sum_q\left(\frac{\partial\mathbf{H}_0^*}{\partial\lambda_q}\right)\text{var}\left(\hat{\lambda}_q\big|\mathbf{X}_q\right)\left(\frac{\partial\mathbf{H}_0^*}{\partial\lambda_q}\right)^T\right]\left[\left(\frac{\partial\mathbf{H}_0^*}{\partial\beta}\right)^{-1}\right]^T \tag{5.14}$$

where $\mathbf{H}_0^* = \mathbf{H}^*\left(\beta_0, \lambda_0\right)$ with β_0 and λ_0 denoting the true values of β and λ, and $\partial\mathbf{H}_0^*/\partial\beta$ and $\text{var}\left(\mathbf{H}_0^*\big|\mathbf{X}\right)$ are defined in the following (5.12) (after setting $\lambda_q = \lambda_{0q}$). Also,

$$\frac{\partial\mathbf{H}_0^*}{\partial\lambda_q} = \left(M_q - 1\right)^{-1}\left(M_q\mathbf{I}_q - \mathbf{1}_q\mathbf{1}_q^T\right)\mathbf{f}_q.$$

Note that M_q denotes the number of units in m-block q, and $\mathbf{1}_q$ denotes the vector of ones of size M_q.

To illustrate the performance of the bias correction methods described so far, Chambers (2009) describes a small-scale simulation study where data were generated for a population of size $N = 2000$ made up of three blocks of size $M_1 = 1500$, $M_2 = 300$ and $M_3 = 200$, respectively, with no linkage errors in m-block 1 and with linkage errors in m-blocks 2 and 3 generated under (5.8) with $\lambda_2 = 0.95$ and $\lambda_3 = 0.7$, respectively. The values of y were generated using the linear model formula

$$y = 1 + 5x + \varepsilon$$

with values of the scalar explanatory variable x independently drawn from the uniform distribution over [0,1] and the errors ε independently drawn from the standard $N(0,1)$ Gaussian distribution. In order to assess the impact of providing estimated correct linkage rates rather than actual values, these rates were estimated based on random audit samples of size $m_q = 20$ drawn independently from each m-block, with the estimate of λ_q then calculated as

$$\hat{\lambda}_q = \min\left[m_q^{-1}\left(m_q - 0.5\right), \max\left(M_q^{-1}, p_q\right)\right],$$

where p_q denotes the proportion of correctly linked pairs identified in the audit sample in m-block q. The estimated variance of $\hat{\lambda}_q$ was calculated as $m_q^{-1}\hat{\lambda}_q\left(1 - \hat{\lambda}_q\right)$. This scenario was independently simulated 1000 times, with values of relative bias and RMSE as well as coverage of Gaussian-type nominal 95% confidence intervals over the 1000 simulations set out in Table 5.1. We see that the naive estimator $\hat{\beta}_{OLS}$ that ignores the linkage errors is substantially biased. In contrast, the alternative estimators $\hat{\beta}_R$, $\hat{\beta}_{LL}$ and $\hat{\beta}_{BL}$ all correct this bias, with $\hat{\beta}_{BL}$ being the most efficient, even when the correct linkage rates are estimated, rather than specified. However, it is also important to note that when correct linkage rates are estimated, we must allow for their contribution to the overall variability of the estimator of the regression parameter. That is, we need to use (5.14), rather than (5.12), when estimating this variability.

Table 5.1   Simulation results for linear regression.

Estimator	Relative bias (%)		Relative RMSE (%)		Coverage (%)	
	Intercept	Slope	Intercept	Slope	Intercept	Slope
Correct linkage rates specified						
$\hat{\beta}_{OLS}$	7.82	−3.19	9.14	8.05	61.9	51.9
$\hat{\beta}_R$	−0.33	0.07	4.84	3.83	95.3	95.0
$\hat{\beta}_{LL}$	−0.33	0.07	4.80	3.77	95.0	95.1
$\hat{\beta}_{BL}$	−0.31	0.07	4.81	3.76	94.4	94.3
Correct linkage rates in m-blocks 2 and 3 estimated from audit sample						
$\hat{\beta}_{OLS}$	8.41	−3.38	9.67	8.42	57.6	46.3
$\hat{\beta}_R$	−0.05	0.00	5.28	4.27	96.9	96.0
$\hat{\beta}_{LL}$	0.20	−0.10	5.01	3.99	96.5	96.0
$\hat{\beta}_{BL}$	0.46	−0.21	4.77	3.71	95.5	95.7

Source: Chambers (2009).
Values of relative bias and relative root mean squared error (RMSE), both expressed in percentage terms, as well as the actual coverage rates (as %) for nominal 95% Gaussian confidence intervals.

5.4.2   Logistic regression

The previous subsection used an estimating equation framework to develop methods for correcting the bias induced by linkage errors. An immediate advantage is that these methods are then easily extended to other, not necessarily linear, models. We illustrate this by now briefly describing how the approach can be used to bias-correct logistic regression modelling of linked data. Here, y is a binary response and a common regression model is the linear logistic. That is, the population values y_i of y satisfy

$$y_i | \mathbf{X}_i \sim \text{independent Bernoulli} \{\pi(\mathbf{X}_i)\},$$

where $\pi(\mathbf{X}_i)$ is linear in the logistic scale, that is,

$$\pi(\mathbf{X}_i) = \text{pr}(y_i = 1 | \mathbf{X}_i) = \frac{\exp(\mathbf{X}_i^T \beta)}{1 + \exp(\mathbf{X}_i^T \beta)} = f(\mathbf{X}_i; \beta).$$

The estimating equation approach also can be used for the logistic model. Let $\mathbf{f}_q = \mathbf{f}_q(\beta)$ denote the vector of values of $f(\mathbf{X}_i; \beta)$ for the population units in m-block q. Then estimating Equation 5.9 can still be used to estimate β, and as in the linear model case, different weights $\mathbf{G}_q^*$ lead to different estimators of this parameter vector. In particular, the 'BLUE-type' efficient weights (5.11) in this case are of the form

$$\mathbf{G}_q^*(\beta) = \left[\mathbf{T}_{Aq} \frac{\partial \mathbf{f}_q}{\partial \beta} \right]^T \left(\text{var}(\mathbf{y}_q^* | \mathbf{X}_q) \right)^{-1},$$

where $\partial \mathbf{f}_q / \partial \beta = \mathbf{D}_q(\beta) \mathbf{X}_q$ with $\mathbf{D}_q(\beta) = \text{diag} \left[f(\mathbf{X}_i; \beta) \{1 - f(\mathbf{X}_i; \beta)\} \right]$.

Note that the formulae (5.12) and (5.14) for the asymptotic variance of the solution $\hat{\beta}^*$ to (5.9) still apply, with appropriate adjustments to allow for the different functional form of $\mathbf{f}_q$ in the logistic case (see Chambers (2009)).

5.5   Regression analysis using incomplete binary-linked data

We now turn to the more realistic situation where a sample of records from one register (here $\mathbf{X}$) is linked to the records in another register (here $\mathbf{y}$). In this situation, we need to allow for multiple sources of variability – the population variability associated with the regression relationship of interest, sampling variability, variability induced because of linkage errors and finally variability because not all records in $\mathbf{X}$ (and in particular not all sample records) are actually linked.

In order to deal with these different sources of variability, we need to make some assumptions. The first is not contentious and corresponds to an assumption of non-informative sampling within m-blocks. That is:

Non-informative sampling: Let S_q denote the random variable corresponding to the labels of the records in $\mathbf{X}_q$ selected to be in sample. Then S_q and $\mathbf{y}_q$ are independent given $\mathbf{X}_q$.

Note that non-informative sampling is not ignorable in general, and typically, we will need to use sample weights w_i to estimate population quantities. In what follows, we assume that these weights are available for all sampled records from $\mathbf{X}$.

Our second assumption extends the concept of non-informative linking to the sample case.

Non-informative sample linking: Given that one-to-one binary linking within each m-block q can be characterised by a random permutation matrix $\mathbf{A}_q$, then $\mathbf{A}_q$ is independent of both $\mathbf{y}_q$ and S_q given $\mathbf{X}_q$.

Note that implicit in this non-informative sample linking assumption is the idea that all records from $\mathbf{X}_q$ are potentially 'linkable', thus ensuring that $\mathbf{A}_q$ exists. Furthermore, this assumption implies that the linkage errors in the sampled records have the same stochastic behaviour as linkage errors overall, so we can treat the sampled component of $\mathbf{A}_q$ as a fixed component of this matrix.

Finally, we make the following assumption about the records that cannot be linked.

Ignorable non-linking: Within each m-block q, linkage (correct or incorrect) of a record (sampled or non-sampled) from $\mathbf{X}_q$ with a record from $\mathbf{y}_q$ is at random.

This represents our most contentious assumption, since it is usually the case that non-linkage is associated with records that are more likely to be incorrectly linked. However, under the assumption that the ELE linkage error model (5.8) is true, linkage errors within an m-block are all equally likely, and so assuming that the distribution of non-links within an m-block is random is not unreasonable.

Taken together, the aforementioned three assumptions allow us to condition on the actual sampled records that are linked when developing an appropriate modification to the complete linkage estimating Equation 5.9 for this case. To this end, let $\mathbf{X}_{sq}$ be the set of sampled records in $\mathbf{X}_q$, with $\mathbf{X}_{slq}$ denoting the records in $\mathbf{X}_{sq}$ that are linked to records in $\mathbf{y}_q$ and $\mathbf{X}_{suq}$ denoting the records in $\mathbf{X}_{sq}$ that cannot be linked to records in $\mathbf{y}_q$. Similarly, let $\mathbf{X}_{rq}$ denote the non-sampled records in $\mathbf{X}_q$, with a corresponding partition into $\mathbf{X}_{rlq}$ and $\mathbf{X}_{ruq}$. Here, $\mathbf{X}_{rlq}$ denotes the set of non-sampled records that would have been linked to records in $\mathbf{y}_q$ if in fact all records in $\mathbf{X}_q$ had been linked, and $\mathbf{X}_{ruq}$ denotes the corresponding set of non-sampled records that would not have been linked.

Under the one-to-one linkage assumption, $\mathbf{y}_q^*$ can then also be theoretically divided into four groups, namely, $\mathbf{y}_{slq}^*$, $\mathbf{y}_{suq}^*$, $\mathbf{y}_{rlq}^*$ and $\mathbf{y}_{ruq}^*$, and (5.2) can be modified to accommodate non-linkage of sampled records by writing

$$
\mathbf{y}_q^* = \begin{pmatrix} \mathbf{y}_{slq}^* \\ \mathbf{y}_{suq}^* \\ \mathbf{y}_{rlq}^* \\ \mathbf{y}_{ruq}^* \end{pmatrix} = \begin{bmatrix} \mathbf{A}_{slsl,q} & \mathbf{A}_{slsu,q} & \mathbf{A}_{slrl,q} & \mathbf{A}_{slru,q} \\ \mathbf{A}_{susl,q} & \mathbf{A}_{susu,q} & \mathbf{A}_{surl,q} & \mathbf{A}_{suru,q} \\ \mathbf{A}_{rlsl,q} & \mathbf{A}_{rlsu,q} & \mathbf{A}_{rlrl,q} & \mathbf{A}_{rlru,q} \\ \mathbf{A}_{rusl,q} & \mathbf{A}_{rusu,q} & \mathbf{A}_{rurl,q} & \mathbf{A}_{ruru,q} \end{bmatrix} \begin{pmatrix} \mathbf{y}_{slq} \\ \mathbf{y}_{suq} \\ \mathbf{y}_{rlq} \\ \mathbf{y}_{ruq} \end{pmatrix} = \begin{bmatrix} \mathbf{A}_{sl,q} \\ \mathbf{A}_{su,q} \\ \mathbf{A}_{rl,q} \\ \mathbf{A}_{ru,q} \end{bmatrix} \begin{pmatrix} \mathbf{y}_{slq} \\ \mathbf{y}_{suq} \\ \mathbf{y}_{rlq} \\ \mathbf{y}_{ruq} \end{pmatrix}. \tag{5.15}
$$

Similarly, (5.3) can be partitioned as

$$
E\left(\mathbf{A}_q \mid \mathbf{X}_q\right) = \mathbf{T}_{Aq} = \begin{bmatrix} \mathbf{T}_{slsl,Aq} & \mathbf{T}_{slsu,Aq} & \mathbf{T}_{slrl,Aq} & \mathbf{T}_{slru,Aq} \\ \mathbf{T}_{susl,Aq} & \mathbf{T}_{susu,Aq} & \mathbf{T}_{surl,Aq} & \mathbf{T}_{suru,Aq} \\ \mathbf{T}_{rlsl,Aq} & \mathbf{T}_{rlsu,Aq} & \mathbf{T}_{rlrl,Aq} & \mathbf{T}_{rlru,Aq} \\ \mathbf{T}_{rusl,Aq} & \mathbf{T}_{rusu,Aq} & \mathbf{T}_{rurl,Aq} & \mathbf{T}_{ruru,Aq} \end{bmatrix} = \begin{bmatrix} \mathbf{T}_{sl,Aq} \\ \mathbf{T}_{su,Aq} \\ \mathbf{T}_{rl,Aq} \\ \mathbf{T}_{ru,Aq} \end{bmatrix}. \tag{5.16}
$$

5.5.1   Linear regression using incomplete sample to register linked data

We now develop the estimating equation approach for incomplete sample to register linked data in the context of the linear regression model (5.1). In this case, the observed linked data in m-block q is $\left(\mathbf{y}_{slq}^{*}, \mathbf{X}_{slq} \right)$, and the analogue of estimating Equation 5.9 is

$$\mathbf{H}_{sl}^{*}(\beta) = \sum_{q} \mathbf{G}_{slq}^{*} \left(\mathbf{y}_{slq}^{*} - E\left(\mathbf{y}_{slq}^{*} \middle| \mathbf{X}_{slq} \right) \right) = 0, \tag{5.17}$$

where

$$
\begin{aligned}
E\left(\mathbf{y}_{slq}^{*} \middle| \mathbf{X}_{slq} \right) &= \mathbf{T}_{sl,A_{q}} E\left(\mathbf{y}_{slq} \middle| \mathbf{X}_{slq} \right) \\
&= \mathbf{T}_{sl,Aq} E\left(\mathbf{X}_{q} \middle| \mathbf{X}_{slq} \right) \beta \\
&= \left(\mathbf{T}_{slsl,Aq} \mathbf{X}_{slq} + \mathbf{T}_{slsu,Aq} E\left(\mathbf{X}_{suq} \right) + \mathbf{T}_{slrl,Aq} E\left(\mathbf{X}_{rlq} \right) + \mathbf{T}_{slru,Aq} E\left(\mathbf{X}_{ruq} \right) \right) \beta.
\end{aligned}
$$

Given our assumptions and assuming that linkage errors follow the ELE model,

$$\mathbf{T}_{slsl,Aq} = \left[\frac{\lambda_{q} M_{q} - 1}{M_{q} - 1} \right] \mathbf{I}_{slq} + \left[\frac{1 - \lambda_{q}}{M_{q} - 1} \right] \mathbf{1}_{slq} \mathbf{1}_{slq}^{T},$$

$$\mathbf{T}_{slsu,Aq} = \left[\frac{1 - \lambda_{q}}{M_{q} - 1} \right] \mathbf{1}_{slq} \mathbf{1}_{suq}^{T},$$

$$\mathbf{T}_{slrl,Aq} = \left[\frac{1 - \lambda_{q}}{M_{q} - 1} \right] \mathbf{1}_{slq} \mathbf{1}_{rlq}^{T},$$

$$\mathbf{T}_{slru,Aq} = \left[\frac{1 - \lambda_{q}}{M_{q} - 1} \right] \mathbf{1}_{slq} \mathbf{1}_{ruq}^{T},$$

and so

$$\mathbf{T}_{sl,Aq} E\left(\mathbf{X}_{q} \middle| \mathbf{X}_{slq} \right) = \left[\frac{\lambda_{q} M_{q} - 1}{M_{q} - 1} \right] \mathbf{X}_{slq} + \left[\frac{1 - \lambda_{q}}{M_{q} - 1} \right] \mathbf{1}_{slq} E\left(\mathbf{1}_{q}^{T} \mathbf{X}_{q} \middle| \mathbf{X}_{slq} \right).$$

Evaluating the second term on the right-hand side above represents a problem for a secondary analyst, since such a person, by definition, does not have access to $\mathbf{X}_{q}$. However, the components of the unknown conditional expectation in this term are just the m-block totals of the columns of $\mathbf{X}_{q}$. Under complete linkage, these totals can be estimated by sample-weighted sums of the corresponding columns of $\mathbf{X}_{sq}$. Under incomplete linkage, our assumption of ignorable non-linkage within m-blocks leads to modified sample-weighted estimates based on the columns of $\mathbf{X}_{slq}$ of the form

$$\hat{E}\left(\mathbf{1}_{q}^{T} \mathbf{X}_{q} \middle| \mathbf{X}_{slq} \right) = \tilde{\mathbf{w}}_{slq}^{T} \mathbf{X}_{slq}.$$

where

$$\tilde{\mathbf{w}}_{slq} = \left(\frac{M_{sq}}{M_{slq}}\right)\mathbf{w}_{slq} \tag{5.18}$$

Here, $\mathbf{w}_{slq}$ denotes the vector of sample weights associated with the linked sample records, and M_{sq}, M_{slq} denote the number of sampled records and the number of linked sample records in m-block q, respectively. Substituting (5.18) back in (5.17) leads to the modified estimating equation for this case:

$$\mathbf{H}_{sl}^*(\beta) = \sum_q \mathbf{G}_{slq}^*\left(\mathbf{y}_{slq}^* - \tilde{\mathbf{T}}_{slsl,Aq}\mathbf{X}_{slq}\beta\right) = 0, \tag{5.19}$$

where

$$\tilde{\mathbf{T}}_{slsl,Aq} = \left[\frac{\lambda_q M_q - 1}{M_q - 1}\right]\mathbf{I}_{slq} + \left[\frac{1-\lambda_q}{M_q - 1}\right]\mathbf{1}_{slq}\tilde{\mathbf{W}}_{slq}^T.$$

The general solution to (5.19) is of the form

$$\hat{\beta}_{sl}^* = \sum_q \left(\mathbf{G}_{slq}^*\tilde{\mathbf{T}}_{slsl,Aq}\mathbf{X}_{slq}\right)^{-1}\mathbf{G}_{slq}^*\mathbf{y}_{slq}^*. \tag{5.20}$$

Furthermore, an efficient estimator of β in this case is defined by substituting $\mathbf{G}_{slq}^* = \left[\tilde{\mathbf{T}}_{slsl,Aq}\mathbf{X}_{slq}\right]^T\left(\mathrm{var}\left(\mathbf{y}_{slq}^*\right)\right)^{-1}$ in (5.20), while the asymptotic variance of (5.20) can be obtained by using similar arguments as in previous section.

In particular, using Taylor series approximation, this asymptotic variance is given by the familiar sandwich formula

$$\mathrm{var}\left(\hat{\beta}_{sl}^*\middle|\mathbf{X}_{sl}\right) \approx \mathbf{D}_{sl}^{-1}\left[\sum_q \mathbf{G}_{slq}^*\,\mathrm{var}\left(\mathbf{y}_{slq}^*\middle|\mathbf{X}_{slq}\right)\left(\mathbf{G}_{slq}^*\right)^T\right]\left(\mathbf{D}_{sl}^{-1}\right)^T \tag{5.21}$$

where

$$\mathbf{D}_{sl} = \partial\mathbf{H}_{sl}^*(\beta_0)/\partial\beta = \sum_q \mathbf{G}_{slq}^*\tilde{\mathbf{T}}_{slsl,Aq}\mathbf{X}_{slq}.$$

See Kim and Chambers (2012a) for a general formula for $\mathrm{var}\left(\mathbf{y}_{slq}^*\middle|\mathbf{X}_{slq}\right)$. Here, we note that for the linear regression case, we then have the approximation

$$\mathrm{var}\left(\mathbf{y}_{slq}^*\middle|\mathbf{X}_{slq}\right) \approx \mathrm{diag}\left[\sigma^2 + \left(1-\lambda_q\right)\left\{\lambda_q\left(f_i - \bar{f}_{slq}\right)^2 + \bar{f}_{slq}^{(2)} - \left(\bar{f}_{slq}\right)^2\right\}\right].$$

Furthermore, a consistent estimator of σ^2 is

$$\hat{\sigma}^2 = M_{slq}^{-1}\left(\sum_q \left(\mathbf{y}^*_{slq} - \hat{\mathbf{f}}_{slq}\right)^T \left(\mathbf{y}^*_{slq} - \hat{\mathbf{f}}_{slq}\right) - 2\sum_q \left(\hat{\mathbf{f}}_{slq}\right)^T \left[\mathbf{I}_{slq} - \tilde{\mathbf{T}}_{slsl,q}\right]\hat{\mathbf{f}}_{slq}\right).$$

As in the complete linkage case, replacing λ_q by an estimate $\hat{\lambda}_q$ in the earlier development leads to an increase in the asymptotic variance. In particular, (5.21) then becomes

$$\operatorname{var}\left(\hat{\beta}^*_{sl}\big|\mathbf{X}_{sl}\right) = \mathbf{D}_{sl}^{-1}\left[\sum_q \mathbf{G}^*_{slq}\left[\operatorname{var}\left(\mathbf{y}^*_{slq}\big|\mathbf{X}_{slq}\right) + \Phi_{slq}\right]\left(\mathbf{G}^*_{slq}\right)^T\right]\left(\mathbf{D}_{sl}^{-1}\right)^T$$

where $\Phi_{slq} = \phi_{slq}\operatorname{var}\left(\hat{\lambda}_q\big|\mathbf{X}_{slq}\right)\phi_{slq}^T$ with

$$\phi_{slq} = \left[\left(M_{slq} - 1\right)^{-1}\left(M_{slq}\mathbf{I}_{slq} - \mathbf{1}_{slq}\tilde{\mathbf{w}}^T_{slq}\right)\right]\mathbf{X}_{slq}\beta.$$

When $\hat{\lambda}_q$ is calculated using the data obtained in an audit subsample of size m_{slq} selected randomly from the known links in m-block q, then

$$\operatorname{var}\left(\hat{\lambda}_q\big|\mathbf{X}_{slq}\right) = m_{slq}^{-1}\lambda_q\left(1 - \lambda_q\right).$$

See Kim and Chambers (2012a) for more details, including simulation results that are in line with those reported in Table 5.1. Note that these authors also briefly discuss the case where the non-linkage is informative.

5.6 Regression analysis with multi-linked data

As noted at the start of this chapter, linked datasets created using multiple sources are now common. Secondary analysis of these multi-linked datasets is the focus of this section. As in the previous section, we concentrate on development of bias-corrected estimation methods for the parameters of the linear model (5.1). We also restrict the number of linked data sources to three, since this suffices to illustrate the basic ideas. In particular, we consider the situation where the linear regression model of interest is

$$\mathbf{y} = \mathbf{X}_1\beta_1 + \mathbf{X}_2\beta_2 + \varepsilon = \mathbf{X}\beta + \varepsilon = \mathbf{f} + \varepsilon, \tag{5.22}$$

where the components of the error vector ϵ are independently distributed as $(0, \sigma^2)$ and $\mathbf{y}$, $\mathbf{X}_1$ and $\mathbf{X}_2$ denote three separate population registers covering the same population. Without loss of generality, we assume that $\mathbf{X}_1$ includes an intercept term. Extension to four or more registers is straightforward but notationally messy.

Without loss of generality, we assume that $\mathbf{y}$ and $\mathbf{X}_2$ are each separately linked to $\mathbf{X}_1$. We also initially assume that these linkages are complete, resulting in the linked dataset $\left(\mathbf{y}^*, \mathbf{X}_1, \mathbf{X}_2^*\right)$. The extension to the incomplete linkage case, where a sample of records from $\mathbf{X}_1$ is linked to $\mathbf{y}$ and $\mathbf{X}_2$, is addressed in the following subsection.

5.6.1   Uncorrelated multi-linking: Complete linkage

Under complete linkage, the values in $\mathbf{y}^*$ and $\mathbf{X}_2^*$ satisfy (5.6), where $\mathbf{A}_q$ and $\mathbf{B}_q$ are unobserved random permutation matrices of order M_q. Since then $\mathbf{B}_q^T \mathbf{B}_q = \mathbf{I}_q$, it follows that $\mathbf{X}_{2q} = \mathbf{B}_q^T \mathbf{X}_{2q}^*$ and so (5.22) implies

$$\mathbf{y}_q^* = \mathbf{A}_q \left[\mathbf{X}_{1q} \beta_1 + \mathbf{B}_q^T \mathbf{X}_{2q}^* \beta_2 \right] + \mathbf{A}_q \varepsilon_q. \tag{5.23}$$

We see from (5.23) that it is the regression of $\mathbf{y}^*$ on $\mathbf{X}^* = \left[\mathbf{X}_1 \ \mathbf{X}_2^* \right]$ which is of interest, since it is $\mathbf{X}^*$ rather than $\mathbf{X}$ that is observed. An immediate implication is that all assumptions about non-informative behaviour are given $\mathbf{X}^*$ in what follows. In particular, we now assume non-informative uncorrelated multi-linkage given $\mathbf{X}^*$. This corresponds to assuming:

$\mathbf{A}_q$ and ε_q are independently distributed given $\mathbf{X}_q^* = \left[\mathbf{X}_{1q} \ \mathbf{X}_{2q}^* \right]$.

$\mathbf{A}_q$ and $\mathbf{B}_q^T$ are independently distributed given $\mathbf{X}_q^* = \left[\mathbf{X}_{1q} \ \mathbf{X}_{2q}^* \right]$.

Under these assumptions,

$$E\left(\mathbf{A}_q \mathbf{B}_q^T \big| \mathbf{X}_q^* \right) = E\left(\mathbf{A}_q \big| \mathbf{X}_q^* \right) E\left(\mathbf{B}_q^T \big| \mathbf{A}_q, \mathbf{X}_q^* \right) = E\left(\mathbf{A}_q \big| \mathbf{X}_q^* \right) E\left(\mathbf{B}_q^T \big| \mathbf{X}_q^* \right).$$

Furthermore, if both $\mathbf{A}_q$ and $\mathbf{B}_q$ can be modelled as ELE, then

$$\begin{aligned}
\mathbf{T}_{Aq} &= E\left(\mathbf{A}_q \big| \mathbf{X}_q^* \right) = \left(\lambda_{Aq} - \gamma_{Aq} \right) \mathbf{I}_q + \gamma_{Aq} \mathbf{1}_q \mathbf{1}_q^T, \\
\mathbf{T}_{Bq} &= E\left(\mathbf{B}_q \big| \mathbf{X}_q^* \right) = \left(\lambda_{Bq} - \gamma_{Bq} \right) \mathbf{I}_q + \gamma_{Bq} \mathbf{1}_q \mathbf{1}_q^T = E\left(\mathbf{B}_q^T \big| \mathbf{X}_q^* \right),
\end{aligned} \tag{5.24}$$

where λ_{Aq} is the rate of correct linkage between $\mathbf{y}_q^*$ and $\mathbf{X}_{1q}$ and λ_{Bq} is the rate of correct linkage between $\mathbf{X}_{2q}$ and $\mathbf{X}_{1q}$.

Now, from (5.22), (5.23) and (5.24),

$$E\left(\mathbf{Y}_q^* \big| \mathbf{X}_q^* \right) = E\left(\mathbf{A}_q \big| \mathbf{X}_q^* \right) E\left(\mathbf{X}_{1q} \beta_1 + \mathbf{B}_q^T \mathbf{X}_{2q}^* \beta_2 \big| \mathbf{X}_q^* \right) = \mathbf{T}_{Aq} \left(\mathbf{X}_{1q} \beta_1 + \mathbf{T}_{Bq} \mathbf{X}_{2q}^* \beta_2 \right) = \mathbf{T}_{Aq} \mathbf{X}_q^E \beta$$

where $\mathbf{X}_q^E = \left[\mathbf{X}_{1q} \ \mathbf{T}_{Bq} \mathbf{X}_{2q}^* \right]$. For this case, estimating Equation 5.9 becomes

$$\mathbf{H}^* (\beta) = \sum_q \mathbf{G}_q^* \left(\mathbf{y}_q^* - \mathbf{T}_{Aq} \mathbf{X}_q^E \beta \right) = 0 \tag{5.25}$$

with solution

$$\hat{\beta}^* = \sum_q \left(\mathbf{G}_q^* \mathbf{T}_{Aq} \mathbf{X}_q^E \right)^{-1} \mathbf{G}_q^* \mathbf{y}_q^*.$$

Furthermore, the optimal weight to use in (5.25) is

$$\mathbf{G}_q^* = \left[\frac{\partial E\left(\mathbf{y}_q^* \big| \mathbf{X}_q^* \right)}{\partial \beta} \right]^T \left(\mathrm{var}\left(\mathbf{y}_q^* \big| \mathbf{X}_q^* \right) \right)^{-1} = \left(\mathbf{T}_{Aq} \mathbf{X}_q^E \right)^T \left(\mathrm{var}\left(\mathbf{y}_q^* \big| \mathbf{X}_q^* \right) \right)^{-1}.$$

The asymptotic sandwich variance formula (5.12) still holds, except that now

$$\frac{\partial \mathbf{H}^*(\beta)}{\partial \beta} = \sum_q \left(\mathbf{G}_q^* \mathbf{T}_{Aq} \mathbf{X}_q^E \right).$$

Evaluation of (5.12) in this case requires an expression for $\mathrm{var}\left(\mathbf{y}_q^* \middle| \mathbf{X}_q^* \right)$. Put $\mathbf{f}_{2q}^* = \mathbf{X}_{2q}^* \beta_2 = \left(f_{2q,i}^* \right)$ and let $\mathbf{f}_q^E = \mathbf{X}_q^E \beta = \left(f_{q,i}^E \right)$. Following the development in Kim and Chambers (2012b), we can show that

$$\mathrm{var}\left(\mathbf{y}_q^* \middle| \mathbf{X}_q^* \right) = \sigma^2 \mathbf{I}_q + \mathbf{V}_{Aq} + \mathbf{V}_{Cq}, \tag{5.26}$$

where $\mathbf{V}_{Aq}$ is the component of variance due to linkage errors between $\mathbf{X}_{1q}$ and $\mathbf{y}_q$ and $\mathbf{V}_{Aq}$ is the component of variance due to linkage errors between $\mathbf{X}_{1q}$ and $\mathbf{X}_{2q}$. Here,

$$\mathbf{V}_{Aq} = \left(1 - \lambda_{Aq}\right) \mathrm{diag}\left[\left\{ \lambda_{Aq} \left(f_{q,i}^E - \overline{f}_q^E \right)^2 + \overline{f}_q^{E(2)} - \left(\overline{f}_q^E \right)^2 \right\} \right]$$

with $\overline{f}_q^E = M_q^{-1} \sum_{i=1}^{M_q} f_{q,i}^E$ and $\overline{f}_q^{E(2)} = M_q^{-1} \sum_{i=1}^{M_q} \left(f_{q,i}^E \right)^2$. Furthermore,

$$\mathbf{V}_{Cq} = \left(1 - \lambda_{Bq}\right) \mathrm{diag}\left[\left(M_q - 1\right)^{-1} \left\{ \left(\lambda_{Aq} M_q - 1\right) d_i + M_q \left(1 - \lambda_{Aq}\right) \overline{d}_q \right\} \right],$$

where $d_i = \lambda_{Bq} \left(f_{2q,i}^* - \overline{f}_{2q}^* \right)^2 + \overline{f}_{2q}^{*(2)} - \left(\overline{f}_{2q}^* \right)^2$ with $\overline{f}_{2q}^* = M_q^{-1} \sum_{i=1}^{M_q} f_{2q,i}^*$ and $\overline{f}_{2q}^{*(2)} = M_q^{-1} \sum_{i=1}^{M_q} \left(f_{2q,i}^* \right)^2$.

Finally, we note that an unbiased estimator of σ^2 for this case is

$$\hat{\sigma}^2 = N^{-1} \left(\sum_q \left(\mathbf{y}_q^* - \mathbf{f}_q^E \right)^T \left(\mathbf{y}_q^* - \mathbf{f}_q^E \right) - 2 \sum_q \left(\mathbf{f}_q^E \right)^T \left(\mathbf{I}_q - \mathbf{T}_{Aq} \right) \mathbf{f}_q^E \right).$$

In practice, of course, λ_{Aq} and λ_{Bq} will not be known and will be estimated (e.g. using an audit sample). We omit a detailed development for this situation, however, since it represents a special case of the results presented in the next subsection. It suffices to observe that there is then an extra component of variance in (5.26) due to the variability associated with these estimates.

5.6.2   Uncorrelated multi-linking: Sample to register linkage

The situation considered here is the multi-linkage equivalent of that considered in Section 5.5.1, and so notation introduced there is used without further comment. Within each m-block q, the linked sample data are $\left(\mathbf{y}_{slq}^*, \mathbf{X}_{1slq}^*, \mathbf{X}_{2slq}^* \right)$, where we implicitly assume that the records in $\mathbf{X}_{1sq}$ are independently matched to records in $\mathbf{y}_q$ and $\mathbf{X}_{2q}$. Similarly to (5.16), we can partition $\mathbf{T}_{Bq}$ as

$$\mathbf{T}_{Bq} = \begin{bmatrix} \mathbf{T}_{slsl,Bq} & \mathbf{T}_{slsu,Bq} & \mathbf{T}_{slrl,Bq} & \mathbf{T}_{slru,Bq} \\ \mathbf{T}_{susl,Bq} & \mathbf{T}_{susu,Bq} & \mathbf{T}_{surl,Bq} & \mathbf{T}_{suru,Bq} \\ \mathbf{T}_{rlsl,Bq} & \mathbf{T}_{rlsu,Bq} & \mathbf{T}_{rlrl,Bq} & \mathbf{T}_{rlru,Bq} \\ \mathbf{T}_{rusl,Bq} & \mathbf{T}_{rusu,Bq} & \mathbf{T}_{rurl,Bq} & \mathbf{T}_{ruru,Bq} \end{bmatrix} = \begin{bmatrix} \mathbf{T}_{sl,Bq} \\ \mathbf{T}_{su,Bq} \\ \mathbf{T}_{rl,Bq} \\ \mathbf{T}_{ru,Bq} \end{bmatrix}^T.$$

The analogue to the linked sample data-based estimating Equation 5.17 is then

$$\mathbf{H}_{sl}^{*}\left(\beta\right)=\sum_{q}\mathbf{G}_{slq}^{*}\left(\mathbf{y}_{slq}^{*}-\tilde{\mathbf{T}}_{sl,Aq}\mathbf{X}_{slq}^{E}\beta\right)=0 \tag{5.27}$$

where

$$\tilde{\mathbf{T}}_{sl,Aq}=\left[\frac{\lambda_{Aq}M_{q}-1}{M_{q}-1}\right]\mathbf{I}_{slq}+\left[\frac{1-\lambda_{Aq}}{M_{q}-1}\right]\mathbf{1}_{slq}\tilde{\mathbf{w}}_{slq}^{T}$$

and

$$\mathbf{X}_{slq}^{E}=\left[\mathbf{X}_{1slq}\ \mathbf{T}_{sl,Bq}\mathbf{X}_{2q}^{*}\right].$$

However, the term $\mathbf{T}_{sl,Bq}\mathbf{X}_{2q}^{*}$ in the definition of $\mathbf{X}_{slq}^{E}$ above cannot be evaluated without access to $\mathbf{X}_{2q}^{*}$. Consequently, we replace it by its linked sample-weighted estimate $\tilde{\mathbf{T}}_{sl,Bq}\mathbf{X}_{2slq}^{*}$ where

$$\tilde{\mathbf{T}}_{sl,Bq}=\left[\frac{\lambda_{Bq}M_{q}-1}{M_{q}-1}\right]\mathbf{I}_{slq}+\left[\frac{1-\lambda_{Bq}}{M_{q}-1}\right]\mathbf{1}_{slq}\tilde{\mathbf{w}}_{slq}^{T}.$$

Put

$$\tilde{\mathbf{X}}_{slq}^{E}=\left[\mathbf{X}_{1slq}\ \tilde{\mathbf{T}}_{sl,Bq}\mathbf{X}_{2slq}^{*}\right].$$

A computable version of estimating Equation 5.27 is then

$$\mathbf{H}_{sl}^{*}\left(\beta\right)=\sum_{q}\mathbf{G}_{slq}^{*}\left(\mathbf{y}_{slq}^{*}-\tilde{\mathbf{T}}_{sl,Aq}\tilde{\mathbf{X}}_{slq}^{E}\beta\right)=0$$

with solution

$$\hat{\beta}_{sl}^{*}=\sum_{q}\left(\mathbf{G}_{slq}^{*}\tilde{\mathbf{T}}_{sl,Aq}\tilde{\mathbf{X}}_{slq}^{E}\right)^{-1}\mathbf{G}_{slq}^{*}\mathbf{y}_{slq}^{*}. \tag{5.28}$$

As usual, the optimal weights for use in (5.28) are of the form

$$\mathbf{G}_{slq}^{*}=\left(\tilde{\mathbf{T}}_{sl,Aq}\tilde{\mathbf{X}}_{slq}^{E}\right)^{T}\left(\operatorname{var}\left(\mathbf{y}_{slq}^{*}\left|\mathbf{X}_{slq}^{*}\right.\right)\right)^{-1}.$$

The asymptotic variance of $\hat{\beta}_{sl}^{*}$ is of the usual sandwich form:

$$\operatorname{var}\left(\hat{\beta}_{sl}^{*}\left|\mathbf{X}_{sl}^{*}\right.\right)\approx\left[\frac{\partial\mathbf{H}_{sl}^{*}}{\partial\beta}\right]^{-1}\operatorname{var}\left(\mathbf{H}_{sl}^{*}\left|\mathbf{X}_{sl}^{*}\right.\right)\left(\left[\frac{\partial\mathbf{H}_{sl}^{*}}{\partial\beta}\right]^{-1}\right)^{T}, \tag{5.29}$$

where

$$\frac{\partial \mathbf{H}_{sl}^*}{\partial \beta} = \sum_q \mathbf{G}_{slq}^* \tilde{\mathbf{T}}_{sl,Aq} \tilde{\mathbf{X}}_{slq}^E$$

and

$$\text{var}\left(\mathbf{H}_{sl}^* \middle| \mathbf{X}_{sl}^*\right) = \sum_q \mathbf{G}_{slq}^* \text{var}\left(\mathbf{y}_{slq}^* \middle| \mathbf{X}_{slq}^*\right) \left(\mathbf{G}_{slq}^*\right)^T.$$

Furthermore, it can be shown that

$$\text{var}\left(\mathbf{y}_{slq}^* \middle| \mathbf{X}_{slq}^*\right) = \sigma^2 \mathbf{I}_{slq} + \mathbf{V}_{(sl)Aq} + \mathbf{V}_{(sl)Cq},$$

where

$$\mathbf{V}_{(sl)Aq} \approx (1 - \lambda_{Aq}) \text{diag} \left[\lambda_{Aq} \left(\tilde{f}_{slq,i}^E - \overline{\tilde{f}}_{slq}^E \right)^2 + \overline{\tilde{f}}_{slq}^{E(2)} - \left(\overline{\tilde{f}}_{slq}^E \right)^2 \right]$$

with $\tilde{\mathbf{f}}_{slq}^E = \tilde{\mathbf{X}}_{slq}^E \beta = \left(\tilde{f}_{slq,i}^E \right),$ $\overline{\tilde{f}}_{slq}^E = M_{slq}^{-1} \sum_{i=1}^{M_{slq}} \tilde{f}_{slq,i}^E$ and $\overline{\tilde{f}}_{slq}^{E(2)} = M_{slq}^{-1} \sum_{i=1}^{M_{slq}} \left(\tilde{f}_{slq,i}^E \right)^2.$

Put $\mathbf{f}_{2slq}^* = \mathbf{X}_{2slq}^* \beta_2 = \left(f_{2slq,i}^* \right).$ Then

$$\mathbf{V}_{(sl)Cq} \approx (1 - \lambda_{Bq}) \text{diag} \left[(M_q - 1)^{-1} \left\{ (\lambda_{Aq} M_q - 1) \tilde{d}_i + M_q (1 - \lambda_{Aq}) \overline{\tilde{d}}_{slq} \right\} \right]$$

where $\overline{\tilde{d}}_{slq} = M_{slq}^{-1} \sum_{i=1}^{M_{slq}} \tilde{d}_i,$ $\tilde{d}_i = \lambda_{Bq} (f_{2slq,i}^* - \overline{f}_{2slq}^*)^2 + \overline{f}_{2slq}^{*(2)} - \left(\overline{f}_{2slq}^* \right)^2$ with $\overline{f}_{2slq}^* = M_{slq}^{-1} \sum_{i=1}^{M_{slq}} f_{2slq,i}^*$
and $\overline{f}_{2slq}^{*(2)} = M_{slq}^{-1} \sum_{i=1}^{M_{slq}} \left(f_{2slq,i}^* \right)^2.$

Proof of the asymptotic variance expression (5.29) is in Kim and Chambers (2012b). These authors also consider the situation where λ_{Aq} and λ_{Bq} are replaced by independently estimated values $\hat{\lambda}_{Aq}$ and $\hat{\lambda}_{Bq}$, respectively. In this case, they show that $\text{var}\left(\mathbf{H}_{sl}^* \middle| \mathbf{X}_{sl}^*\right)$ in (5.29) is replaced by

$$\text{var}\left(\mathbf{H}_{sl}^* \middle| \mathbf{X}_{sl}^*\right) + \frac{\partial \mathbf{H}_{sl}^*}{\partial \lambda_{Aq}} \text{var}\left(\hat{\lambda}_{Aq} \middle| \mathbf{X}_{sl}^*\right) \left(\frac{\partial \mathbf{H}_{sl}^*}{\partial \lambda_{Aq}}\right)^T + \frac{\partial \mathbf{H}_{sl}^*}{\partial \lambda_{Bq}} \text{var}\left(\hat{\lambda}_{Bq} \middle| \mathbf{X}_{sl}^*\right) \left(\frac{\partial \mathbf{H}_{sl}^*}{\partial \lambda_{Bq}}\right)^T,$$

where

$$\frac{\partial \mathbf{H}_{sl}^*}{\partial \lambda_{Aq}} = \sum_q \mathbf{G}_{slq}^* \left[(M_q - 1)^{-1} \left(M_q \mathbf{I}_{slq} - \mathbf{1}_{slq} \tilde{\mathbf{w}}_{slq}^T \right) \right] \tilde{\mathbf{f}}_{slq}^E$$

and

$$\frac{\partial \mathbf{H}_{sl}^*}{\partial \lambda_{Bq}} = \sum_q \mathbf{G}_{slq}^* \tilde{\mathbf{T}}_{sl,Aq} \left[(M_q - 1)^{-1} \left(M_q \mathbf{I}_{slq} - \mathbf{1}_{slq} \tilde{\mathbf{w}}_{slq}^T \right) \right] \mathbf{f}_{2slq}^*.$$

In order to illustrate the gains from using (5.28) instead of standard OLS to estimate β in a multi-linking situation, we reproduce in Table 5.2 simulation results presented in Kim and Chambers (2012b). Here, $\hat{\beta}_{LL}$ corresponds to (5.28) with $\mathbf{G}_{slq}^* = \tilde{\mathbf{T}}_{sl,Aq} \tilde{\mathbf{X}}_{slq}^E$, and $\hat{\beta}_{BL}$ corresponds

Table 5.2 Simulation values of relative bias and relative RMSE (both expressed in percentage terms) for linear model parameter estimates under uncorrelated sample to population multi-linkage.

Estimator	Relative bias (%)		Relative RMSE (%)		Coverage (%)	
	λ known	λ unknown	λ known	λ unknown	λ known	λ unknown
Estimation of intercept coefficient						
$\hat{\beta}_{OLS}$	129.75	129.75	130.98	130.98	0.0	0.0
$\hat{\beta}_{LL}$	0.61	4.25	17.69	33.48	96.0	100.0
$\hat{\beta}_{BL}$	0.71	7.13	8.70	18.16	97.9	100.0
Estimation of x_1 coefficient						
$\hat{\beta}_{OLS}$	−10.08	−10.08	10.23	10.23	0.0	0.0
$\hat{\beta}_{LL}$	−0.08	−0.37	1.65	3.41	96.8	100.0
$\hat{\beta}_{BL}$	−0.09	−0.72	0.80	1.81	97.8	100.0
Estimation of x_2 coefficient						
$\hat{\beta}_{OLS}$	−19.90	−19.90	20.17	20.17	0.0	0.0
$\hat{\beta}_{LL}$	−0.12	−0.67	3.24	5.00	96.6	100.0
$\hat{\beta}_{BL}$	−0.07	−0.84	1.64	2.82	98.8	100.0

Source: Kim and Chambers (2012b).
Empirical coverages (expressed in percentage terms) of normal theory-based nominal 95% confidence intervals based on estimated asymptotic variances are also shown.

to (5.28) with $\mathbf{G}^*_{slq}$ set to its optimal value $\left(\tilde{\mathbf{T}}_{sl,Aq}\tilde{\mathbf{X}}^E_{slq}\right)^T \left(\text{var}\left(\mathbf{y}^*_{slq}\middle|\mathbf{X}^*_{slq}\right)\right)^{-1}$. These results are based on a population-level linear regression model of the form

$$y = 1 + 3x_1 + 0.7x_2 + \varepsilon$$

with the values of x_1 drawn from the normal distribution with mean 2 and variance 4 and with the values of ϵ independently drawn from the $N(0,1)$ distribution. The values of x_2 were generated as $x_2 = 1 + 2z + \gamma$ where the distribution of z is the same as the distribution of x_1 and where the values of γ were independently drawn from the $N(0,1)$ distribution. There were three m-blocks. Each m-block consisted of 2000 records, with 1000 randomly sampled. Only half of these sampled records could be linked, however. The correct linkage rates between x_1 and y were such that $\lambda_{A1} = 1$, $\lambda_{A2} = 0.95$ and $\lambda_{A3} = 0.75$. Similarly, the correct linkage rates between x_1 and x_2 were such that $\lambda_{B1} = 1$, $\lambda_{B2} = 0.85$ and $\lambda_{B3} = 0.8$. There were a total of 1000 simulations. The impact of estimating correct linkage rates was assessed by using two independent audit samples in each m-block, where each audit sample was of size 25. The large gains from using (5.28), preferably with optimal weighting, are clear.

5.6.3   Correlated multi-linkage

For notational simplicity, we omit explicit reference to conditioning in this subsection, though this is still necessary for non-informative multi-linking. Our main focus instead is extending the results in the previous subsection to accommodate the reasonable observation that multi-linkage errors are generally correlated. For example, if some records in $\mathbf{X}_1$ are incorrectly linked to records in $\mathbf{y}$, then it is highly likely that these records will be also incorrectly linked to records in $\mathbf{X}_2$. The limiting case, of course, is where $\mathbf{y}$ and $\mathbf{X}_2$ correspond to the same population register. In general, therefore, we need to consider a conditional model for the distribution of $\mathbf{B}_q$ given $\mathbf{A}_q$. Let $\mathbf{x}_{i,1q}$ denote the ith record in $\mathbf{X}_{1q}$, with $\mathbf{x}_{i,2q}$ and $y_{i,q}$ defined similarly. Define the joint probability

$$\phi_q = \mathrm{pr}\left\{\left(\mathbf{x}_{i,1q},\mathbf{x}_{i,2q}\right) \text{correctly linked and} \left(\mathbf{x}_{i,1q},y_{i,q}\right) \text{correctly linked}\right\},$$

and assume that ϕ_q does not depend on i. Like the ELE assumption, this is a practical assumption for a secondary analyst, since if ϕ_q varies with i, then it is highly likely that this information will be confidential and hence not available to a secondary analyst.

In order to model $E(\mathbf{B}_q|\mathbf{A}_q)$, put $\lambda_{(B|A)q} = \lambda_{Aq}^{-1}\phi_q$. Note that under uncorrelated multi-linkage, $\lambda_{(B|A)q} = \lambda_{Bq}$. If both $\mathbf{A}_q$ and $\mathbf{B}_q$ satisfy an ELE model, we can then show that

$$\mathbf{T}_{(B|A)q} = E\left(\mathbf{B}_q \middle| \mathbf{A}_q\right) = \left(\lambda_{(B|A)q} - \gamma_{(B|A)q}\right)\mathbf{I}_q + \gamma_{(B|A)q}\mathbf{1}_q\mathbf{1}_q^T, \tag{5.30}$$

where $\gamma_{(B|A)q} = (M_q - 1)^{-1}(1 - \lambda_{(B|A)q})$. It follows that

$$E\left(\mathbf{A}_q\mathbf{B}_q\right) = E\left(\mathbf{A}_q\right)E\left(\mathbf{B}_q \middle| \mathbf{A}_q\right) = \mathbf{T}_{Aq}\mathbf{T}_{(B|A)q},$$

and we can proceed by replacing all occurrences of $\mathbf{T}_{Bq}$ in the preceding two subsections by $\mathbf{T}_{(B|A)q}$ defined by (5.30). Consequently, all the theory developed for uncorrelated multi-linkage carries directly over to the correlated multi-linkage case once this substitution is made. See Kim and Chambers (2013) for a complete development of this case, including the necessary adjustments to the asymptotic variance of $\hat{\beta}_{sl}^*$ when λ_{Aq} and ϕ_q are simultaneously estimated from the same sample.

5.6.4   Incorporating auxiliary population information

The phenomenon of non-linkage implies that as the number of contributing population registers increases, the size of the final multi-linked dataset will decrease. This has implications for the efficiency of the bias-corrected estimators developed in the preceding subsections, since we then expect to see an increase in their bias due to these smaller (and less representative) samples. In large part, this is because we have assumed that the only information about the underlying population available to a secondary analyst is contained in the multi-linked dataset itself, that is, the analyst does not have access to any further information about the contributing population registers. Key register-based summations contributing to these estimators are approximated by weighting sums of linked sample data, leading to a decrease in the efficiency of the bias correction.

In this subsection, we show how having access to marginal information from contributing population registers can help alleviate this problem. In doing so, we note that the extent of the marginal information that a linking agency can release will depend on confidentiality considerations. However, for the purposes of our development, we shall assume that, in addition to the multi-linked dataset $\left(\mathbf{y}^{*}_{slq}, \mathbf{X}_{1slq}, \mathbf{X}^{*}_{2slq} \right)$, the mean values $\bar{y}_{q}$, $\bar{\mathbf{x}}_{1q}$ and $\bar{\mathbf{x}}_{2q}$ of the analysis variables within each m-block are also made available to the analyst. Note that we assume correlated multi-linkage in what follows, so all occurrences of the subscript B in the references we give in the following are replaced by the subscript $(B \mid A)$.

Let $\bar{\mathbf{x}}_{q} = \left[\bar{\mathbf{x}}^{T}_{1q}\ \bar{\mathbf{x}}^{T}_{2q} \right]^{T}$ denote the vector of column averages of the matrix $\mathbf{X}_{q}$. We start by observing that under the ELE model, the vector of column averages of the matrix $\mathbf{X}^{E}_{q} = \left[\mathbf{X}_{1q}\ \mathbf{T}_{(B \mid A)q} \mathbf{X}^{*}_{2q} \right]$ is equal to $\bar{\mathbf{x}}_{q}$. Consequently, we can replace $\mathbf{X}^{E}_{slq}$ in estimating Equation 5.27 by

$$\mathbf{X}^{E}_{slq} = \left[\mathbf{X}_{1slq} \left(\lambda_{(B \mid A)_{q}} - \gamma_{(B \mid A)_{q}} \right) \mathbf{X}^{*}_{2slq} + M_{q} \gamma_{(B \mid A)_{q}} \mathbf{1}_{slq} \bar{\mathbf{x}}^{T}_{2q} \right].$$

Furthermore, the term $\tilde{\mathbf{T}}_{sl,Aq} \mathbf{X}^{E}_{slq} \beta$ in this equation can then also be replaced by

$$E \left(\mathbf{y}^{*}_{slq} \middle| \mathbf{X}^{*}_{slq}, \bar{\mathbf{x}}_{q} \right) = \left\{ \left(\lambda_{Aq} - \gamma_{Aq} \right) \mathbf{X}^{E}_{slq} + M_{q} \gamma_{Aq} \mathbf{1}_{slq} \bar{\mathbf{x}}^{T}_{q} \right\} \beta.$$

That is, there is no need for sample weighting when calculating $\mathbf{H}^{*}_{sl}(\beta)$ if we have access to the m-block means of the variables defining $\mathbf{X}_{1}$ and $\mathbf{X}_{2}$. In addition, if we know the m-block mean $\bar{y}_{q}$, we can go further, because we can then add an extra term to this estimating function. This term represents the average residual defined by the non-sampled, non-linked records, which we collectively denote by r below and for which we can now calculate the m-block specific average value:

$$\bar{y}^{*}_{rq} = M^{-1}_{rq} \left(M_{q} \bar{y}_{q} - M_{slq} \bar{y}^{*}_{slq} \right).$$

Here, $M_{rq} = M_{q} - M_{slq}$ and M_{slq} denotes the number of linked sample records in m-block q. Kim and Chambers (2013) show that $E \left(\bar{y}^{*}_{rq} \middle| \bar{\mathbf{x}}_{q} \right) = \bar{\mathbf{x}}^{*}_{rq} \beta$, where

$$\bar{\mathbf{x}}^{*}_{rq} = M^{-1}_{rq} \left[M_{q} \left(1 - M_{slq} \gamma_{Aq} \right) \bar{\mathbf{x}}_{q} - M_{slq} \left(\lambda_{Aq} - \gamma_{Aq} \right) \bar{\mathbf{x}}^{E}_{slq} \right].$$

That is, access to auxiliary population data consisting of the m-block average values of the analysis variables allows us to replace (5.27) by the *calibrated* estimating equation $\mathbf{H}^{*}_{cal}(\beta) = 0$, where

$$\mathbf{H}^{*}_{cal}(\beta) = \sum_{q} \left(\mathbf{G}^{*}_{slq} \left[\mathbf{y}^{*}_{slq} - \left\{ \left(\lambda_{Aq} - \gamma_{Aq} \right) \mathbf{X}^{E}_{slq} + M_{q} \gamma_{Aq} \mathbf{1}_{slq} \bar{\mathbf{x}}^{T}_{q} \right\} \beta \right] + \bar{\mathbf{G}}^{*}_{rq} \left\{ \bar{y}^{*}_{rq} - \bar{\mathbf{x}}^{*T}_{rq} \beta \right\} \right). \quad (5.31)$$

Here, $\bar{\mathbf{G}}_{rq}^*$ denotes a suitable weight for the additional term on the right-hand side of (5.31). Kim and Chambers (2013) suggest that we put

$$\bar{\mathbf{G}}_{rq}^* = M_{rq} \bar{\mathbf{x}}_{rq}^{*T} \left(\bar{V} \left(\mathbf{y}_{slq}^* \big| \mathbf{X}_{slq}^* \right) \right)^{-1}$$

where $\bar{V} \left(\mathbf{y}_{slq}^* \big| \mathbf{X}_{slq}^* \right)$ is the mean of the diagonal elements of $\text{var}\left(\mathbf{y}_{slq}^* \big| \mathbf{X}_{slq}^* \right)$. These authors also develop expressions for the asymptotic variance of the solution to this calibrated estimating function, both for the case where the parameters of the linkage error distribution are known and also when they are estimated from an independent audit sample. Finally, we note that simulation results presented in this reference indicate that the main gain in using the calibrated estimating function (5.31) compared with ignoring this calibration information is when linked sample sizes in the m-blocks are small.

5.7 Conclusion and discussion

In this chapter, we focus on methods for bias correction of linked data analysis that are feasible for a secondary analyst, that is, one without access to the complete record of the matching process. Such an analyst must perforce make assumptions about the distribution of linkage errors in the linked dataset. Here, we advocate use of the ELE model for this distribution, since this seems to be a very simple way of characterising linkage errors, in the sense that it only requires specification of the correct linkage rate within homogeneous groups of linked records. Other more complex models may be appropriate in more complex linking exercises, and further work is necessary for these situations.

Given the ELE model holds, the theory outlined in Chambers (2009) and Kim and Chambers (2012a; 2012b; 2013) seems promising. In particular, the simulation results reported in these papers indicate effective bias correction as well as good efficiency in a wide variety of linked data scenarios, including sample to register linkage and correlated multi-linked data. The use of an estimating equation approach also means that these methods can be applied widely. In this context, we note that a recent extension of the ELE model to variance components estimation using linked two level data is reported in Samart and Chambers (2014). The capacity to easily integrate auxiliary information about the datasets being linked represents another advantage of the estimating equation approach, and some preliminary results on the advantages of having access to this auxiliary data are presented in Kim and Chambers (2013).

Two issues remain however. The first is that all the methods that have been developed so far for the analysis of probability-linked data have at their core the assumption that the linking is non-informative. That is, the error distribution for the population model of interest and the linkage error distribution are independent within m-blocks. It is not difficult to construct scenarios where this is not the case. Development of appropriate bias correction methods for such cases remains an open question.

The second issue is potentially more serious and concerns bias due to non-linkage, that is, where it is impossible to find suitable matches for records in the different registers being linked. Non-linkage is a very common problem, and in the development set out in Sections 5.4 and 5.5, it is assumed that non-linkage is at random within m-blocks. This is a strong assumption, and extending the theory developed in these subsections to include more plausible non-linkage mechanisms is necessary. In this context, we observe that non-linkage is very similar to non-response, and so strategies that are effective for dealing with non-response may prove useful here as well. In particular, a strategy that weights the linked sample data by the inverse of the estimated joint probability of being sampled and then being linked (based on an appropriate model for this joint probability) is essentially equivalent to a propensity-weighting strategy for dealing with survey non-response. This strategy is well worth exploring in future research in this area.

6

Record linkage: A missing data problem

Harvey Goldstein[1,2] and Katie Harron[3]

[1] Institute of Child Health, University College London, London, UK
[2] Graduate School of Education, University of Bristol, Bristol, UK
[3] London School of Hygiene and Tropical Medicine, London, UK

6.1 Introduction

The focus of this chapter is on record linkage as a tool for providing information on variables required for a statistical analysis. It is assumed that the data analyst has a primary data file, for example, derived from a survey, clinical trial, registry or administrative database. There are certain variables of interest (VOIs) that are required for purposes of statistical modelling, but that are not recorded in the primary file. These VOIs reside instead in one or more secondary or linking files to which the analyst has access. It is assumed that the information in the linking files corresponds to the same individuals, or a well-defined subset, of those in the primary file. The aim is to transfer the values of the VOI from the individuals in the linking file to the corresponding individuals in the primary file and that this will be carried out by 'linking' each primary file individual record to the 'correct' VOI value in the linking file.

This record linkage process is viewed as a means to an end, namely, to carry out the appropriate statistical analysis. Thus, for example, the process of linkage can sustain ambiguity about whether a primary file record actually links to the 'correct' linking file record, for example, by retaining the possibility of several links, so long as appropriate information about the associated variable values can be transmitted. This perspective departs from the traditional record linkage one where the emphasis is upon identifying the correct linking record and forming static links between files. Where this cannot be ascertained unambiguously, a choice of a single record is nevertheless made, and most of the theoretical apparatus supporting what is known as 'probabilistic record linkage' (PRL), as discussed elsewhere in

Methodological Developments in Data Linkage, First Edition. Edited by Katie Harron, Harvey Goldstein and Chris Dibben.
© 2016 John Wiley & Sons, Ltd. Published 2016 by John Wiley & Sons, Ltd.

this volume, is devoted to optimising such a choice. Naturally, in some cases, for example, where there are administrative concerns, the emphasis may lie largely with the correct linking rather than statistical analysis, in which case techniques such as PRL will still be appropriate.

In this context, we first set out the case for viewing record linkage as a missing data problem, developing our approach for the case where there is a single primary and a single linking file and then discussing extensions. We then provide an example based on linkage of electronic health records for the purposes of statistical analysis.

Figure 6.1 shows a simple data structure that explains the essence of our approach. The set A variables are those to be transferred from the linking file to the primary file. Prior to linkage, the values of the set A variables are set to 0, indicating a missing value. Some of the set B variables are also missing. For purposes of analysis, we would like to change all the 0s to Xs, that is, to fill in the missing values. With suitable assumptions, we can carry out a statistical analysis where the 0s become converted to Xs via a suitable 'missing data' algorithm such as multiple imputation (MI), the details of which we will elaborate later. For the set A variables, this is not possible since every record has all values missing. If, however, we were able straightforwardly to unequivocally link some (preferably most) of the records from the primary file with those in the linking file (e.g. using what are often referred to as deterministic linkage methods), we would then have a structure such as that in Figure 6.2. In this figure, Records 2 and 3 have been linked unequivocally, and values of the set A variables have been transferred to the primary file. Records 1 and 4 were unable to be linked unequivocally, and values for the set A variables in these records remain missing.

Record	Set A variables		Set B variables		
1	0	0	X	X	X
2	0	0	X	0	X
3	0	0	X	X	0
4	0	0	0	0	X

Figure 6.1 Primary data file with four records where the set B variables are recorded and the set A variables are located in a linking file. X represents a recorded variable value and 0 a missing value. Initially, all the set A variables are missing and also some set B variables are missing as shown.

Record	Set A variables		Set B variables		
1	0	0	X	X	X
2	X	X	X	0	X
3	0	X	X	X	0
4	0	0	0	0	X

Figure 6.2 Primary data file with four records where the primary record file set B variables are recorded and the set A variable values for records 2 and 3 have been correctly transferred, unequivocally, via deterministic linkage with a linking file. X represents a variable with known value and 0 a missing value.

We now see that this is simply another missing data structure, and we can apply our existing missing data algorithms to obtain consistent estimates for our statistical models. In fact, in many cases, as we will show, such an analysis will be adequate, without invoking any further linkage complexity. In the following sections, we shall briefly refer to existing PRL methods, show how these can be elaborated to improve performance using prior-informed imputation (PII) and discuss further extensions.

6.2 Probabilistic Record Linkage (PRL)

The essence of PRL (see Chapter 2) is as follows. Identifying or matching variables on the individuals in both the primary file and the linking file is used to 'link' the same individual recorded in both files. In some cases, hopefully the majority, the link is unequivocal and we can carry across the relevant variable values from the linking file to the primary file. In other cases, there is some uncertainty about the link, due to missing or incorrect data in the matching variables. In these cases, a set of weights are estimated, based on the number of matches and discriminatory power of the matching variables. We note at this point that even where there is a 'perfect match' with agreement on all matching variables, such as age, name, date of birth, etc., we may still encounter linkage problems. This might occur because the set of matching variables is insufficiently discriminatory so that several linking file records match a primary file record or because there may be errors in both files that produce incorrect but coincidentally identical values. The second possibility is likely to be very rare and is typically ignored. In the first case with traditional PRL methods, a choice will have to be made to select one of the chosen records to link, possibly at random. This implies that in some cases the wrong record will be chosen, so that the procedure itself is biased. As we show in the following text, however, this can often be avoided or mitigated using PII.

Fundamental to PRL is the ascertainment of match weights. For each primary file record that is not unequivocally linked (on all matching variables), there will be in general several associated linking file records, that is, those that agree on at least one of the matching variables. We refer to these as 'candidate' records. For each of these primary file records, there will be a given pattern g of matching variable agreement values. For example, for three binary matching variables, we may observe a pattern $g = \{1,0,1\}$ indicating {match, no match, match}.[1] We compute the probability of observing each pattern of matching variable values:

(a) Given that the candidate record is the correct match: $P(g|M)$

(b) Given that the candidate record is not the correct match: $P(g|NM)$

These probabilities are known as the m- and u-probabilities (conditional probabilities). The traditional PRL procedure then computes $R = P(g|M)/P(g|NM)$ and a weight $W = \log_2(R)$, so that for primary file record i and candidate record j, we obtain the weight w_{ij}. Initial estimates of $P(g|M)$ and $P(g|NM)$ can be obtained given a set of certain matches or can be based on other datasets. The probabilities can be updated as more matches and non-matches are

---

[1] We may also encounter missing matching variable values. In this case, the primary file record match status will always be equivocal. Linkage will take place using the remainder of matching variables (assuming missingness is at random). Alternatively, match weights can be derived for missing values (i.e. matching variables are no longer binary but can take three values – agree, disagree, missing).

allocated in an iterative procedure (Yancey, 2004). In practice, probabilities are determined separately for each matching variable and summed, essentially assuming that the probabilities associated with the matching variables are independent: estimating the joint probabilities is typically regarded as too complicated. If the dataset is large, it may be more efficient to divide the individuals into mutually exclusive blocks (e.g. age groups) and only consider matches within corresponding blocks. $P(g|M)$ and $P(g|NM)$ may be allowed to vary between the blocks (e.g. age group (Newcombe, 1995)).

The PRL methods propose a cut-off threshold for W, so that matches with W above this threshold are accepted as true matches. This threshold is typically chosen to minimise the percentage of 'false positives'. Where several candidates exceed the threshold, the record with the highest weight is chosen. If no candidate record reaches the threshold, then no link is made. Thus, at the end of the process, the linked file will have some records with missing variable values where links have not been made. We could then apply standard MI as described previously, although this appears to be very rare in applications (McGlincy, 2004).

Variations on this procedure occur when the linking is one to many or many to many. For example, we may wish to link a birth record to several admission episodes for an individual within a single hospital linking file. In such a case, we could proceed by first linking the episodes in the linking file (de-duplication) so that each individual is represented by a single (longitudinal) record and then linking these records to those in the primary file. We may also have a many-to-many case where, for example, multiple, unmatched educational events such as test scores for individuals are to be linked to a set of unmatched health records. Again, we might proceed by de-duplication of data within the educational and within the health files and then linking between files.

There are certain problems with PRL. The first is the assumption of independence for the probabilities associated with the individual matching variables. For example, observing an individual in any given ethnic group category may be associated with certain surname structures, and hence, the joint probability will not simply be the product of the separate probabilities for ethnicity and surname. We shall return to this issue later and propose a way of dealing with it. The second problem is that, typically, records that cannot be matched above a weight threshold are excluded from data analysis, reducing efficiency, although as suggested previously, this strictly is not necessary. The third problem occurs when the errors in one or more matching variables are associated with the values of the linking file variables to be transferred for analysis (see Chapter 4). Thus, Lariscy has shown that certain ethnic group surnames are more error prone than others, and this can lead to biased inferences for associated variables such as mortality rates (Lariscy, 2011).

6.3 Multiple Imputation (MI)

The use of MI for handling missing data in either response or predictor variables in statistical models is a common technique, and because it forms the basis for the PII method that we shall describe, we now outline how it operates. Further details can be found, for example, in Carpenter and Kenward (2012).

MI is used to replace missing values with a set of imputed values in the model of interest (MOI), for example, a regression model. For each missing value, the posterior distribution of the value is computed, conditionally on the other variables in the MOI and any auxiliary variables, and a random draw taken from this distribution. Auxiliary variables are those that are associated with the responses in the imputation model but do not appear in the MOI. It is assumed that each missing value is missing at random (MAR), that is, randomly missing given the remaining variables in the MOI and any auxiliary variables used. The standard application assumes that all the variables in the MOI have a joint normal distribution. In practice, this involves setting up a model where the responses are variables with any missing data and predictors include other variables in the MOI and any auxiliary variables with fully known values. Generally, however, we cannot assume multivariate normality, for example, where some variables are categorical. Goldstein et al. (2009) propose a procedure that we refer to by the authors' initials GCKL and which provides a means of dealing with this by transforming all variables to multivariate normality, carrying out the imputation and then transforming back to corresponding non-normal variable scales (Goldstein et al., 2009). A description of such a 'latent normal model' is given in Appendix A.

In practice, an MCMC algorithm is used to sample a value from the conditional posterior distribution, for each value missing, so that after every cycle of the algorithm, we effectively have a complete dataset consisting of a mixture of imputed and known data values. The algorithm is used to generate a number, n, of such complete datasets that are, as far as possible, independent by choosing MCMC cycles sufficiently far apart; in practice, a distance apart of 250–500 will often be satisfactory. The value of n should be large enough to ensure the accuracy of the final estimates, which are obtained by fitting the MOI to each completed dataset and averaging over these according to the so called 'Rubin's rules' (Rubin, 1987). A value of 5 is often used, although between 10 and 20, completed datasets has been found by GCKL to be needed for multilevel data.

Where the MOI is multilevel, the multilevel structure should also be used in the imputation model. More recently, Goldstein et al. extend this so that quite general models can be fitted within a single MCMC chain, rather than producing multiple datasets for analysis (Goldstein, Carpenter and Browne, 2014). In what follows, we shall assume standard MI, although this more recent procedure will generally be faster as well as allowing more general models to be fitted.

6.4 Prior-Informed Imputation (PII)

In PRL, the acceptance of a record as linked is determined by the weights W that depend on $P(g|M)$ and $P(g|NM)$. In PII, we work instead with the probability of a match given the matching variable pattern, $P(M|g)$. For primary file record i and a candidate record j, denote this by $\pi_{m,ij}(g)$. For primary file record i, by default, we scale these probabilities to add to 1.0, and these scaled values are denoted by $\pi_{ij}(g)$. This assumes that the 'true' matching record belongs to this set of candidate records. We discuss the case when this may not be true in the following text. In practice, to avoid very large files where many of the probabilities for candidate linking records are very small, a lower threshold can be chosen so that records with probabilities less than this are ignored.

For the set A variables to be transferred from the linking file (Figure 6.1), denote their distribution, conditional on the set B variables, by $f\left(Y^{A|B}\right)$. This conditioning is derived from the joint distribution of the responses and any covariates in the MOI, as well as any auxiliary variables already present in the primary file that may be used to satisfy the MAR assumption. Initial values are derived from the unequivocal records that are transferred, and the conditional distribution is updated at each cycle of the MCMC algorithm. This joint distribution is the latent normal distribution described previously, that is, with suitable transformations as necessary for non-normal variables. We now have a structure such as that in Figure 6.2, and we use an MCMC chain to impute the missing values. For each primary file record i with no unequivocal match, we carry out the following procedure at each iteration.

We compute a modified prior probability, that is, the likelihood component, $f\left(Y^{A|B}\right)$, multiplied by the prior $\pi_{ij}(g)$, for associated (equivocal) linking file record j, namely, $\pi_{ij} \propto f\left(y_{ij}^{A|B}\right)p_{ij}$. These are scaled to add to 1.0 and comprise the modified probability distribution (MPD) for each primary file record, denoted by π_{ij}.

We first note that we should not simply sample records at random according to the MPD since this will result in some incorrect choices of the true record in a similar way to standard probabilistic linkage. Instead, we propose that, as in standard PRL, a threshold is set for accepting a record as a true link. If no record exceeds the threshold, then the data values are regarded as missing and standard MI is used, meaning that, unlike PRL, all records are retained for analysis and no information is discarded. It is also possible that for any given record, we may find a record exceeding the threshold at some iterations, whereas at other iterations, standard MI is used. In general, we would choose only high thresholds to minimise bias. For example, if a value of 0.95 is chosen, this implies that the ratio of the highest to the next highest probability is at least $0.95/0.05 = 20$. Given a high enough threshold, the proposed procedure will produce approximately unbiased estimates. It has the advantage of efficiency over PRL in that all records in the primary file contribute to the estimation. Conditioning on the values of further variables when computing the $f\left(Y^{A|B}\right)$, including the matching variables as auxiliaries, can be expected to make the MAR assumption more reasonable. Incorporating the likelihood component in the MPD can be expected to lead more often to the correct record being the one to exceed a given threshold.

So far, we have assumed that the true matching record is located within the linking file. In some cases, however, this may not be the case. For example, if we wish to match a patient file to a death register in order to record survival status in the primary file, some equivocal records might either indicate that the patient is still alive or that they are dead but not equivocally matched. Assume we know, or have a good estimate, of the mortality rate among our patients, say, π_d. If a proportion of the primary file $\pi_m < \pi_d$ is unequivocally matched records, then the probability that a randomly chosen remaining record in the LDF is not a death from the FOI sample is $\pi_r = 1 - \left(\pi_d - \pi_m\right)$. We therefore multiply the $\pi_{ij}(g)$ by $1 - \pi_r$ and add an extra pseudo-record with probability π_r with an associated code for a surviving patient. If a good estimate of the mortality rate is not available, then a sensitivity analysis might be carried out for a range of plausible values. Alternatively, we assign the pseudo-record with probability $1 - \max\left(\pi_i(g)\right)$.

We have assumed that record linkage is between two files. In practice, however, there may be several files to be linked. Without loss of generality, we can assume that one of these is the main primary file with several linking files. One way to proceed is conditionally. Thus, for each iteration of the algorithm, we first carry out a PII for the primary file and the first linking file, say, linking file$_1$. Then, conditioning on the original set A variables and those carried over from linking file$_1$, we carry out a PII for the augmented primary file and linking file$_2$ and so on. We assume that matching errors across linkages are independent. Alternatively, we can think of forming the joint prior distribution and hence a joint MPD over the complete set of linking files, but this may become impractical when the number of linking files is moderately large.

In some cases, we may have sets of matching variables that are common only to a subset of linking files. Thus, we may wish to match patient records within the same hospital on different occasions, using a local hospital identifier, but which is not available for the main primary file. In this case, we would first carry out a PII choosing one of the hospital linking files as the primary file and then carry out a PII where the combined records are matched to the main file of interest. If there are matching variables common to all three files, then the linkage of the linked hospital records to the primary file will need to consider the matching probabilities associated with the three possible combinations of values across files for each matching variable.

6.4.1   Estimating matching probabilities

In general, the prior probabilities $\pi_{ij}(g)$ are unknown. Given the overall probabilities of a true match occurring and a given observed pattern, these are proportional to the (inverse) probabilities $P(g|M)$ described previously. Thus, we could use these, as derived from a PRL analysis, suitably scaled. Goldstein et al. suggested that the weights w_{ij} could be scaled to add to 1.0 (Goldstein, Harron and Wade, 2012). This uses information about the probability of a non-match and is equivalent to working with the scaled $logit(\pi_{ij}(g))$ values, although in practice this may not make very much difference.

One of the difficulties with the use of PRL estimates is that they will be based upon the assumption of independence. An alternative approach, that avoids this, is to attempt to estimate the joint prior probabilities directly. This would involve empirical evidence about ways in which linking variable errors occur, for example, based upon experimental situations. If a gold-standard dataset is available where the correct matching status is known, then the results of a trial involving coding and recording of records in the files would provide such data. We are currently pursuing research into this.

6.5   Example 1: Linking electronic healthcare data to estimate trends in bloodstream infection

To demonstrate the use of PII and to highlight the importance of accounting for linkage uncertainty within analysis, we provide an example based on linkage between infection surveillance data and national audit data on admissions to paediatric intensive care (Harron et al., 2013). Results from PRL and PII are compared.

6.5.1   Methods

6.5.1.1   Data

Admission data for children admitted paediatric intensive care units from March 2003 are available within the Paediatric Intensive Care Audit Network database (PICANet) (Universities of Leeds and Leicester, 2013). The aim was to link these data to national infection surveillance data collected from hospital laboratories across England and Wales, coordinated by Public Health England. However, identifiers in the national laboratory system are of poor quality, and it was first necessary to evaluate the most appropriate linkage methods. We therefore started with a gold-standard dataset based on validated microbiology data containing well-completed identifiers from two different hospital laboratories for the period between March 2003 and December 2010.

To create the gold-standard linked dataset, we performed deterministic linkage of PICANet data and laboratory records based on unique identifiers: National Health Service (NHS) number, hospital number, name, date of birth and sex. The deterministic linkage was manually verified to ensure there were no false matches or missed matches, and additional data from the hospital IT systems (e.g. examination of previous names) were used to clarify any uncertainties. This process provided a gold-standard dataset in which the true match status of each record pair was known, which could be used to compare other linkage methods.

Matching variables that would be available for linkage of the national infection surveillance data are mostly restricted to date of birth, sex, and Soundex code (an anonymised phonetic code use for reporting surname to the surveillance system) (Mortimer and Salathiel, 1995). To evaluate PRL and PII for linkage of such data, unique identifiers were removed from the microbiology data. Linkage using PRL and PII was then repeated using date of birth, sex and soundex only.

6.5.1.2   VOIs

The purpose of the linkage was to transfer information on whether an admission was associated with an infection. The VOI was therefore a binary variable representing infection. The VOI took a value of 1 for records in the primary file matching a record in the linking file and 0 otherwise.

Outcome measures were the rate of infection per 1000 bed-days and the incidence rate ratio of infection in the first hospital compared with in the second hospital (based on a Poisson regression model including individual-level predictors of infection). Since the match status of each record pair was known in the gold-standard data, match probabilities and match weights were estimated directly from the data.

6.5.1.3   Linkage

For PRL, thresholds for classifying record pairs as links or non-links are typically chosen by manual inspection of record pairs ordered by match weight and examination of the distribution of weights. This manual review is not feasible for national data, firstly due to the large numbers of records, and secondly due to the scarcity of identifying information on records. Alternatively, a single threshold that minimises the effect of error can be chosen, based on known error rates. As error rates are usually unknown, it might be possible to obtain estimates from a subset of gold-standard data where the true match status is known. In this example, a random 10% subset of data where the true match status was known was used to select a threshold that minimised the sum of linkage errors (false matches + missed matches). An alternative would be to choose the threshold that minimised the net error (|false matches − missed matches|).

For PII, records with a match probability greater than 0.9 were classified as unequivocal. For these records, a VOI value of 1 was accepted. For the remaining records, the MPD was derived from the likelihood in the unequivocally linked records and the prior distribution of match probabilities in the candidate linking records. The MPD threshold was also set to 0.9, so that VOI values would be accepted if they exceeded this probability and standard MI would be performed if no value exceeded this threshold.

6.5.2   Results

In the gold-standard data, 1496 (7.1%) of the 20924 admission records extracted from PICANet linked to at least one laboratory record of infection. Based on results from data linked using date of birth, sex and Soundex only, the number of infections was estimated as 1316 (6.3%) using PRL and 1457 (7.0%) using PII.

The rate of infection was 12.88 (95% CI 12.23–13.53) per 1000 bed-days in the gold-standard data, 11.33 (95% CI 10.72–11.95) using PRL and 12.75 (95% CI 11.61–12.89) using PII.

The incidence rate ratio for infection at the first hospital compared with the second hospital was 1.31 (95% CI 1.18–1.46) in the gold-standard data, 1.25 (95% CI 1.12–1.41) using PRL and 1.27 (95% CI 1.14–1.43) using PII.

Figure 6.3 compares the rate of infection estimated using PRL and PII.

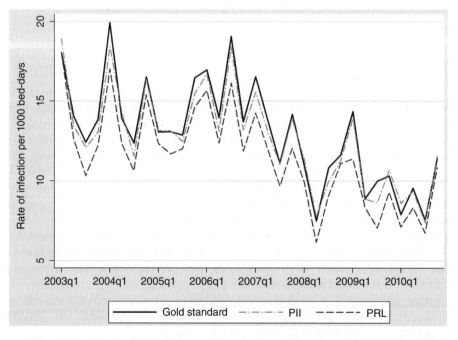

Figure 6.3   Comparison of prior-informed imputation (PII) and probabilistic record linkage (PRL) with gold-standard data: rates of infection by quarter of calendar year.

6.5.3 Conclusions

Even in data with well-completed identifiers, bias was introduced to results due to linkage error. For all outcome measures evaluated, PII provided less biased results than PRL.

6.6 Example 2: Simulated data including non-random linkage error

Example 1 demonstrates that PII can reduce some of the bias resulting from linkage errors using the traditional PRL approach. However, the impact of linkage error can vary according to the expected match rate (the number of primary file records expected to have a match to the linking file). This is because for a given rate of linkage error (false-match rate or missed-match rate), the absolute number of false matches or missed matches is directly related to the number of true matches and non-matches.

The impact of linkage error also depends on the distribution of error. Linkage error can have a large impact on results when the probability of linkage is associated with particular variables or subgroups of data (see Chapter 4). For example, relative outcome measures can be affected by differences in data quality between subgroups (e.g. by hospital or by ethnic group); outcome measures may be underestimated if the outcome is difficult to capture in linked data (e.g. under-representation of vulnerable groups due to missing identifiers (Ford, Roberts and Taylor, 2006; Lariscy, 2011)).

Example 2 demonstrates the performance of PII in different linkage situations (varying identifier error rates and distribution of error) through the use of simulated data.

6.6.1 Methods

6.6.1.1 Simulated data

The primary file was generated by randomly sampling 10 000 values for Soundex, day of birth, month of birth, year of birth and sex from an extract of 112 890 PICANet records. Values for seven predictor variables were randomly sampled from values of variables in the PICANet file. Predictor values were sampled jointly to preserve the association between variables. Identifier values were then brought together with predictor values to create 10 000 complete simulated records in the primary file (Figure 6.4).

The linking file was created by selecting a number of records from the primary file to represent admissions that had experienced an infection. Associations between the predictor variables and the VOI (infection) were induced by selecting records according to the values of their predictor variables. Additional identifier and predictor values were sampled from PICANet and used to create 'non-match' records which were added to the linking file so that, in total, the linking file contained 10 000 records, some of which had a match in the primary file and some of which did not (Figure 6.4).

To represent data quality found in administrative data, identifier errors and missing values were randomly introduced into each identifier in the linking file at a rate of 5%. The process was repeated to produce a set of 25 simulated linking files.

To explore the performance of PII with different match rates, the proportion of true matches was set to 10, 50 or 70% by selecting the corresponding number of records from the primary file to create each linking file.

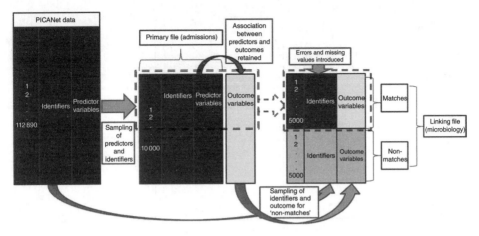

Figure 6.4   Generation of simulated linking files (for 50% match rate example).

To explore the performance of PII for handling non-randomly distributed error, the way in which error was introduced into simulated datasets was varied. Firstly, non-random error was introduced into the simulated datasets according to unit: data from Unit 1 were set to be five times more likely to include error than data from Unit 2. Secondly, error was introduced according to the outcome: linking file records for children with an infection were set to be five times more likely to have error than records for children with no infection.

6.6.1.2 VOIs

The outcome of interest was the rate of infection, and a secondary outcome was the absolute difference in adjusted rates between hospitals. The VOI was therefore the presence of infection, represented as a binary variable. Statistical analysis was performed as described in Example 1.

6.6.2 Results

Overall, most bias was introduced into results when linkage error was distributed non-randomly, that is, associated with either the hospital or with having the outcome (infection). Estimates of the rate of infection were most biased when error was associated with the outcome of infection and PRL provided particularly biased results in this situation (Figures 6.5, 6.6 and 6.7).

The amount of bias introduced also differed according to the underlying match rate. Using PII rather than PRL had the most dramatic benefit for high match rates.

Estimates of the difference in adjusted rates were not substantially affected by linkage error when the error was distributed randomly (Figure 6.8), as error was introduced to each hospital equally and the relative outcome was not affected. However, estimates of the difference in rates were substantially biased by non-random error associated with the hospital, as errors in the data from one hospital led to apparent lower rates and therefore falsely inflated the difference between units (Figure 6.8).

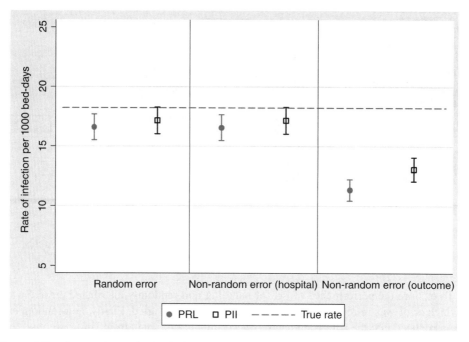

Figure 6.5   Comparison of prior-informed imputation (PII) and probabilistic record linkage (PRL) with simulated data and 10% match rate: rates of infection.

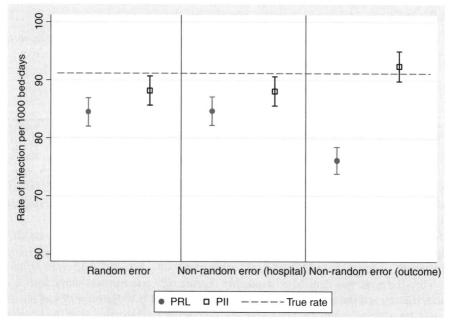

Figure 6.6   Comparison of prior-informed imputation (PII) and probabilistic record linkage (PRL) with simulated data and 50% match rate: rates of infection.

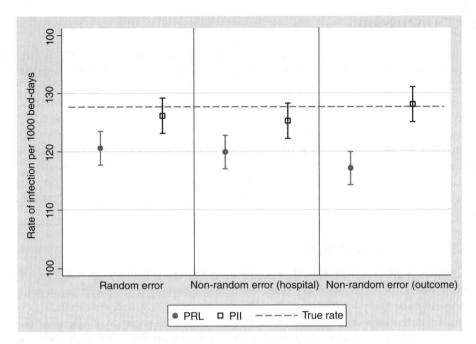

Figure 6.7   Comparison of prior-informed imputation (PII) and probabilistic record linkage (PRL) with simulated data and 70% match rate: rates of infection.

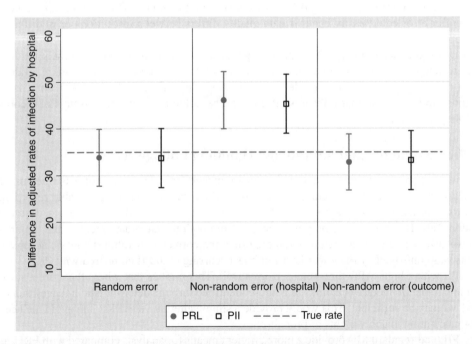

Figure 6.8   Comparison of prior-informed imputation (PII) and probabilistic record linkage (PRL) with simulated data and 70% match rate: difference in adjusted rates of infection by hospital.

6.7   Discussion

Existing methods that aim to adjust for linkage bias are generally limited to the context of regression analysis and rely on a number of assumptions (Chambers et al., 2009; Hof and Zwinderman, 2012; Kim and Chambers, 2011; Scheuren and Winkler, 1997). This chapter describes how viewing record linkage as a missing data problem could help to handle linkage error and uncertainty within analysis. The motivation for using imputation methods for linkage is that the ultimate purpose of linkage is not to combine *records* but to combine information from records belonging to the same individual. Measuring the quality of linkage then shifts from quantifying match rate and linkage error to obtaining correct estimates for the outcomes of interest.

Linkage of simulated datasets with different characteristics (i.e. with non-random error or with different match rates) illustrates that linkage error affects different types of linkage and analysis in complex ways.

6.7.1   Non-random linkage error

Simulations highlighted that when data quality differs by unit (identifier errors more likely to occur in one hospital than another), relative outcome measures (e.g. differences in adjusted rates) were more likely to be affected than absolute measures (e.g. incidence rate). This finding has important implications for analysis of linked data in the presence of linkage error. For example, if linkage error is constant over time, estimated trends should be unaffected, even if absolute rates are over- or underestimated. However, if the aim is to compare groups and linkage error is not constant between these groups, relative outcome measures are likely to be biased, either over-exaggerating differences or biasing to the null. This type of non-random identifier error could easily occur if data quality differs between institutions or in different groups of records (see Chapter 4).

Detailed understanding of the underlying quality of data to be linked could help to identify which populations are most vulnerable to bias due to linkage error. Furthermore, evaluation of linkage quality, for example, through comparing linked and unlinked record, is of utmost importance so that linkage strategies can be tailored for different groups of records (Bohensky et al., 2010).

6.7.2   Strengths and limitations: Handling linkage error

PII was not able to completely avoid bias due to linkage error. The causes of bias when using PII are the same as those occurring when using PRL, that is, matching variable recording errors, missing values or agreement of identifiers between records belonging to different individuals. However, combining information from both the candidate records and the unequivocally linked records means that more often, the correct VOI value should be accepted. This was confirmed by the lower levels of bias occurring with PII compared with PRL.

PII with a high MPD threshold performs well. This implies that where there are a sufficient number of unequivocal links (e.g. those identified through deterministic linkage), standard MI may be sufficient. This would provide a simple alternative to PRL and avoid the need for calculating match weights or probabilities.

PII (and standard MI) provide a more efficient means for analysis compared with PRL, as all records are retained for analysis. A further advantage of PII over PRL is related to standard errors. For probabilistic linkage, standard errors are calculated assuming that there is no error and are therefore falsely small (see Chapter 5). For PII, the process of combining several imputed datasets means that uncertainty occurring during linkage is properly reflected, resulting in slightly larger standard errors compared with probabilistic linkage.

PII also provides advantages over existing methods for linkage bias adjustment. Previously described methods have been limited to simulation studies and have not been adopted in practice, possibly due to their complex nature and a lack of practical guidance for users. Conversely, PII has been evaluated both in simulated data and for the linkage of two large national administrative data sources, and this linkage has been described in practical terms in several papers. Furthermore, PII can be implemented using REALCOM code implemented through the Stat-JR software developed by the University of Bristol (Charlton et al., 2012).

6.7.3   Implications for data linkers and data users

In order for research based on linked data to be transparent, data linkers (including trusted third parties) need to be willing to provide details of the linkage processes used to create linked datasets. Data users need to know what to ask for, in terms of information required to evaluate the quality of linkage. This means that linked data provided should not be restricted to only the highest-weighted link but that information from other candidate links should also be made available to facilitate sensitivity analyses and PII. Furthermore, characteristics of unlinked data should also be provided to allow comparisons with linked data and identification of potential sources of bias.

As the size of datasets to be linked increases, manual review will become infeasible, even where sufficient identifying information is available. In these cases, alternative linkage methods will become even more important. The practicalities of storing multiple candidate links and associated match weights or match probabilities to facilitate sensitivity analyses need to be further explored. Graph databases (as opposed to traditional relational databases) could provide a technical solution to this problem by storing records and links in the form of edges and nodes. This area will be explored in Chapter 7.

Acknowledgements

The authors would like to thank Ruth Gilbert and Angie Wade for all their input to this work. We would also like to thank Berit Muller-Pebody (Public Health England) and Roger Parslow and the PICANet team. We would like to thank all the staff in participating hospitals who have collected data for PICANet or responded to survey questionnaires. We are grateful to the UK Paediatric Intensive Care Society for continued support and to the members of the PICANet Steering Group and Clinical Advisory Group who are listed on the PICANet website http://www.picanet.org.uk/About/.

Appendix A

The latent normal model

For multivariate data with mixtures of response variable types, GCKL show how such a response distribution can be represented in terms of an underlying 'latent' multivariate normal distribution (Goldstein et al., 2009). For ordered categorical variables and for continuously distributed variables, each such variable corresponds to one normal variable on the latent scale. For an unordered categorical variable where just one category is observed to occur, with p categories, we have $p-1$ normal variables on the latent scale. They also show how this can be extended to the multilevel case. An MCMC algorithm is used which samples values from the latent normal distribution.

This representation can be used to fit a wide variety of multivariate generalised linear models with mixed response types, and, after sampling the latent normal variables, reduces to fitting a multivariate normal linear model. The following summary steps are those used to sample values from this underlying latent normal distribution given the original variable values. At each cycle of the MCMC algorithm, a new set of values is selected. Each such sampling step conditions on the other, current, latent normal values.

Normal response

If the original response is normal, this value is retained.

Ordered categorical data

If we have p ordered categories, we have an associated set of $p-1$ cut points, or threshold, parameters on the latent normal scale such that if category k is observed, a sample value is drawn from the standard normal distribution interval defined by

$$(-\infty, 1) \text{ if } k = 1,$$

$$(p-1, \infty) \text{ if } k = p,$$

$$(k-1, k) \text{ otherwise}$$

The threshold parameters are estimated in a further step. In the binary case, this corresponds to a standard probit model.

Unordered categorical data

If we have p unordered categories, then we sample from a standard $p-1$ multivariate normal with zero covariances, as follows. The final category is typically chosen as the reference category. A random draw is taken from the multivariate normal, and if the category corresponding to the maximum value in this draw is also the one which is observed, then the values in that draw are accepted. If all the values in the draw are negative and the last category is the one observed, then the draw is accepted. Otherwise, a new draw is made.

The procedure can be extended, with certain limitations, to discrete distributions, such as the Poisson (Goldstein and Kounali, 2009), and to non-normal continuous distributions for which a normalising transformation exists, such as the Box–Cox family (Goldstein et al., 2009).

After all of these sampling steps have been completed, we obtain a multivariate normal distribution. Where there are missing data values, we can therefore use standard imputation procedures to impute the missing values, on the normal scales, and use the inverse set of transformations to those given previously, in order to provide a randomly imputed value on the original scales.

7

Using graph databases to manage linked data

James M. Farrow
SANT Datalink, Adelaide, South Australia, Australia
Farrow Norris, Sydney, New South Wales, Australia

7.1 Summary

Linked data has traditionally been managed using relational databases and methodologies that for historical reasons have been optimised to minimise the use of memory and persistent storage. This approach discourages exploration of the relationship between linked records because such information is either not retained or, depending on how it is stored, is difficult to exploit.

Linked data naturally form a *graph* or *network*: a collection of *nodes* (the records) connected by *edges* (their relationships). When data about record associations are stored in a traditional *relational* form,[1] that is, in a conventional *relational database*, without regard to the graph nature of the data, it makes the tasks of data management and analysis more difficult.

By storing *record data and the relationships between the records* explicitly in a *graph database* – a technology specifically designed to store 'natural' graph structures and query such information – many shortcomings of the relational approach can be avoided, and new approaches to managing and exploiting linked data are enabled.

Here are compared a relational and a graph-based approach and an overview given of how linked record data can be managed using a graph database based on the experience gleaned in building such a system at SANT DataLink in South Australia: the Next Generation Linkage Management System (NGLMS).

---

[1] It is unfortunate that the term *relational* is the one conventionally used to describe a database format that is less suited to capturing relationships.

Methodological Developments in Data Linkage, First Edition. Edited by Katie Harron, Harvey Goldstein and Chris Dibben.
© 2016 John Wiley & Sons, Ltd. Published 2016 by John Wiley & Sons, Ltd.

7.2   Introduction

In Australia, data linkage is often performed without the benefit of universal identifiers (ID), which can be used to deterministically link datasets. Data comes from different sources, and there is a strong overriding privacy constraint that has led to a practice of separating the (demographic) data attributes used for linkage from the other data used for research. The data custodians supply the demographic portion of the data along with a record ID to *data linkage units* such as SANT DataLink in South Australia. These units determine sets of related records, which are deemed to (probably) relate to the same person and return the related ID to the custodian who then provides only the linked non-demographic data to researchers.

SANT DataLink was set up in 2009 as a consortium. The Australian government has provided financial support through the National Collaborative Research Infrastructure Strategy (NCRIS) and the Population Health Research Network (PHRN).

In 2010, the idea of storing all relationship information as a graph rather than just the outcome of the record clustering process was floated by Dr Tim Churches among record linkage researchers in Australia with some proof-of-concept Python code. Churches noted that 'this approach although infeasible in the 1980s was achievable with modern hardware and computing techniques'.

In 2011, as part of the PHRN Technical Forum, the design of a new linked data management system for South Australia was presented to the assembled nodes of the PHRN from the other states (Farrow and Churches, 2011). The new system was based around a graph approach, storing rich relationship data between records to allow dynamic determination of *clusters* of related records as an improvement upon the existing approach of grouping related records together and assigning them a static cluster ID.

In 2012, the approach was presented in detail to a workshop at the 2012 International Data Linkage Conference and at the conference itself (Farrow, 2012a; 2012c). An informal survey of the assembled representatives of various data linkage units from various national and international jurisdictions revealed that data was still being stored in relational databases, but, tantalisingly, PopData BC was (relationally) storing 'outcome strings': a summary of decisions made during pairwise record comparison (Hills, 2014). A full system architecture and working software using Neo4j for the graph database, PostgreSQL, Java, Python, Groovy and Gremlin was presented at the 2012 PHRN Technical Forum (Farrow, 2012b).

Since its inception, the NGLMS was designed to:

- Separate the data comparison and cluster detection phases of data linkage

- Allow a flexible mix-and-match approach to data linkage by customising which datasets and which comparisons are used for a particular research project

- Allow more flexibility with regard to data privacy and usage restrictions by providing this customisable approach

- Allow a full history of all decisions made regarding record linkage to be retained and to exploit this history by allowing 'historical' extractions to be made, for example, the extraction as it would have appeared if done on a certain date in the past

- Minimise the computational overhead of record and record set delete and update by localising the computation needed, that is, all data does not need to be relinked

- Allow data to be deleted or updated and both the full history of those deletions to be retained and the effects of the deleted/deprecated data to be completely ignored prospectively

- Allow progressively better linkage quality to be achieved over time via incremental data improvements

- Allow custom and possibly multiple extractions of record clusters using different clustering parameters, enabling researches to undertake sensitivity analyses around the linkage process

The NGLMS was designed to meet theses technical challenges, some of which were subsequently listed in Boyd et al. (2014) as desirable features of a modern data linkage system.

A traditional approach to managing data linkage has been to manage record data using relational databases. Typically, the calculation of record similarities and the finding of clusters of related records are conflated into a single compare-and-find-clusters phase possibly followed by a manual or automated 'clerical review' phase to tidy up borderline cluster elements and improve linkage quality (Kendrick and Clarke, 1993). In the absence of reliable 'person ID' identifying individuals, large amounts of computation may have to be performed comparing records to determine clusters of related records. This information is immediately used to determine clusters and then either discarded or stored in a form that does not readily lend itself to further computation.

Although designed to meet the needs of South Australian data linkage, the NGLMS is flexible enough to handle:

- Deterministically and probabilistically linked data

- One-to-one, one-to-many and many-to-many data linkages

- Various topologies of data configuration, for example, full graph or a data population 'spine'

7.2.1   Flat approach

The following section discusses linkage of data where a unique 'person ID' on which to link is not available. This linkage process is well established and so will not be covered in depth (Acheson, 1967; Fellegi and Sunter, 1969; Winkler, 1994).

Consider the sample data in Table 7.1. Linking these records involves comparisons on name, gender, date of birth and other demographic information not shown here such as address, possible aliases, nicknames and middle names (all modified using a generous dose of heuristics to cope with misspellings, bad data entry, incomplete data and so on). Table 7.2 shows the result of taking the data shown above, comparing pairwise fields and summing the weight of the matches for each column into one value for the entire record.

Further review of these weights would set an upper bound on the match value above which the results of the computation are taken as a definite match and a lower bound below which the records are taken as not matching.

This would leave a number of 'uncertain' record pairings in the middle that would need to be classified as matches or non-matches. This might be done automatically with further computation, or it might be done manually with human review of the records involved to determine pairings.

Finally, records would be assigned a cluster ID to indicate a group of related records. This would be written back to each record to create a *master linkage list* or *master linkage file* shown in Table 7.3 and the comparison information discarded or archived for audit purposes.

7.2.2   Oops, your legacy is showing

The core of this approach is based on techniques developed in the 1970s and 1980s and makes various assumptions about the computing environment that are no longer true. A few things have changed in the last 30–40 years when it comes to computing:

- Computer power is no longer as expensive as it once was.

- Memory is no longer scarce and expensive.

- Persistent storage space is no longer scarce and expensive.

In particular, optimising for a case that assumes persistent storage *is* scarce and expensive leads to the approach mentioned previously: cluster ID are assigned, and the vast bulk of the computation – *the expensive part to repeat* – is discarded.

7.2.3   Shortcomings

There are numerous shortcomings to this approach.

Single cluster ID

Each record is *definitively assigned a cluster ID*. This can lead to the perception of the master linkage list as the 'truth', whereas the information captured in the table represents an amalgamation of assumptions at all stages of processing: heuristic matching algorithms, weight

Table 7.1   Sample data for comparison.

Record	Surname	First name	Sex	Date of birth
1	Farnell	Michael	M	3/6/84
2	Farnell	Mike	M	3/6/84
3	Farnelli	Michael	M	3/6/84
4	Farnelli	Mike	M	3/6/84
5	Farnelli	Michael	M	1/6/84
6	Farnelli	M	M	1/1/84
7	Farnell	Mitchell	M	6/3/84
8	Farnell	M	M	6/3/84
9	Farnell	M	M	1/1/84
10	Farnell	Michelle	F	3/6/84
11	Farnell	Matthew	M	3/6/84
12	Farnell	Mikayla	F	3/6/84

Table 7.2 Pairwise comparison of sample data.

Score	Left ID	Right ID	Left surname	Right surname	Left first name	Right first name	Left sex	Right sex	Left DOB	Right DOB	
25.9	3	4	Farnelli	Farnelli	Michael	Mike	M	M	3/6/84	3/6/84	High confidence
25.9	1	2	Farnell	Farnell	Michael	Mike	M	M	3/6/84	3/6/84	
22.5	1	3	Farnell	Farnelli	Michael	Michael	M	M	3/6/84	3/6/84	
22.5	6	9	Farnelli	Farnell	M	M	M	M	1/1/84	1/1/84	
22.5	2	4	Farnell	Farnelli	Mike	Mike	M	M	3/6/84	3/6/84	
22.0	1	4	Farnell	Farnelli	Michael	Mike	M	M	3/6/84	3/6/84	
22.0	2	3	Farnell	Farnelli	Mike	Michael	M	M	3/6/84	3/6/84	
21.6	7	8	Farnell	Farnell	Mitchell	M	M	M	6/3/84	6/3/84	
19.4	3	5	Farnelli	Farnelli	Michael	Michael	M	M	3/6/84	1/6/84	
18.9	4	5	Farnelli	Farnelli	Mike	Michael	M	M	3/6/84	1/6/84	Uncertain
18.4	1	11	Farnell	Farnell	Michael	Matthew	M	M	3/6/84	3/6/84	
18.4	2	11	Farnell	Farnell	Mike	Matthew	M	M	3/6/84	3/6/84	
17.6	1	8	Farnell	Farnell	Michael	M	M	M	3/6/84	6/3/84	
17.6	8	11	Farnell	Farnell	M	Matthew	M	M	6/3/84	3/6/84	
17.6	2	8	Farnell	Farnell	Mike	M	M	M	3/6/84	6/3/84	
17.4	10	12	Farnell	Farnell	Michelle	Mikayla	F	F	3/6/84	3/6/84	
16.6	5	6	Farnelli	Farnelli	Michael	M	M	M	1/6/84	1/1/84	
15.5	1	5	Farnell	Farnelli	Michael	Michael	M	M	3/6/84	1/6/84	
15.4	1	10	Farnell	Farnell	Michael	Michelle	M	F	3/6/84	3/6/84	Low confidence
15.0	2	5	Farnell	Farnelli	Mike	Michael	M	M	3/6/84	1/6/84	
14.9	8	9	Farnell	Farnell	M	M	M	M	6/3/84	1/1/84	
14.4	2	7	Farnell	Farnell	Mike	Mitchell	M	M	3/6/84	6/3/84	
14.4	7	11	Farnell	Farnell	Mitchell	Matthew	M	M	6/3/84	3/6/84	
14.4	1	7	Farnell	Farnell	Michael	Mitchell	M	M	3/6/84	6/3/84	
13.7	3	8	Farnelli	Farnell	Michael	M	M	M	3/6/84	6/3/84	
13.7	4	8	Farnelli	Farnell	Mike	M	M	M	3/6/84	6/3/84	
12.7	5	9	Farnelli	Farnell	Michael	M	M	M	1/6/84	1/1/84	

Table 7.3   'Master linkage table' of sample data.

Record	Surname	First name	Sex	Date of birth	Cluster ID
1	Farnell	Michael	M	3/6/84	1
2	Farnell	Mike	M	3/6/84	1
3	Farnelli	Michael	M	3/6/84	1
4	Farnelli	Mike	M	3/6/84	1
5	Farnelli	Michael	M	1/6/84	1
6	Farnelli	M	M	1/1/84	1
7	Farnell	Mitchell	M	6/3/84	1
8	Farnell	M	M	6/3/84	1
9	Farnell	M	M	1/1/84	1
10	Farnell	Michelle	F	3/6/84	2
11	Farnell	Matthew	M	3/6/84	3
12	Farnell	Mikayla	F	3/6/84	4

assignments, user input and indeed user error. Even the name carries with it this connotation of authority.

There is no easy way to extract from the list different views of the same data. Should a researcher desire matches with higher specificity or higher recall, *all the record comparison computations must be performed again.* Consequently, in the case where manual clerical review is part of the usual workflow, it is likely that manual clerical review would need to be performed again. In addition, *assigning ID to this list is destructive:* information is overwritten and only one value may be maintained at a time. If different views of the world are desired, they must either be created as a one-off, or multiple versions of the 'master' list must be maintained. This approach does not scale well when multiple projects have different clustering requirements.

One size doesn't fit all
Because cluster information is 'baked in' very early in the process, any quality processes attached to record linkage must be done as thoroughly as possible and effectively once for all time when new data is added: it is hard to disentangle groups and work backwards from clusters to individual record comparisons.

Should a researcher desire an interim for preliminary probabilistic linkage to examine the feasibility of a proposed study, datasets and linkage results must nevertheless be thoroughly reviewed lest a poor linkage affect other clusterings in the future or to cover the case where a future researcher might need high-quality linked data. Either this low-quality linkage must be done as a one-off, or the researcher must wait until all quality processes are complete as the master linkage list can become a single point of resource contention between projects.

Please hold, your project is valuable to us…
It may take some time to complete the final review and clustering of a project as the master list approach can obstruct parallelisation of multiple linkages. Linkage projects can queue up awaiting completion as each in turn waits for a time when the master linkage list is free to have

an individual project's new data folded into it. The time window in which the master linkage list may be updated becomes a resource for which all projects must compete for access.

Where linkage is performed between new data and the entire list, the list cannot change from the beginning of the clerical review process until the end in order for results to be consistent. Since the clerical review process may take weeks or more depending on the number of records involved, this can result in long delays.

This is also an argument for performing less manual review. Work has been done which shows that automatic review can achieve at least the same (or better) level of quality and would remove this time-expensive step of contention on the master linkage list. Originally, manual 'clerical review' involved seeking more information that was not available to the linkage process. However, it has since become just a human review of the same data that was available during the linkage process. This would not solve the other issues listed here dealing with the artificial single view of the world.

Uncertainty is lost
The 'master' nature of the list as mentioned introduces an artificial certainty into calculations. Researchers can easily fall into the trap of seeing the list as 'true' and that a 'cluster' is the same as a 'person.'

Information is thrown away/hard to use
Using this approach, the bulk of the computation, the very data of interest – the degree of similarity between records – is thrown away after use or retained but retained in a form unamenable to further computation, for example, a log file or CSV data, or stored as pairwise data relating records in a relational database.

A different approach is needed which better matches the nature of the data involved.

7.3   Graph approach

Such an approach is found in storing the data differently. Storing the data relationally does not adequately capture the underlying nature of the data. It is desirable to capture the *graph* nature of the data: that it is *a network of nodes or vertices (records) connected by edges (comparisons).*

Graph databases are specifically designed to *store and query* information in this form.

7.3.1   Overview of graph concepts

Graph databases capture the way in which data elements relate to one another. For example, consider four individuals, Alice, Bob, Carol and Dave. Alice is friends with Bob, Carol and Dave. Carol works for Bob and is married to Dave. These entities and the relationships between them could be captured in a graph as shown in Figure 7.1.

Here, the entities, all people so far, are captured as *nodes* (also called *vertices*) in the graph, and their relationships are captured as the *edges* between the nodes.

Note that some relationships are *bidirectional* and some are *unidirectional*. Alice and Carol are friends with each other, but sadly, it appears that although Alice is friends with Dave, Dave does not consider himself friends with Alice.

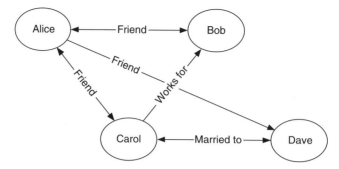

Figure 7.1   Alice, Bob, Carol and Dave and their relationships.

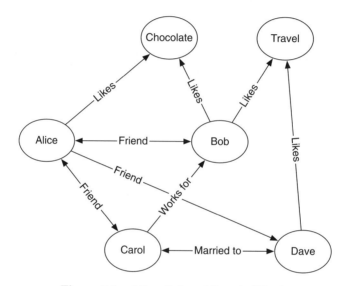

Figure 7.2   Alice, Bob and Dave's 'likes'.

Typically, although so far this graph is *homogeneous* (having all the elements of the same type), graph databases in general are not constrained to being *homogeneous*. In most conventional relational databases, all records in a table have the same number of attributes (columns), essentially forcing them to have the same type. In a graph database, typically nodes can be *heterogeneous* and vary in type. To continue the example, Alice and Bob like chocolate and Bob and Dave like travel as shown in Figure 7.2. Again, note these relationships are unidirectional: Bob likes chocolate, but clearly, it makes no sense to say chocolate likes Bob.

Further, since they like travel, Bob and Dave have visited a few cities as shown in Figure 7.3.

Although only the name of each node has been shown so far, nodes are free to have their own attributes, as are edges as shown in Figure 7.4.

It's worth noting that a *directed acyclic graph (DAG)* is a special case of graph where all edges are directional and no cycles are present (a path through the graph that returns to the same node).

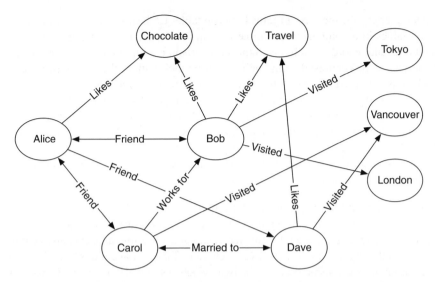

Figure 7.3   Bob, Carol and Dave's travel experience.

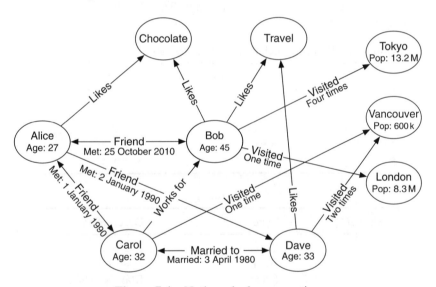

Figure 7.4   Node and edge properties.

7.3.2   Graph queries versus relational queries

Having constructed the graph to capture the relationships between entities, the graph may be queried. These queries consist of traversals of the graph topology. For example:

- Which friends of Alice like chocolate? (Bob)

- Who has a friend that has visited Tokyo? (Alice)

- Is there anyone that likes chocolate and travel? (Bob)

- Who has a friend who has a friend who has visited London? (Carol)

Relational queries take the form of joins between tables of data. Prototypically, a column (or subset of values in a column) in one table is found to match against values in a column of another table, and records which match this comparison are returned as the result of a query. Such queries can be optimised using indices, but by their nature, they are expensive, that is, slow, when used to traverse graph structures stored in relational databases.

Each step along an edge in a graph that has been represented relationally requires a join operation. Typical traversals of a graph using graph algorithms can involve hundreds if not thousands of such steps and quickly become prohibitively slow using relational database queries.

A *graph database* is designed to store data in a manner that facilitates such queries. Edge information is directly associated with a vertex, and as a result, operations which step from vertex to vertex are computationally optimised.

Example: People who bought this also bought

As a more detailed example of a graph query, consider information on purchases made by customers to an online store. In a relational representation, there might be one table representing customers, another containing details of products as in Table 7.4 and a third 'join' table essentially capturing the relationship between the two: which customers bought which products.

In a simplified form, this might be: In a graph database, the two types of entity, 'customer' and 'product', are both stored as nodes in the graph. The PURCHASE relationship is captured by the edges between the nodes (Figure 7.5).

Table 7.4   Product purchases as relational tables.

Customers		
Customer ID	Surname	First name
1	Smith	David
2	Jones	Mike
3	Laurie	Stephen

Products		
Product ID	Type	Description
1	Book	*The Hobbit*
2	Book	*Inheritor*
3	DVD	Blake's 7, Season 1
4	Book	*The Anabasis*

Purchases		
Purchase ID	fk_customer_id	fk_product_id
1	1	1
2	1	3
3	2	1
4	2	2
5	3	2
6	3	4

It is important to note the same information is being captured in both scenarios. The logical data model is the same, but it is given a different concrete expression in each case.

In the case where a customer is thinking of purchasing product #2 *Inheritor*, to find which other products were purchased by people who bought this product, one can follow the 'PURCHASE' links *backwards* to find the purchasers and then *forwards* to find the products purchased (Figure 7.6).

As the number of links to be traversed increases, the advantage of storing the information in a graph-based store over a relational store becomes more and more pronounced. The graph-based store is optimised for just such an operation, whereas in a relational database, the traversal is effected by means of repeated SELECT and/or JOIN statements.

One of the operations used to identify a cluster of similar linked records is *transitive closure* in which links are followed while a certain condition is met. This can involve the examination of many links.

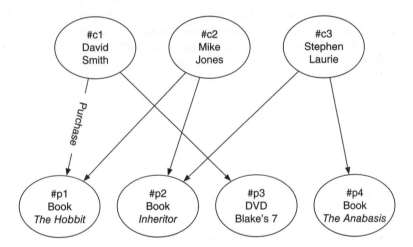

Figure 7.5   Product purchases as a graph.

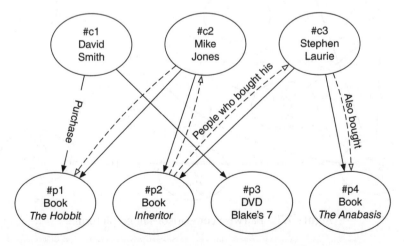

Figure 7.6   Traversing the purchase graph to find similar purchases.

7.3.3   Comparison of data in flat database versus graph database

To store linked records in a graph database, records are stored as nodes of the graph and the results of comparisons between records, that is, the similarities between records are stored as edges between records. In other words, each pairwise comparison that might be performed ends up corresponding to an edge in the graph between records.

The comparison of records performed in Table 7.2 would give rise to the graph in Figure 7.7 wherein, for ease of identification, the high-confidence, low-confidence and uncertain links have been shown in different styles and weights.

Transitive closure approach to cluster identification
Transitive closure is an operation on a set, where an operation is repeated on elements of a set and the results of the operation added back to the set. The process is repeated until no more elements are added to the set.

This can be used to find clusters of similar records. By starting at any one node (record), all the records 'similar' to that record (for some predefined level of similarity) can be found by moving out from that node only following links which have a weight above the desired similarity threshold. Later, the case will be covered where different sets of edges have been inserted using different comparison schemes and different weights. For now, assume all comparisons have been performed using the same comparison metrics and single threshold suffices to determine similarity.

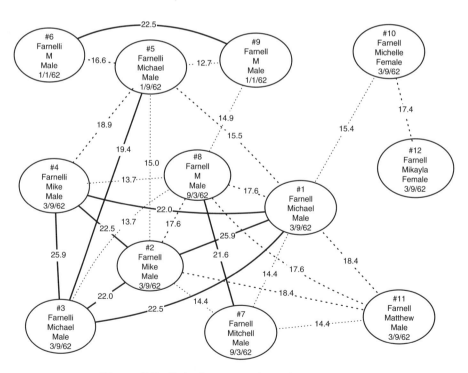

Figure 7.7   Pairwise comparisons in graph form.

In the previous graph example, consider starting at node #1 and using a threshold of 19 (this choice will ensure only the high-confidence links are traversed). In this process, a cluster corresponds to a set of records, and the cluster is built up from an initial starting node or *seed node*. The initial starting set containing record #1 is written as {#1}.

Starting with the set {#1}, all edges with a weight greater than 19 are traversed; this leads to nodes #2, #3 and #4, so they go into the set {#1, #2, #3, #4}. Following links out from these nodes, links to nodes already visited can be safely skipped, that is, there is no need to return to node #1 as it has already been visited. Examining the newly added nodes in turn, 'interesting' links (links with a weight >19) out from #2 only lead to #1, #3 and #4 (all of which are already in the result set). As well, links from #4 only lead to #1, #2 and #3, all of which have been visited already in this process. Following links from #3 leads to #1, #2, #4 and #5, of which #5 is new, so it goes into the result set, giving {#1, #2, #3, #4, #5}. In the next pass, there is nowhere to go from #5 that does not result in visiting an already visited node. Therefore, this is the final cluster of related records: {#1, #2, #3, #4, #5}.

Had different thresholds been used, this cluster would have been different. A higher threshold would have given rise to a smaller cluster containing records of greater similarity. A lower threshold would have given rise to a larger cluster containing more difference between records.

Using a threshold of 25 starting at #1 gives a cluster consisting of just {#1, #2}. Using 16 as the threshold gives {#1, #2, #3, #4, #5, #6, #8, #9, #11}. Algorithm 7.1 shall be revisited later in a more general form, but for now, consider it as an overview of the process used to find a group of 'similar' records given a starting record.

7.3.4   Relaxing the notion of 'truth'

One side effect of this approach is that *there is no explicit cluster ID*. The approach removes the notion of a single definitive interpretation of a group of records as belonging to or even 'being' a particular individual.

For the master linkage file or database approach, where 'person' ID or keys are assigned to individual records, it can be seductive to consider the information in the 'master' list as true. Even the name 'master list' lends itself to this interpretation, and yet these groupings are

Algorithm 7.1   Transitive closure of similarity

```
Place the starting node into a set (of one) called the pending set
While the pending set is not empty
    Pick any node in the pending set and make it the current node
    Remove the current node from the pending set
    Add the current node to the result set
    Find all the edges from the current node where weight > threshold
    Take the nodes at the ends of the edges as the new candidate set
    Remove from the new candidate set all nodes already in the result set
    Add the nodes remaining in the candidate set into the pending set
    Repeat (until the pending set is empty)
```

often arrived at via probabilistic processes where different choices along the data processing path can give rise to different final results.

Clearly, it is desirable to capture the underlying truth as much as possible. However, short of reviewing all comparison against external authoritative data sources, there will remain an element of probabilistic matching, especially in the presence of data entry errors and in the absence of reliable deterministic linkage fields.

Where deterministic linkage fields are available, the graph approach can still be used to manage data as it accommodates the frequently encountered need to mix data for which such unique identifying key fields are available with additional datasets for which such information is not available. Since many different link types can be stored in the same graph, the admixture of these different datasets presents no problem.

7.3.5   Not a linkage approach *per se* but a management approach which enables novel linkage approaches

The use of a graph is not a linkage approach *per se* (in the same way the use of a relational database is not a 'linkage approach') but an implementation choice designed to meet data management needs. Storing the data as a graph in a graph database provides advantages to both the management of data and the analysis of data, opening an avenue to novel linkage approaches and quality metrics.

In order to manage the data more effectively, different sets of data are kept distinct and tracked within the database.

Different datasets
First, exactly as different datasets are tracked in a relational system, datasets and subsets of datasets are still able to be managed separately.

For example, the NGLMS separates data from different data providers and data deliveries from each provider. The data is *not* just poured into the graph as one large pool of records.

Tracking data in this way allows projects to be constructed conventionally around which datasets are to be a part of a project, for example, hospital separations, cancer registry records and death records. Datasets may further be subdivided according to additional criteria as usual, for example, records from 2000 to 2010, all individuals in the cancer registry with breast cancer and so forth.

The conventional necessary flexibility is preserved using the graph approach.

Different linkage sets
In addition, the graph approach allows different sets of linkage information to be employed in a project, even different choices of thresholds to other projects using the same datasets.

Because cluster identification is a result of the threshold choices made and these choices are not 'baked in' to the data by the assignment of a 'person' ID, individual projects are free to choose thresholds appropriate to their needs.

The construction of a project thus consists of:

- A decision on which datasets are to be used for linkage

- A decision on which datasets are to be used for extraction

- A decision on which linkage sets are to be used

- A decision on which thresholds are to be used with those linkage sets

As multiple linkages can exist *non-destructively* in the graph database *at the same time*, parallel investigations of different linkage strategies and their effect on linkage results and quality can be undertaken. Should a linkage run prove to have suboptimal results or be based on erroneous assumptions, it may simply be ignored until a new run is effected of the desired quality. At this point, the appropriate linkage information may be 'switched on' and included in projects.

7.3.6   Linkage engine independent

This approach is not dependent on where the links are coming from. Weighted or unweighted links can come from any source:

- A computer programme, for example, linkage software and heuristic cluster detection

- A human, for example, clerical review processes and quality feedback

- Other systems, for example, other linked data stores

Link types: Weighted/unweighted
The linkage information stored in the graph can be of many different types:

- Weighted comparisons (probabilistic links) from a linkage engine

- Weighted comparisons using different schemes from different linkage engines

- Results of static comparisons between records (deterministic links)

- Clerical review results

- Genomic similarity

- Familial and tribal/clan kinship structures

7.3.7   Separates out linkage from cluster identification phase (and clerical review)

Storing pairwise information in a graph separates out the linkage, review and cluster identification phase.

7.4   Methodologies

The methodologies we discuss here are a simplification of the processes used with the NGLMS at SANT DataLink. They cover:

- Data loading
- Deterministic linkage

- Probabilistic linkage

- Clerical review

- Final cluster extraction

The processes described here deal with data coming from deterministic processes and probabilistic processes. Some are created through automated processes and some from human interaction. However, *the graph approach is not tied to any particular source or sources of linkage information or methodology*. It is an approach to managing data produced by other processes – be they automated or manual, deterministic, probabilistic or heuristic or batch or interactive. Whereas one data linkage unit may add 'clerical review links' as a result of manual processes to clean up clusters, another might add 'automated review links' to disentangle inconsistent graph topologies as a result of computer analysis of records in a cluster or as a result of analysis of a cluster's graph topology itself.

7.4.1   Overview of storage and extraction approach

As discussed previously, the NGLMS stores data subsets and comparison information separately and as identifiable collections of data. Part of a data analysis exercise (called a project in NGLMS terminology) involves the decision as to which datasets and which sets of comparison information are to be included when identifying clusters.

One way of considering this is as a collection of layers of data which are turned on or off on a project-by-project basis.

Figure 7.8 shows a project consisting of two sets of data records and two sets of linkage information:

- Two record sets: A and B

- A set of links constructed after a self-linkage or de-duplication of record set A in order to find similar records within that dataset

- A set of links *between* A and B in order to identify similar records between the datasets

The final 'view of the world' used in this project is the composition of these pieces of information. When identifying clusters of records in these two datasets, only the two specified sets of links will be taken into account. When traversing the graph, only edges belonging to participating link sets and nodes belonging to participating record sets take part in the traversal.

Defining 'extraction' as the cluster formation step, different linkage strategies may be compared, for example, by repeating extractions from this project but varying the AB cross-linkage layer or by swapping out one set of links and swapping in another set and performing another extraction.

Threshold parameters can vary, the results of different linkage runs can be swapped in and out, and different approaches compared efficiently without having to rerun a combined linkage and cluster detection step.

After comparison of different strategies, sets of links deemed useful may be retained for use in other projects, and less successful link sets may be discarded.

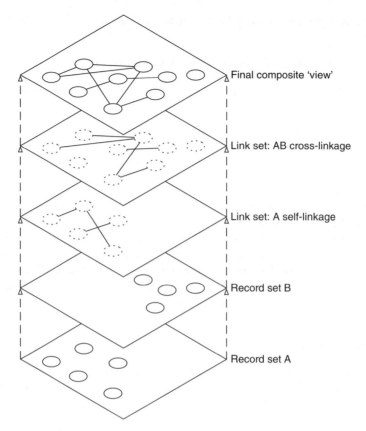

Figure 7.8 Composing a project from records and links.

7.4.2 Overall management of data as collections

In the NGLMS, record data are held as identifiable discrete sets of information in a loose two-tier organisational structure:

1. Logical collections of data, for example, birth data, cancer registry data and educational data, conceptually from an identifiable data provider or custodian

2. Data 'segments' which form part of logical collections such as a batch of records received from a data provider that share similar analysis characteristics, for example, a batch of records from a data custodian all with the same fields or of similar quality

Data segments are organised so as records within a data segment are similar enough to be linked using the same linkage parameters, for example, they are of similar quality or share the same set of linkage attributes and may be compared using the same linkage strategies. However, this is purely an organisational mechanism. Linkage may be performed on subsets (or compositions) of data segments, and projects are not forced to use an entire segment when only a subset of records is needed.

Linkage information is similarly held as identifiable discrete sets of links. Some examples include:

- Static (deterministic) links identified when data is first loaded

- Probabilistic links, for example, created as a result of self-linkage within data segments or between data segments

- Links arising from clerical review during a particular task or for a particular research project

Each data segment and each set of linkage data may be used as a layer when constructing a project as in Figure 7.8.

All data entering the system are time stamped. Record and link data in the NGLMS are write once, read many – that is, they are never changed in place, so there is no risk of data becoming out of step and inconsistent as a result of being stored in more than one place.

By never deleting older data and having data time stamped, historical extractions can always be performed again if necessary with exactly the same results. When performing a graph traversal, any edge or node with a date later than the date of interest is ignored, thus ensuring the traversal is exactly the same as performed previously.

7.4.3   Data loading

Data is cleaned and standardised in the same fashion as though it were going to be loaded into a conventional relational database. In fact, the same data, once cleaned, are loaded both into the graph database and into a relational database for other purposes.

The graph storage does not force data to adhere to a rigid schema. That is not to say it is disorganised: the NGLMS has a subset of columns to which incoming column names are normalised if the names differ, but any extra attributes on a record are also inserted into the database as is.

As an example of attribute normalisation, consider an attribute representing a date of birth. Incoming datasets may have this as a column labelled as 'birth', 'birth date', 'birthday', 'date of birth' or 'DOB'. In the NGLMS, the attribute name is standardised to 'dateOfBirth'. A core set of 17 or so attribute names are normalised in this fashion, and other attributes are inserted as is. An external data dictionary is maintained of concepts and column names to be used to capture data in the system. Note that this normalisation of the *name* of the attribute is separate to any normalisation or standardisation of the attribute value itself.

Some records and record sets may therefore be 17 attributes 'wide', and some may be 24 or 40 attributes wide depending on the data coming from the data provider. Standard linking takes place on a core set of attributes, but individual linkage strategies between specific datasets may take advantage of any extra information if necessary.

Typically, data arrives in a CSV file or similar and after cleaning is loaded into the graph database. At this point, each incoming record from the upstream data source is assigned an ID. This becomes its permanent ID for the lifetime of the data in the system. This ID *always* refers to this version of the data. If new data arrives later which supersedes older data, the new data is given a separate new ID, and a special type of link indicating it supersedes older data is inserted into the system between the records. Because this link has two ends, the other end indicates that the older record has been superseded.

7.4.4 Identification of equivalence sets and deterministic linkage

As a first step after loading the data, a round of deterministic linkage is performed. In the NGLMS, this is a deterministic linkage on up to 17 attributes to find records that may be considered exact matches. These records are linked using a link type that identifies this exact match relationship, and only one representative record from the resulting subset of 'identical' records is used in further probabilistic linkage strategies.

This approach is a processing decision within the SANT DataLink linkage unit, and there is no requirement in general for these data to be excluded during later linkage. In the SANT DataLink case, because so many linkage fields are being used for deterministic linkage (encompassing all the fields used for probabilistic linkage), it is a highly conservative approach with the side affect that all records in the identified equivalence set would link the same way. They are therefore excluded in order to cut down on the number of links generated not because the system could not cope with them capacity-wise but because they were deemed to add no new useful information to the comparison graph.

This is illustrated in Figure 7.9, where (on the left) a group of identical (for matching purposes) records X, X′ and X″ exists. When these records are not excluded, their similarity gives rise to a large number of links in the graph which essentially add no new information. In additional, when retrieved for clerical review, the reviewer is presented with a sequence of identical records that make it harder to ascertain the records that do differ within a cluster presented for review.

On the right, these records have been identified and joined using a link type that indicates their equivalence for matching purposes, and only a single record X (taken as being representative of the equivalence set) used for further matching. During review, only X is presented to the reviewer, but during later extraction, by following the equivalence links, all records including X′ and X″ can be returned as part of any identified cluster which includes the representative node X.

In other cases where deterministic linkage takes place but other fields are present that do not take part in the deterministic linkage process (but that may be used to perform probabilistic matching against other datasets), it would be desirable to not exclude these fields from further linkage efforts.

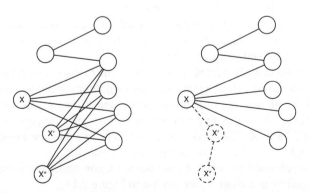

Figure 7.9   Linkage without (left) and with (right) equivalence links.

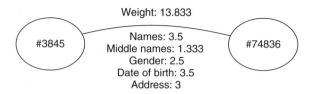

Figure 7.10   Weighted edge with weight vector.

7.4.5   Probabilistic linkage

To perform probabilistic linkage, records are extracted from the graph database and fed to a linkage engine, and the resulting pairwise comparisons are loaded back into the graph database as a link set. There are a few noteworthy points about this process.

First, there is no need to identify clusters of similar records at this point. The usual blocking (or any other appropriate technique) can be done to optimise the number of comparisons that need to be made, but the output of this step is not which records are related but *how* the records are related.

Not only is the weighted comparison total loaded into the database, but the entire *weight vector* can be loaded in as an attribute of the weighted link edge for later use as in Figure 7.10.

These weight components may be used later in analysis to find why certain edges had weights that were higher or lower than expected. This is similar to storing an *outcome vector* providing more details as to which fields matched, partially matched or failed to match in the comparison between records (Hills, 2014) and indeed since edges may have arbitrary attributes may be combined with such an approach.

Analyses can be performed to provide some *default thresholds* for the linkage set. Individual project compositions may override these with project-specific thresholds, but each link set also has a fallback position of default thresholds, which make sense for that particular set.

7.4.6   Clerical review

Typically, probabilistic linkage gives rise to the need to choose cut-off points on weights below which links are considered to be too tenuous and are ignored and above which links are considered to be sufficiently strong and accepted.

Sometimes, a single cut-off point is chosen. In other cases, a lower threshold and an upper threshold are chosen, and comparisons whose weights fall between these thresholds are considered 'uncertain' and worthy of further review.

If the link weights are considered in relation to whether the link represents a 'correct' association between records, given a good matching algorithm, usually most high weights are correctly identified with matches (true positives) and most low weights are correctly associated with non-matches (true negatives); however, some higher weights may imply a match where none should be made (false positives), and some matches are associated with lower weights which might cause them to be missed (false negatives).

If the edges are grouped by match status (match vs. non-match) and collected by weight, then we typically arrive at a chart or plot similar to Figure 7.11.

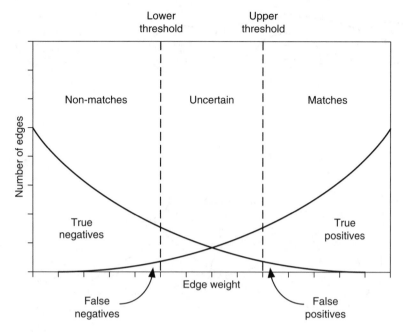

Figure 7.11   Match weight histogram with cut-off thresholds.

Figure 7.11 illustrates a choice of two thresholds in order to minimise false negatives and false positives. In doing so, the choice leaves a number of edges with uncertain match status. Resolving these uncertain matches into definite matches or non-matches may be a manual or automated process. It is desirable to choose these thresholds both to minimise the number of false positives and negatives and to minimise the number of uncertain edges that need to be reviewed. Competing requirements may relax some of these conditions, for example, false positives may not be so much of an issue, or perhaps there might be a desire to achieve as few false positives and negatives as possible, regardless of the number of uncertain links that would need to be reviewed as a result.

Without entering deeply into the debate over the merits of manual versus automated review of these uncertain or indeterminate links, it is worth noting that some jurisdictions practise heavy manual review, while others have investigated automated approaches with commensurate levels of quality when compared to the manual approaches.

A graph-based storage *supports both approaches equally well* and, in fact, can greatly facilitate both, for example, by removing bottlenecks in the manual case and by exposing the graph topology for further analysis in the automated case.

7.4.7   Determining cut-off thresholds

Several methods of determining these cut-off points exist. Here, we consider two approaches, a manual and an automated approach, both of which exploit the graph nature of the data either directly or indirectly.

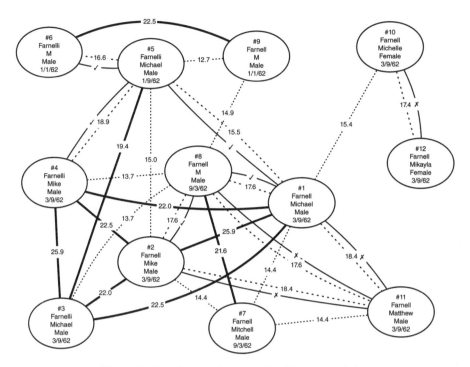

Figure 7.12   Comparison graph with review links.

Manual threshold determination **via** *clerical review and sampling*

The details of how the graph is curated to effect clerical review will be presented presently, but for now, it is enough to say that the result of clerical review (either automated or manual) is to add additional edges to the graph confirming or rejecting an uncertain edge. As clerical review progresses, one may create the histogram in Figure 7.11 by extracting from the graph all edges for which a clerical review edge has been added as a companion, using the decision associated with the review edge to determine match status. A confirming edge is a match, a rejecting edge is a non-match, and weights are categorised accordingly. Figure 7.12 shows this pairing of weighted links with clerical review links.

By taking a few large clusters extracted from the graph with a low threshold (perhaps lower than ultimately might be necessary) and performing clerical review on those large clusters of related and unrelated records by breaking them into smaller clusters of definitely related records, clerical review links are written back to the graph as both confirming and rejecting edges. By choosing appropriate clusters for review at various boundary weights, a sampling of the distribution of edge weights may be made along with the determination of match status.

Once enough sampling has been performed by manual review, cut-off thresholds may be chosen according to need, and a more comprehensive clerical review can take place with the chosen lower and upper thresholds in place.

Automated threshold determination from an examination of graph topology

Another approach is to consider the graph topology itself. Groups of related records are well connected (each record connects to many other records in the cluster), and it takes very few edge traversals to move from one record to another in the cluster because of this well connectedness.

By choosing a succession of cut-off values, extracting clusters and examining the topology of the clusters extracted for given cut-off values (are they well connected and cohesive vs. do they contain nodes only loosely connected to the main body of the cluster), one may determine a cut-off value at which point most clusters are well connected and cohesive.

7.4.8   Final cluster extraction

Before discussing the final extraction step, it will be helpful to revisit the cluster identification algorithm presented in Algorithm 7.1 in a more general form. This time, the algorithm will be presented taking into account which datasets and which linkage sets and thresholds are to be used.

Some additional parameters are needed:

- *Data segments:* A collection of datasets participating in the extraction

- *Quality parameters:* A collection of linkage sets along with thresholds for each set

- *Threshold:* The particular named threshold being used in this extraction

To give a concrete example based on Figure 7.8:

- The *data segments* being used would be:

  - Record set A

  - Record set B

- The *quality parameters* being used might be:

  - Self-linkage A with thresholds {lower=14, upper=24}

  - Cross-linkage AB with thresholds {lower=12, upper=25}

- And using the 'upper' *threshold*

Algorithm 7.1 is now presented in a more general form taking into account these extra parameters. This version also returns all edges that form part of the cluster.

Algorithm 7.2 can be adapted to also track and return edges that would lead out of the cluster over the boundary of the cluster by saving edge sets that would otherwise be 'of no interest'. These edges that are of 'no interest' – in other words, the edges that fall below the similarity threshold – are the very edges that stop the traversal and define the boundary of the cluster and thus exit the cluster.

The algorithm can also be adapted to ignore all nodes and edges added to the graph after a certain time by the addition of appropriate filtering steps at (†) before the node and edge tests.

7.4.9   Graph partitioning

Graph partitioning is a repeated application of cluster identification in Algorithm 7.2 to take a set of nodes and partition it into a set of clusters of nodes.Note that *result clusters* are a set of clusters, not a set of nodes. That is to say Algorithm 7.3 takes a set of nodes $N = \{n_1, n_2, n_3, \ldots, n_m\}$

Algorithm 7.2   Cluster identification (general form)

```
Call a collection of data sets the data segments
Call a collection of linkage sets and thresholds the quality parameters
Call the name of the threshold to use the threshold
Call an optional set of nodes the limiting nodes
Place the starting node into a set (of one) called the pending nodes
Create an empty set of nodes called the result nodes
Create an empty set of edges called the result edges
While the set of pending nodes is not empty
    Pick any node in the pending nodes and make it the current node
    Remove the current node from the pending nodes
    Add the current node to the result nodes
    If the clustering operation is limited and the current node is not
                                    in the set of limiting nodes:
        Do nothing and check for the next pending node (next loop
        iteration)
    Take all the edges from the current node call the current edges
    (†)
    Remove current edges that don't lead to a node in the data
    segments
    Remove current edges not in the quality parameters link sets
    // the next section makes a decision about whether to follows this edge
    // it can be extended with different edges types as appropriate
    // herein is considered CR links and weighted edge links
    For each group of edges in the current edges grouped by destination node:
        If the group contains any clerical review (CR) links:
            If the latest CR link is BREAK:
                Skip this edge group and go to next edge group
            If the latest CR link is FORCE:
            Add the destination node to the new node candidates
            Add the current edges to the result edges
            Go to the next edge group
            If the latest CR link is IGNORE:
            Ignore all CR decisions made about this edge
            Fall back to looking at weights and thresholds
        For each candidate edge in the current edges
            Determine which linkage set the candidate edge belongs to
            If the weight of the candidate edge is > the looked up
                            threshold for the identified linkage
                            set in the quality parameters:
            Add the destination node to the new node candidates
            Add the current edges to the result edges
            Go to the next edge group
        If there is no threshold for the identified linkage set
                        in the quality parameters and
                        the edge weight > the threshold in
                        the linkage set's defaults:
            Add the destination node to the new node candidates
```

```
          Add the current edges to the result edges
          Go to the next edge group
       Otherwise the edge is of no interest
   Remove from the new node candidates all nodes already in the
   result nodes
   Add the nodes remaining in the candidate set into the pending
   nodes
   Repeat (until the set of pending nodes is empty)
Return the result nodes and the result edges
```

Algorithm 7.3   Partitioning a set of nodes into clusters

```
Take a set of nodes to be partitioned called the pending set
Create an empty set of clusters called the result clusters
While the pending set is not empty:
   Pick any node in the pending set and make it the seed node
   Apply Algorithm 7.2 to the seed node to get a cluster
   Take all nodes in the cluster out of the pending set
   Add the cluster to the result clusters
   Repeat (until the pending set is empty)
```

and partitions it into a set of clusters $P = \{(C_1, E_1), (C_2, E_2), ..., (C_k, E_k)\}$ where each cluster, as mentioned previously, is a set of nodes within the cluster and a set of edges joining those nodes.

Note that C_1 to C_k form a partitioning of N. Each n_i $(1 \le i \le m)$ is in only one C_j $(1 \le j \le k)$ and the union of C_1 to C_k covers N. None of C_1 to C_k is an empty set:

- $\forall A, B \in \{C_1,,...,,C_k\} : A \neq B \Rightarrow A \cap B = \varnothing$

- $\bigcup_{C \in \{C_1,...,C_k\}} C = N$

- $\varnothing \notin \{C_1,...,C_k\}$

This partitioning algorithm is used significantly in two situations:

1. To partition a collection of records into clusters on final extraction

2. To partition a review cluster into sub-clusters for review

The first of these is straightforward: all the records in a project are partitioned into clusters once clerical review has finished. It does not matter whether the 'upper' or 'lower' threshold is used for this extraction since at this point clerical review is complete and thus by definition all 'uncertain' links (those lying between the 'upper' and 'lower' thresholds) have been replaced by clerical review links either affirming or rejecting the links.

The second covers the case where a cluster is presented for clerical review. In this case, a cluster has already been identified in a previous set by cluster identification using Algorithm

7.2 and the 'lower' threshold. Before presenting the list of records to be reviewed to a reviewer, the list is partitioned according to the 'upper' threshold to group together records for which a high confidence of match is deemed already to exist.

7.4.10   Data management/curation

The NGLMS takes the approach of only ever *adding* data to the graph. Clerical review decisions are superseded if necessary but never removed. This allows data extractions/clustering that may have been performed in the past to be repeated later with the same result (by ignoring all data added and actions performed after a given time stamp).

The links in a link set layer are never removed. Instead, clerical review links encapsulating decisions about the nodes at the ends of the links are added. For example, should two nodes joined by an 'uncertain' edge be deemed to be related, a FORCE edge is added to confirm the match of those two nodes. Should they be deemed to not match, they are separated by adding a BREAK edge. As edges are not removed, a third edge type IGNORE is also available to indicate that all clerical review decisions up to this point should be ignored.

Returning to Figure 7.7, clerical review links might be added as in Figure 7.12 as part of the clerical review process, giving rise to a final clustering (for the given thresholds) that matches the original 'master' groupings of Table 7.3. Clerical review links are shown as either confirming (✓) or rejecting (✗) relationships between nodes.

7.4.11   User interface challenges

Although the review process is manipulating the graph topology, it may not be desirable to present the graph directly to a reviewer especially when reviewers may be used to looking at tables of records presented in a row-based format.

This presents the need to convert decisions about which nodes belong together into decisions about which edges to confirm or reject.

The clerical review process consists of determining which records belong together (either through manual inspection or automated calculation and heuristics) and then 'changing' the graph by overlaying clerical review links to make the graph capture the desired statements about record matches.

We're managing links (edges) but reviewers see records (nodes)
Consider Figure 7.7. On extracting a cluster at a lower threshold of 15.5 to extract a 'review' cluster starting at node #1, the cluster is extracted. This might be presented to the user as in Table 7.5.

The reviewer examines these records and decides on the groupings in Table 7.6.

After making these review decisions, the following 'clusters' need to be 'written back' to the graph: {#1, #2, #3, #4, #5, #6, #7, #8, #9} and {#11}.

Review links are added to the graph by considering the desired cluster in relation to the current graph topology, *confirming* all uncertain edges with the cluster by the addition of FORCE links and *rejecting* all edges that cross out of the cluster to be by the addition of BREAK links.

Table 7.5   Initial records for clerical review.

Surname	First name	Sex	DOB
Farnell	Michael	M	3/6/84
Farnell	Mike	M	3/6/84
Farnelli	Michael	M	3/6/84
Farnelli	Mike	M	3/6/84
Farnelli	Michael	M	1/6/84
Farnelli	M	M	1/1/84
Farnell	Mitchell	M	6/3/84
Farnell	M	M	6/3/84
Farnell	M	M	1/1/84
Farnell	Michelle	F	3/6/84
Farnell	Matthew	M	3/6/84
Farnell	Mikayla	F	3/6/84

Table 7.6   Grouped records after clerical review.

Group 1			
Surname	First name	Sex	DOB
Farnell	Michael	M	3/6/84
Farnell	Mike	M	3/6/84
Farnelli	Michael	M	3/6/84
Farnelli	Mike	M	3/6/84
Farnelli	Michael	M	1/6/84
Farnelli	M	M	1/1/84
Farnell	Mitchell	M	6/3/84
Farnell	M	M	6/3/84
Farnell	M	M	1/1/84

Group 2			
Surname	First name	Sex	DOB
Farnell	Matthew	M	3/6/84

If the cluster {#1, #2, #3, #4, #5, #6, #7, #8, #9} is considered (Figure 7.13), it can been seen that all uncertain links ($15.5 \leq$ weight ≤ 19) have been confirmed within the cluster and rejected where they would cross out of the cluster and bring in other nodes.

The algorithm to effect this is slightly more complicated than the cluster extraction. To create appropriate clerical review links, the graph is traversed, and uncertain links are 'fixed' as previously discussed to bring them into agreement with the clusters to be created. As the graph is traversed, a set of links to be added is compiled (Algorithm 7.4).

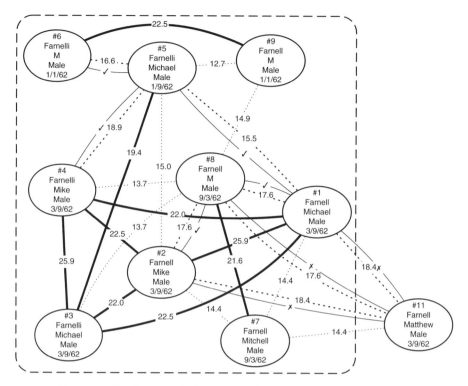

Figure 7.13   Reviewed cluster boundary and clerical review links.

The core of the determination of whether or not to add a review link and which type of review link to add can be done by recourse to a lookup table (Table 7.7) based on:

- The current clerical review state of the edge bundle: FORCE, BREAK and none

- The current confidence level of the weighted links: none, low, uncertain and high

- Whether the edges cross the cluster boundary: 1 (crossing) and 2 (internal)

The review state and confidence level can be determined by querying an appropriately constructed EdgePolicy object (see Algorithm 7.8).

An edge crossing value can be calculated as

$$|\{\text{from node}, \text{to node}\} \cap \text{desired nodes}|$$

When both nodes are in the desired nodes set, this will have a value of 2; if only one node is in the set and the other outside it, this will results in a value of 1.

Clerical review on clusters is repeated until there are no links remaining with weights within the uncertain region that do not have a corresponding review decision.

Algorithm 7.4   Determination of clerical review links


```
Call a collection of nodes the boundary nodes, any edges leaving
                    this set will not be modified
Call a collection of nodes to be a cluster the desired cluster nodes
Call a collection of data sets the data segments
Call a collection of linkage sets and thresholds the quality
parameters
Call the name of the lower threshold to use the lower threshold
Call the name of the upper threshold to use the upper threshold
Create a copy of set of the desired cluster nodes called the pending
nodes
Create an empty set called the seen nodes
Create an empty set called the seen edges
Create an empty set called the edges to add
Create new partitioning visitor initialised with the data segments,
  the quality parameters and the lower threshold
Limit the partitioning visitor to only work on the desired cluster
nodes
While the set of pending nodes is not empty
    Pick any node in the pending nodes and make it the current node
    Remove the current node from the set of pending nodes
    If the current node is in seen nodes
        Do nothing and check for the next pending node (next loop
        iteration)
    Find the cluster with the current node (using the partitioning
    visitor)
    Retrieve the found cluster nodes of this cluster
    Retrieve the found cluster edges of this cluster
    Add found cluster nodes &cap; desired cluster nodes to seen
    nodes
    Group all the edges together by source and destination nodes
    // i.e. bundle all the edges between two nodes together
    For each (from node, edges, to node) bundle:
        If either from node or to node is in desired cluster
        nodes and &not; to node is in boundary nodes and in data
        segments:
            if {from node, to node} is in seen edges:
                do nothing, this has been examined coming the other way
            add {from node, to node} to seen edges
            // see below for more detail of the next 5 steps
            determine the current clerical review state of this edge
            bundle
            determine the current confidence level of this edge bundle
            determine the crossing state of this edge bundle
            based on this triplet of values decide if an edge is to be
            added
            add the edge to edges to add
```

```
// If at this point there are no pending nodes but the cluster
// is not complete pick a random node in the remainder and add a
clerical
// review link to it, add it into the pending pool and continue
if pending nodes is empty and seen nodes ⊉ desired nodes:
    set done nodes to be desired nodes ∩ seen nodes
    pick a start node at random from the done nodes
    set remaining nodes to be desired nodes – seen nodes
    pick an end node at random from the remaining nodes
    add a link FORCE(start node, end node) to edges to add
    addend node to pending nodes
```

Table 7.7 Decision link lookup table for clerical review.

Confidence	Existing review link	Crossing state	New decision
High	FORCE	Internal	—
High	FORCE	Crosses	BREAK
High	BREAK	Internal	IGNORE
High	BREAK	Crosses	—
High	—	Internal	—
High	—	Crosses	BREAK
Uncertain	FORCE	Internal	—
Uncertain	FORCE	Crosses	BREAK
Uncertain	BREAK	Internal	FORCE
Uncertain	BREAK	Crosses	—
Uncertain	—	Internal	FORCE
Uncertain	—	Crosses	BREAK
Low	FORCE	Internal	—
Low	FORCE	Crosses	—
Low	BREAK	Internal	IGNORE
Low	BREAK	Crosses	—
Low	—	Internal	—
Low	—	Crosses	—
—	FORCE	Internal	—
—	FORCE	Crosses	BREAK
—	BREAK	Internal	IGNORE
—	BREAK	Crosses	—
—	—	Internal	—
—	—	Crosses	—

7.4.12   Final cluster extraction

To perform final cluster extraction (and 'final' here is really a misnomer: cluster extraction can be performed at any time), all the records of interest in the required datasets to be 'linked' are partitioned by choosing thresholds and applying Algorithm 7.3. At this point, each cluster so extracted can be assigned a unique ID.

By recording each extraction, a *difference report* may be generated to compare two different clustering.

Reusing cluster ID

The question arises, 'can cluster ID be reused from one extraction to another?' This question can arise for different reasons. For example:

- A researcher may want to know the minimal set of changes from one extraction to another so as not to have to retrieve all new data from data custodians.

- A researcher may wish to compare 'individuals' in one study with 'individuals' in another study and identify the same 'individuals'.

This last is actually not as straightforward as researchers often think. Just because two clusters share many records *does not* indicate that they are necessarily records relating to the same individual. The intuition that they are 'mostly the same' leads reasoning astray. Consider the case where records in a first extraction were incorrectly placed in a cluster and a subsequent extraction corrected this error, or consider the case where a cluster which contained records relating to two individuals was separated into two separate clusters: which new cluster corresponds to the (non-existent) 'individual' in the first cluster?

The expectations that record clusters are the same as individuals are fostered by the 'master' linkage table approach. In reality, there is very little that can be said about extractions beyond:

1. New records *which were not present anywhere in a first extraction* may have been added to a cluster in a second extraction, that is, new records have been added.

2. Records which were present in a cluster in a first extraction may be *absent from all clusters in a second extraction*, that is, the records have vanished.

3. Records have moved between clusters.

In the first two cases, an argument can be made for reusing cluster ID from the first extraction in a second extraction.

In the third case, *no statement can be made about the equivalence of clusters in the first and second extractions*.

The most flexible approach is to simply provide a change report saying which clusters a record is in for the two extractions and defer the decision as to what this 'means' to the researcher.

7.4.13   A typical end-to-end workflow

A typical end-to-end workflow using the graph approach is as follows:

- Data is cleaned.

- Data is added to system, assigning ID.

- Deterministic links are calculated and equivalence links added to database.

- Self-linkage is performed and de-duplication layer(s) added to database.

- Cross-linkage is performed and cross-linkage layer(s) added to database.

- Thresholds are identified.

- Clusters containing non-reviewed edges within thresholds are identified.

- These clusters are reviewed/resolved (manually or automatically).

- Result cluster extraction(s).

- Cluster ID assigned and change reports generated.

- Data provided/returned to client or custodian.

7.5   Algorithm implementation

Considering all of the aforementioned operations in more detail, there are some basic queries and operations on the graph that suffice to support the previous processes.

We presented here the essence of routines that may be used to traverse and manage the link information stored in a graph. These routines are presented in a code-like manner, which should be readily mapped onto specific programming languages and graph database application programming interfaces. We do not aim to cover all the processing possibilities but handle the core aspects of:

- Graph traversal

- Graph partitioning

- Graph curation for clerical review

The algorithmic fragments presented here are presented in a form that delegates much of the decision-making to customisable code instances. These code instances can be easily replaced with alternatives adapted to other purposes.

7.5.1   Graph traversal

It will be noticed that aspects of these algorithms have a basic structure that involves traversal of the graph and may be implemented in the form of the *visitor* design pattern (Gamma et al., 1994) to effect this traversal.

In the *visitor* pattern, a common algorithm to visit all elements of a structure, for example, all elements in an array or all elements in a tree, is used to apply a *visitor* function or function object to each element. For example, when applying operations to all elements of an array, the loop, which starts at the beginning and goes on until the end and then stops, is common to each application, but the function to be applied may vary.

In this graph case, we will implement a *traverse* operation that repeatedly takes a node from a pool of nodes and 'visits' that node by passing it off to a *visitor* object, which implements the action to be applied to that node. This action is repeated until the pool is empty.

The *visitor* object keeps track of the state of the traversal, implements the operation to be applied to each node and collects any results.

This basic *traverse* operation is shown in Algorithm 7.5.

Here, the traversal is passed a set of seed nodes (which may be a single node) and a visitor object to apply to the graph. The visitor object encapsulates the set-up and clean-up of the

Algorithm 7.5   traverse() the graph using a visitor

```
deftraverse(seedNodes, visitor) {
    visitor.initialise(seedNodes)
    while (visitor.hasPending()) {
        node = visitor.next()
        visitor.visit(node)
    }
    visitor.end()
}
```

Algorithm 7.6   findCluster() using a visitor and traverse()

```
deffindCluster(seedNode, dataSegments, qualityParameters, threshold)
    {
    partitioningVisitor = new PartitioningVisitor(dataSegments,
                                    qualityParameters, threshold)
    traverse({seedNode}, partitioningVisitor)
    return partitioningVisitor.getNodes(), partitioningVisitor.
    getEdges()
}
```

traversal in *initialise()* and *end()*, respectively; makes the decision as to whether to continue traversing the graph because there are unvisited nodes in *hasPending()*; and performs the actual work of visiting a node in *visit()*.

Various strategies for visiting a graph may be implemented by varying the visitor object without having to re-implement the visitation steps over and over.

The visitor object itself accumulates the results of the operation and may be queried at the end to extract the information accumulated.

7.5.2   Cluster identification

The detail of a visitor will be shown presently, but first, here is the *traverse* operation used with a visitor that performs the core of the partitioning step to find a cluster.

The elements of Algorithm 7.6 that map onto Algorithm 7.2 should be readily identifiable. The *findCluster* operation expands a single seed node into a cluster of nodes by working outwards along the graph edges following edges of interest. 'Of interest' is ascertained by the partitioning visitor to be edges which either:

• Have an explicit FORCE clerical review link present or

• Have a probabilistic link with a weight above a threshold

7.5.3   Partitioning visitor

The *PartitioningVisitor* is an object that makes decisions during the graph traversal and accumulates a list of nodes and edges seen in the process. It is parameterised by the datasets, linkage sets and thresholds that take part in the calculations. Although it is really a collection of algorithmic fragments, it is presented here as Algorithm 7.7.

7.5.4   Encapsulating edge following policies

Decisions about whether or not to follow a particular set of edges from one node to another are handled by delegation to an *EdgePolicy* object (Algorithm 7.8). This object takes a collection of edges that connect two nodes, some quality parameters and the name of a threshold. A decision as to whether the edge should be 'followed' is then made, thereby resulting in the decision as to whether the second node is 'related' to the first.

7.5.5   Graph partitioning

As presented previously in a general form in Algorithm 7.3, a set of nodes can be partitioned into clusters by repeatedly finding clusters until there are no nodes remaining. Algorithm 7.9 covers this process in more detail.

7.5.6   Insertion of review links

The insertion of review links is accomplished using a ReviewVisitor that traverses the graph and accumulates a list of edges to be created to 'fix' the graph to its new state as it goes (Algorithm 7.10).

Finally, the routine to actually perform review operations, which takes a collection of clusters to create and alters the graph accordingly, is shown in Algorithm 7.11.

7.5.7   How to migrate while preserving current clusters

One nice side effect of implementing review in this way is that it provides a mechanism for transferring legacy cluster information from a 'master linkage table' to a linkage graph.

After performing Algorithm 7.12, the graph will mirror the state of the 'master linkage table'. If relinking was performed or previous linkage information was retrieved from archival storage and used to create the graph before migration, then very rich data will be available henceforth.

7.6   New approaches facilitated by graph storage approach

Having the comparison data persist and be available for calculations and separating the comparison and cluster identification steps lead to several novel advantages:

- Multiple 'linkages' may coexist for one dataset.

- Linkages may be turned on and off at will.

Algorithm 7.7   Partitioning visitor

```
classPartitioningVisitor:
    // save our parameters of interest for later reference
    defPartitioningVisitor(dataSegments, qualityParameters,
                            threshold, followEquivalenceLinks) {
        save dataSegments for later reference
        save qualityParameters for later reference
        save threshold for later reference
        save followEquivalenceLinks for later reference
        set limitingNodes to be empty
    }

    // setup for a traversal
    definitialise(seedNodes) {
        save seedNodes for later reference
        set pendingNodes = seedNodes
        set seenEdges to the empty set
        set resultNodes to the empty set
        set resultEdges to the empty set
    }

    defhasPending() {
        return whether pendingNodes is not empty
    }

    defnext() {
        remove a node from pendingNodes and return it
    }

    // there exists two 'visit' routines, one for nodes and one for
    edges
    // this 'visit a node' routine assembles all the edges out of a
    node
    // grouped by destination and for each destination checks to see
    // if that destination is in one of our sets of interest and
    // if it is calls the 'visit edges' routine with the current and
    // destination nodes and all the edges between
    defvisit(node) {
        add node to resultNodes
        if limitingNodes is not empty and node is in limitingNodes:
            return
        find all (edge, destination node) pairs from node
        group these pairs by destination node
        // in other words take something like
        // (e, n) (f, n) (g, n) (h, m) (i, m)
        // and turn it into
```

```
    // {n: (e, f, g), m: (h, i)}
    for each destination node and the edges to that node:
        if the destination node is in dataSegments:
            visitEdges(node, edges, destination node)
}

defvisitEdges(fromNode, edges, toNode) {
    if {fromNode, toNode} is in seenEdges:
        do nothing and return
    add {fromNode, toNode} to seedEdges
    // EdgePolicy object encapsulate decisions about whether or
    not
    // to follow a cluster of edges; it examines things like
    clerical
    // review links and weights and thresholds
    create an edgePolicy object = &not;
                    new EdgePolicy(edges, followEquivalenceLinks)
    if edgePolicy(qualityParameters, threshold) says to follow  the
    edges or toNode is in seedIds {
        add the edges to resultEdges
        if toNode isn't already in resultNodes:
            add toNode to pendingNodes
    }
}

// clean up
defend() {
}
```

- Different clusterings may be performed at different thresholds.

- Graph topology rather than just a list of records may be supplied downstream.

- More advanced cluster analysis techniques (which may be more expensive computationally) may be applied to sub-graphs rather than the whole graph.

- Other link types may be added to the database other than weighted field match links.

7.6.1 Multiple threshold extraction

Using a 'master linkage table' approach, only one view of the world is usually possible. Threshold and matching decisions happen long before data is handed out to researchers, and they are hard to revisit or provide alternatives for without relinking and/or keeping multiple copies of the master table with different cluster ID.

Using a graph-based approach multiple extractions can be performed without having to relink data merely by varying the thresholds supplied during the cluster extraction step.

Algorithm 7.8   Edge policy

```
classEdgePolicy:
    defEdgePolicy(edges, followEquivalenceLinks=false) {
        save edges for later reference
        save followEquivalenceLinks for later reference
    }

    // return a clerical review decision if one is present in the
    edges
    defgetCr() {
        if there is a clerical review decision in the saved edges:
            return the latest clerical review decision
        return NULL
    }

    // check to see whether the edges saved in this edge policy
    object
    // should be followed, the option to honour or ignore clerical
    review
    // links is available, by default they are honoured
    defwouldFollow(qualityParameters, threshold, withCr=true) {
        if withCr is true {
            get the latest crDecision by calling getCr()
            if crDecision is FORCE:
                return true
            if crDecision is BREAK:
                return false
            if crDecision is IGNORE:
                ignore all CR decisions and continue deliberations
        }
        if followEquivalenceLinks is true and there is an equivalent
        edge:
                return true
        for each weighted linkage edge in edges:
            if the linkage set the edge belongs to is in
            qualityParameters and edge.weight > the threshold for that
            set in qP:
            return true
        // otherwise
        return false
    }

    defgetConfidence(qualityParameters, lowThreshold, highThreshold)
    {
        // this routine looks at the weighted linkage edges in the
        saved edges
```

```
        // and returns 'high', 'uncertain', or 'low' depending on
        where the
        // weights lie in relation to the given thresholds
        //
        // this is used when filtering out clusters needing review
}
```

Algorithm 7.9   partition() a group of nodes by repeatedly finding clusters

```
defpartition(nodes, dataSegments, qualityParameters, threshold,
                            followEquivalenceLinks, review) {
    // review is a flag to indicate partition should only return
    clusters
    // which have either edges needing review or which contain a
    BREAK edge
    // (indicating an inconsistency)
    pending = {}
    results = []
    done = {}
    pVisitor = new PartitioningVisitor(dataSegments, ¬
    qualityParameters, threshold, followEquivalenceLinks)
    add all nodes to pending
    for (seed in pending) {
        if (seed in done):
            continue
        traverse({seed}, pVisitor)
        cluster = [pVisitor.getNodes(), pVisitor.getEdges()]
        if (!review) {
            candidate = true
        } else if (cluster contains uncertain links or BREAK links) {
            candidate = true
        } else {
            candidate = false
        }
        if (candidate):
            add cluster to results
        add all nodes in cluster[0] to done
    }
    return results
}
```

High specificity versus high recall

As mentioned previously, raising the thresholds increases specificity by returning smaller clusters containing records that are more similar to each other. Conversely, lowering the thresholds increases sensitivity and returns fewer larger clusters.

Algorithm 7.10   Review visitor


```
classReviewVisitor:
    // save our parameters of interest for later reference
    defReviewVisitor(boundaryNodes, dataSegments, qualityParameters,
    lowThreshold, highThreshold) {
        save boundaryNodes for later reference
        save dataSegments for later reference
        save qualityParameters for later reference
        save lowThreshold for later reference
        save highThreshold for later reference
        create pVisitor = new PartitioningVisitor(dataSegments,
                                     qualityParameters, lowThreshold)
    }

    definitialise(desiredNodes) {
        save desiredNodes for later reference
        set pendingNodes to be a copy of desiredNodes
        set seenNodes to be empty
        set seenEdges to be empty
        set edgesToAdd to be empty
        pVistor.setLimitingNodes(desiredNodes)
    }

    defhasPending() {
        return whether pendingNodes is not empty
    }

    defnext() {
        remove a node from pendingNodes and return it
    }

    // node visitor
    defvisit(node) {
        if (node is in seenNodes)
            return
        traverse({node}, pVisitor)
        clusterNodes = pVisitor.getNodes()
        clusterEdges = pVisitor.getEdges()
        add clusterNodes to seenNodes
        group clusterEdges by destination node
        // in other words take something like
        // (e, n) (f, n) (g, n) (h, m) (i, m)
        // and turn it into
        // {n: (e, f, g), m: (h, i)}
        for each destination node and the edges to that node {
            if {node, destination node} intersects with desiredNodes {
                // i.e. if one of the nodes is in desiredNodes
```

```
                    if destination node is in boundaryNodes and
                            destination node is in dataSegments {
                    visitEdges(node, edges, destination node)
            }
        }
}
// If, at this point, we have no pending nodes left but the
cluster
// is not complete, add a new clerical review link between a
random
// node in the cluster so far and a random node in the remainder
and
// then add the new node into the pending pool and continue
if (!pendingNodes and !(seenNodes contains all desiredNodes)) {
        done = desiredNodes &cap; seenNodes
        fromNode = a random node from done
        remaining = desiredNodes - seenNodes
        toNodes = a ranomd node from remaining
        addCrLink(fromNode, toNode, 'FORCE')
        add toNode to pending Nodes
    }
}


// edge visitor
def visitEdges(fromNode, edges, toNode) {
    if {fromNode, toNode} in seenEdges:
        return
    add {fromNode, toNode} to seenEdges
    ep = new EdgePolicy(edges)
    confidence = ep.getConfidence(qualityParameters,
                                    lowThreshold, highThreshold)
    cr = ep.getCr()
    if cr is IGNORE:
        cr = NULL
    crossingState = |{fromNode, toNode} ∩ desiredNodes|
    decision = getAction(confidence, cr, crossingState) // lookup
    table
    if (decision):
    addCrLink(fromNode, toNode, decision)
}

def addCrLink(fromNode, toNode, decision) {
add [fromNode, toNode, decision] to edgesToAdd
}
```

Algorithm 7.11   review() pushes new cluster boundaries back into the graph

```
defreview(clusters, dataSegment, qualityParameters,
    lowThreshold, highThreshold, edgeAdder) {
    set boundaryNodes to all the nodes in clusters
    reviewVisitor = new ReviewVisitor(boundaryNodes, dataSegments,
                    qualityParamenters, lowThreshold, highThreshold)
    for each cluster in clusters {
        traverse(cluster, reviewVisitor)
        // the edgeAdder object actually adds the edges
        edgeAdder.addEdges(reviewVisitor.getEdgesToAdd())
        }
}
```

Algorithm 7.12   Legacy cluster migration

```
Import all data sets into the graph
Relink all data if so designed to a required level of quality (no
    review)
For each cluster already identified in the master linkage table:
    Write that cluster back to the graph using Algorithm 7.11
```

Return to researchers not a single result but results 'bracketing' desired thresholds giving 'bounds' on calculations
This opens up the possibility of returning to researchers not just one extraction but, say, three extractions:

1. An extraction with lower thresholds and higher sensitivity but lower specificity

2. The conventional extraction

3. An extraction with higher thresholds and higher specificity but lower sensitivity

Such an approach allows the researcher to conduct sensitivity analyses around the record linkage process and even to include variance due to record linkage into the reporting of their results rather than only focussing on variance due to sampling error and treating the record linkage as having no errors or variance. The approach allows calculation to be performed with the linkage information retained by the system instead of working backwards from the result to impute characteristics of the input (Harron et al., 2012; 2014).

7.6.2   Possibility of returning graph to end users

It has been proposed that instead of just returning which records for a cluster to end users, an entire graph topology could be returned which would allow end users greater flexibility in analysing data.

While this is a laudable idea, two caveats immediately present themselves:

1. End users may be ill equipped to handle richer data.

2. Handing out richer data may compromise privacy.

This is not to say provision of a graph should be avoided or forbidden, but as with the handing out of any data should be an exercise performed after due consideration of the risks and benefits.

Workflow considerations

It is true that handing out richer data may facilitate richer analyses by end users. However, end users may be ill equipped to handle richer data having been predominantly used to handling record-based data.

New tools and techniques may need to be provided to end users along with education regarding graph concepts and advantages.

Privacy considerations

The data that says how related records are to one another is exactly the kind of data one needs to perform certain types of re-identification.

Consider de-identified data that has been returned in graph form. By taking similar data and clustering it independently using similar comparison techniques (the techniques need not be identical), a second graph of the identifiable data with a similar topology to the graph of the de-identified data may be prepared. The two graphs can then be mapped onto one another, and some re-identification may be possible.

Note that this is a problem with handing out graph data to end users: *it is not a problem with the graph approach when all data is held securely.*

As with any re-identifiable data, there are strategies and techniques that already deal with the re-identification problem, including combinations of obfuscating data, trusting researchers, legal and professional consequences to misbehaviour, secure computing environments and so on.

Neither of the aforementioned caveats should necessarily stop the provision of a graph topology to end users, but such provision should be done after weighing the pros and cons of doing so.

7.6.3   Optimised cluster analysis

Some cluster analysis techniques are computationally expensive, comparing every record against every other record for which edge relationships exists. By breaking the graph into small portions, time and computational effort can be saved.

Instead of applying expensive $O(n^2)$ operations to the entire graph, a coarse breakdown of the graph can be made using transitive closure of similarity and then more computationally intensive methods applied to the sub-clusters to break them into smaller clusters.

For example, a coarse breakdown would find roughly similar records. A topological analysis would then find well-connected regions, construct clusters and break off loosely connected regions into separate clusters. This is similar to the approach taken in Finney et al. (2011) but applied to smaller clusters (although note that in that system, the data appears to be stored relationally).

In general, since no record comparison is being performed during cluster extraction, cluster extraction is O(n): the partitioning of a set of nodes into clusters takes an amount of time on average proportional to the number of nodes being partitioned, that is, a set of records can be partitioned into clusters in a single pass through the set.

7.6.4   Other link types

So far, only weighted comparison edges, clerical review edges and equivalence edges have been discussed explicitly. However, just as the node types may be heterogeneous, so may the link types, and as many link types as desired may be added to the graph along with suitable extensions to the EdgePolicy strategy implementation.

Familial and social relationships
Family, clan, tribal and other social structure information can be added to the graph with the addition of suitable link types. Work is underway at SANT DataLink to encapsulate both Western and Aboriginal and Torres Strait Islander familial relationships.

Such links may not necessarily be used as part of conventional linkage, but their presence allows new types of linkages and data comparisons to be made. It also allows, for example, the different records for mother and child in, say, perinatal datasets to be associated with one another using an appropriately specific link type.

This is a complex issue necessitating extremely flexible link types, in which the NGLMS is well suited to handle having been designed with it in mind. Relationships can vary with the context of that relationship and the same relationship name used for different relationships, for example, the specification of a *gestational/birth* context is appropriate for capturing information regarding parturition events. It is significant to note that the gestational/birth mother may be different to the genetic mother in the case of surrogacy and different to the legal mother in the case of adoption.

Genetic similarity/genomic information
Genomic information may be inserted into the graph database as weighted edges representing genetic similarity.

Geolocation and temporal information
A spatial layer may be added to the graph indicating physical proximity, or a spatio-temporal aspect added to the graph indicating when and where individuals might have come into contact. Such information is important during outbreak tracking. Indeed, the dynamic nature of the graph approach is idea for the fluid and rapidly evolving data management demands of communicable disease outbreak detection, investigation and control.

Arbitrary link types
As mentioned, the edge types are not constrained. Providing that a policy is devised to say what they *mean* and therefore how they behave, any relational information may be captured in the graph.

7.7   Conclusion

A graph-based approach to linked data management provides advantages over a relational approach with no loss of functionality given a suitable choice of graph implementation.

Some of the advantages are:

- A greater degree of parallelism in handling data.

- Multiple 'linkages' may coexist for one dataset.

- Linkages and datasets may be included or 'turned on and off' ad hoc.

- The full history of data may be retained.

- Historical linkages and their effects may be removed.

- Different clusterings may be performed at different thresholds.

- Graph topology rather than just a list of records may be supplied downstream.

- More advanced cluster analysis techniques (which may be more expensive computationally) may be applied to sub-graphs rather than the whole graph.

- Other link types may be added to the database other than weighted field match links.

The computer science relating to graphs is mature, and the technology relating to graph storage is readily available in both commercial and free, proprietary and open-source form (see Buerli (2012)) although this omits some recent graph offerings such as Titan (Aurelius, 2012–2014).

Conversion from a 'master list' approach to a 'graph approach' can be done with no loss of existing clusterings.

A relational approach to storing data is useful where data 'columns' often need to be summarised, for example, the total of all sales or the average of a subset of all ages, but it is less useful for highly connected data where the connections between data items are of interest. Such queries over relationally stored data often have a high complexity and thus an associated time cost because of the way queries must be expressed. There is often also a large space cost since in order to speed up queries the large amount of data is loaded into memory. By storing the data in a graph form which explicitly captures and therefore allowed the exploitation of relationship information, the system is optimised for queries based around how records are related to one another, and both time and memory costs can be kept lower. It is worth noting that while the cost of space may be less significant as storage capacity increases and storage costs come down, where algorithms have a significant time complexity, the cost of algorithms and processes that take a long time to complete can result in significant real-world costs. When space is not an issue, reducing the time cost of algorithms leads to greater benefits than reducing space costs.

As more and more data are collected and linked, more modern, scalable and flexible storage and algorithmic techniques will need to be brought to bear to cope with the explosion of available data. Whereas algorithms based on relational structures and comparisons have a complexity greater than linear complexity, the graph partitioning algorithms have a complexity that is linear on the number of nodes involved. The graph-based approach most naturally represents and allows the exploitation of which it is most desirable to capture the relationship between data items.

Acknowledgements

The author would like to acknowledge Dr Tim Churches for reviewing the text and Chris Radbone and SANT DataLink.

The SANT DataLink activities are part of an initiative of the Australian government being conducted as part of the Population Health Data Linkage Network (National Collaborative Research Infrastructure Strategy 2013 (PHRN, 2013)).

8

Large-scale linkage for total populations in official statistics

Owen Abbott, Peter Jones and Martin Ralphs
Office for National Statistics, London, UK

8.1 Introduction

The population and housing census can be considered as one of the 'pillars' of national statistical systems (Valente, 2012). Traditionally, extensive data collection fieldwork was used. This is still the case in many countries. However, some nations operate a population register, allowing them to move away from expensive large-scale data collection. This chapter reviews approaches to linking records in support of censuses carried out using traditional methods and by linking administrative data across population registers. It considers new and emerging challenges for record linkage in the context of official statistics, in particular the trend for the increased use of administrative sources to replace or complement survey data.

The global economic climate has resulted in pressure on the public sector to maximise efficiency. National Statistical Institutes (NSIs) across the world are facing the challenge of maintaining quality with reduced resources. This is combined with a global trend of falling response rates in official surveys, particularly in the context of socio-demographic statistics (e.g. see Parry-Langdon, 2011). The result is a drive to make increased use of administrative data. It is hoped that such data might present opportunities for improving the quality or timeliness of estimates, facilitating greater efficiencies and reducing respondent burden that is a feature of official surveys. Governments collect and hold data about individuals as a necessary function of providing public services. Such data are referred to as 'administrative data' and include benefit claimant records, tax records and registers of births and deaths among many others. Such data are already being used within the production of official statistics in many countries. For example, the National Health Service Central Register is a key source for estimates of internal migration in the United Kingdom, the Australian Taxation Office data are used to estimate wages and earnings for small areas in Australia (Australian Bureau of

Methodological Developments in Data Linkage, First Edition. Edited by Katie Harron, Harvey Goldstein and Chris Dibben.
© 2016 John Wiley & Sons, Ltd. Published 2016 by John Wiley & Sons, Ltd.

Statistics, 2013), and in many of the Nordic countries, administrative registers provide the majority of data for population censuses (Valente, 2012).

Many countries are exploring or implementing alternative models of census data collection (e.g. see Dygaszewicz, 2012; Federal Statistical Office, 2012a; ONS, 2014a). Since the 1970s, census outputs have been derived from sets of linked registers in countries where administrative registers are used to record key information. This approach, pioneered in the Nordic countries, has the advantage of eliminating the response burden for citizens and potentially providing data annually (Valente, 2012). The key enabler is the availability of a complete population register together with a unique personal identifier, used for linking registers. The main limitation is that data available as inputs to the process are restricted to the available variables in the public registers. In addition, these often do not directly measure the variable of interest, for instance, the exact International Labour Organisation definition of unemployment. In some cases (notably in the Netherlands), administrative data are linked to survey data sources to enable estimation or mass imputation of missing variables (Schulte-Nordholt, 2009).

This chapter first discusses the use of record linkage technology in traditional censuses, including a case study from the 2011 England and Wales Census where the Census was linked to a post-enumeration survey to assess Census coverage. The chapter then reviews the different approaches taken in countries which operate a population register instead of large data collections to derive population-level statistics. Finally, the challenges for the future of record linkage in official statistics are demonstrated through the research being undertaken by the Office for National Statistics (ONS) to explore population-level linkage of anonymised records.

8.2   Current practice in record linkage for population censuses

8.2.1   Introduction

Linkage methods have been applied to many different aspects of traditional census taking. Uses include the collection operation, evaluating collected data or as an input to analyses using census data. Examples of use in the census operation include the 2011 England and Wales Census construction of an address register through linking a number of address sources (ONS, 2012a) and the 2011 Canadian Census using income tax data to provide personal income details (where responders had indicated that they were content for their data to be linked).

Censuses are linked to other data sources for a wide range of analytical applications. The UK Censuses are linked to social surveys to estimate weights for survey non-response bias adjustments to all survey outputs throughout the intercensal period (Weeks et al., 2013). Australia, New Zealand and the United Kingdom use longitudinal studies, which link samples from successive censuses and administrative data, to permit in-depth studies into ageing, social mobility and cancer incidence. Projects to link the census to other data are also undertaken, such as the New Zealand Census-Mortality Study (Blakely, Woodward and Salmond, 2000) which used anonymous census data in a probabilistic linkage.

Evaluating collected data is where linkage is used most frequently. The US Census Bureau have used linkage methods for de-duplication since the 1990 Census (see Chapter 2),

Statistics Canada linked their census at individual level to administrative records in order to evaluate the coverage of the census, and the Basque Statistics Office linked their 2001 Census to the Labour Force Survey to validate economic activity variables (Legarrete and Ayestaran, 2004). Another common application is linking census returns to a post-enumeration survey to measure the coverage of the Census, usually using some form of capture–recapture methodology (see Brown, 2000; Hogan, 1992). The following section provides a case study of the linkage strategy used for this purpose in the 2011 England and Wales Census.

8.2.2   Case study: the 2011 England and Wales Census assessment of coverage

No census is perfect and inevitably some individuals are missed, for example, people in hospital or temporarily overseas. This undercount does not usually occur uniformly across all geographical areas, or across subgroups of the population (such as age and sex groups). Many census takers put in place procedures to measure undercount and over-count (cases where persons are counted incorrectly), for example, the Canadian Reverse Record Check (Dolson, 2010).

The 2011 England and Wales Census included a coverage assessment process to measure the population that was missed, mainly using a large post-enumeration survey called the Census Coverage Survey (CCS). The methodology described by Abbott (2009) included a capture–recapture approach (also referred to as dual system estimation) to estimate the population, treating the Census and the CCS as two independent attempts to count the population in a given area. Capture–recapture was developed initially for estimating the size of wildlife populations (see Petersen, 1896), requiring the identification of those observed in both capture processes. In the census context, this means that the census records must be linked to those captured by the coverage survey to identify those that were in both. The estimate of the total population T for a sampled area is then

$$\hat{T} = \frac{cs}{m} \tag{8.1}$$

where c is the census total for an area, s is the survey total for the same area and m is the number of linked records in that area. This estimate is unbiased provided a number of assumptions are met, including zero linkage errors. False positive and false negative linkage errors cause bias in the population estimates. A false positive link rate of $\xi\%$ will give rise to an error in the estimate of approximately $-\xi\%$, and a false negative link rate of $\psi\%$ will lead to a $\psi\%$ bias in the estimates (Brown, 2000). This is clearly undesirable, and therefore, the linkage strategy must be designed to achieve extremely low error rates. For instance, the ONS (2013a) reports a target of less than 0.1% false positive errors. In the absence of a unique identifier such as that from a population register, this presents a particular challenge.

However, the Census and CCS questionnaires and data processing procedures can be designed with this aim in mind. For instance, the collection and capture of forenames and surnames, dates of birth and the accurate geocoding of addresses all provide data for efficient computer-based linkage. Quality standards for data capture and coding can be set. In addition, the questionnaires themselves can also be made available to a team of clerical staff who can deal with the more difficult or marginal decisions which can help minimise error rates. It was not feasible in terms of time and cost to perform a clerical linkage exercise for all records contained in the CCS sample due to its size (350 000 households). A combination of automatic and clerical linkage strategies was used.

Such an approach was used in both the 2001 and 2011 England and Wales Censuses. A hierarchical strategy for linking the CCS to the Census was developed for the 2001 Census by Baxter (1998). The strategy was designed with the aim of minimising linkage errors. Firstly, a deterministic method (exact linkage) was used to link those records with identical information. Probabilistic score-based[1] linkage was then used both to determine those links that are certain enough not to require clerical resolution and to narrow the clerical exercise by presenting potential candidates for clerical resolution. The thresholds for automatically linking were derived by clerical inspection of samples of candidate pairs across the probability distribution. The thresholds were chosen conservatively so that the probability of errors was extremely small. Clerical effort was then focussed on cases that fell below the thresholds. A final stage of clerical linkage identified the status of the remaining unlinked records. All of these phases took advantage of the hierarchical data structure by using the relationship between individual records and households. The extensive clerical checking is essentially what makes this strategy different from those where a larger error rate can be tolerated, and therefore, more computer-based links can be accepted without expensive clerical checking.

The remainder of this section will focus on the probabilistic methods used in 2001 and 2011 for the automated part of the strategy. The ONS (2012b) provides more information on the clerical aspects.

There were two main phases of Census to CCS linkage: at the household level and the individual level. Within these phases, there were a number of iterations using different blocking variables, linkage variables and linkage functions. A degree of flexibility was required to enable potential links to be considered even if they were excluded in an early first stage. Table 8.1 shows an overview of the automatic linkage process.

8.2.2.1   The 2001 Census: the use of Copas–Hilton

For the 2001 Census, the approach outlined by Copas and Hilton (1990) was used. The idea behind the Copas–Hilton approach is to study the distribution of errors that are likely to arise in the variables within files intended for linkage. The distribution of errors can be studied

Table 8.1   Process-level view of Census to CCS automatic linkage.

Step	Description
1	Input variables go through the standardisation process
2	Exact linkage at the household level
3	Probabilistic linkage of unlinked households
4(i)	Exact linkage of individuals within the set of linked households
4(ii)	Exact linkage of individuals within the set of unlinked households
5(i)	Probabilistic linkage of residual individuals belonging to linked households
5(ii)	Probabilistic linkage of residual individuals belonging to unlinked households
6	The residual units that are not linked are submitted for clerical review

[1] Score-based linking in this chapter refers to the derivation of a numerical score which indicates the strength of agreement. This could be, for example, from a probabilistic framework or a string comparison metric.

using (large) 'training data', consisting of pairs of records, each pair known to correspond to the same individual. Copas and Hilton (1990) suggested a number of modelling approaches, each dependent on the structure of the underlying linkage variable. The fitted models can then be used in the specification of a record linkage algorithm for multiple variables, assuming statistical independence between fields in order to combine the information to provide a global measure of the evidence for a link.

Two models were used: the likelihood ratio and the Hit–Miss model. These models were fitted to training data, and the resulting parameters used to estimate the likelihood of agreement between each variable for record pairs. The likelihood ratios were summed, assuming independence, to provide an overall score indicating the strength of records being the same individual. This score was compared against a threshold to indicate whether a record pair should be linked or reviewed clerically.

Likelihood ratio model

This was used when a linkage variable contained only a few possible outcomes, for example, gender, marital status and tenure. A probabilistic weight was estimated using training data for every possible outcome combination for a linkage variable. For example, a terraced house was more likely to be incorrectly recorded as semi-detached than as detached for a true record pair. The gender of an individual however is less likely to be encoded incorrectly, reflected by a lower probability weight for that event.

The likelihood ratio for a linkage variable was estimated directly using a large linked file obtained from the 1999 Census rehearsal. The rehearsal data were sufficiently representative, containing examples of true and false candidate record pairs. Likelihood ratios were estimated by examining the correspondence of true to false record pairs for each possible variable outcome using these training data. These parameters were updated as real 2001 Census data were fully linked.

This approach to parameter estimation was only feasible for linkage variables with few outcomes. A large sample was required which contained a sufficient number of examples for each possible outcome. Poor estimation of each outcome combination would impact on the accuracy of the model for linkage.

Hit–Miss model

When a linkage variable had a large number of possible outcomes (e.g. day or month of birth), the Hit–Miss model was used. Hit–Miss is a probability model for how potential typographical errors between paired records relating to the same underlying individual true pair occur. The distribution of a hit (two records link on a variable), a miss (two records disagreeing on a variable) and a blank (missing value in either or both records) was modelled. As with the likelihood model, a large linked file was required to estimate the distribution of hit, miss and blanks for true and false record pairs.

Assumptions

The Copas–Hilton approach is dependent on a number of assumptions. The first key assumption is that there will be a sufficient sample of representative data in order to estimate the model parameters directly. This sample requires a sufficient number of true links and non-linked record pairs. A second problem with the Copas–Hilton approach is over-fitting, that is, the problem of estimating the probabilistic linkage model well to one set of records to the detriment of making good predictions from another. There were problems of over-fitting in

2001 where the linkage variable weights converged to predict true linked pairs for a specific demographic of England and Wales. In areas of high diversity, the linkage model provided poor predictive power due to over-fitting. As a result, increased clerical linkage was required. Lastly, the Copas–Hilton approach was not a well-studied or applied method. The 2001 Census was one of the first examples of its application.

8.2.2.2   The 2011 Census: the use of Fellegi–Sunter

Following evaluation of the 2001 Census approach, the choice of probabilistic framework was explored with a view to using a Fellegi–Sunter model. There is a large body of research and practical application of this model (see Chapter 2 of this volume). One of the attractions was that this could overcome some of the Copas–Hilton issues discussed previously.

A solution to the problems of parameter estimation and model over-fitting is to adopt an automated approach such as Expectation–Maximisation (EM). At present, there is not a well-defined EM procedure for the Copas–Hilton models. The problem of parameter estimation for the Fellegi–Sunter and the wider naïve Bayes models has been studied in depth (see Chapter 2 of this volume).

Previous international census experience shows that there are five conditions when EM will work well (see Chapter 2): (i) the proportion of links (M) is greater than 0.05; (ii) the classes of links (M) and non-links (U) are well separated; (iii) typographical error within variables is low; (iv) there must be a sufficient number of linkage variables that overcome errors in others (e.g. a large number of good linkage variables); and (v) the estimated parameters provide good classification rules. All five conditions were expected for the 2011 Census, and so on that basis, a Fellegi–Sunter approach was implemented.

For the probabilistic linkage of households, the blocking strategy used was to firstly block on postcode (a postcode contains around 20 households, and postcode is generally well recorded) and as a second pass block on groups of local authorities (LAs) and the Soundex code of the household representative's surname. The second pass allowed for postcode errors but limited the comparison space to similar surnames. Within these blocks, the linkage variables were:

(a) *Address name or number*

   Given the postcode level blocking, this will normally be a unique identifier. Exceptions are where more than one household/address shares an address point. Overall, it is a powerful linking variable with few instances of misreporting, bad data capture or missing information. The effectiveness of this variable was increased by sorting the alphanumeric characters into alphabetical order and linking on each of the first three characters individually. This allows for partial agreement where one digit has been wrongly coded (e.g. 17 and 17A) and for variations in format (e.g. flat 5 84, 5/84, 84/5 will all be sorted as 4, 5, 8).

(b) *Soundex of head of household's surname*

   This was also a very powerful linking variable, truncated to a maximum of four characters. Different value-specific weights were used for England, Scotland, Wales and Northern Ireland to capture the variation in frequency of surnames.

(c) *Accommodation type*

This variable only had seven possible values, such as 'semi-detached', but it did help to distinguish otherwise similar households.

(d) *Number of people in household*

Although the number of three- or four-person households in an area is likely to be high, the more unusual household sizes helped to distinguish between households.

Linkage variables were chosen that were independent, not also used for blocking, and not used in the subsequent analysis of census coverage (e.g. year of birth or sex) to minimise the risk of matching error patterns being correlated with coverage rates. Lookup files were created to contain the weights for each variable and name frequency lists, calculated from 2001 Census data. For some variables, regional variation was significant enough to use different weights in different areas, for example, to capture surname variation between England and Wales.

For the probabilistic linkage of individuals, linked households were considered first. Comparing individuals within linked households limited potential comparisons for each individual to no more than four or five. This hierarchical linkage allowed for greater confidence in links so thresholds were lower than those used in the household linkage. The probabilistic process compared individuals outside of linked households at a later stage, but if a potential link was found, this was never automatically linked, but sent for clerical review. The linkage variables for individuals were:

(a) *Name*

Forename and surname were both used. Using forename as well as surname was important because individuals are linked while blocking on households where individuals are likely to have the same surname. Using forename did not completely eliminate the problem as in some cases a mother and daughter or father and son have the same forename.

(b) *Date of birth*

Year of birth could not be used for matching as age was an analysis variable. However, day and month were both used separately. With the obvious exception of twins, it was unusual for any two people in the same household to have the same birthday. Same-sex twins share the same demographic characteristics so incorrectly linking one with the other will not affect the estimation process. Different-sex twins could cause an error but were picked up by clerical checks of close links.

(c) *Marital status*

This variable had a limited number of possible values; however, it helped to distinguish between cases such as a father and son who had the same forename and same birthday or where only partial information was available.

(d) *Relationship to head of household*

This variable provided additional information for borderline cases, provided the algorithm used to identify the head of household worked consistently.

Updating thresholds

As linked Census and CCS data became available, the household and individual-level thresholds were updated. Within the automatic linkage process, scores were normalised to a 0–1 scale. The initial automatic linking thresholds were set at 0.95 at household level and 0.88 at individual level. The linkage algorithm was applied without the command to automatically process any matches. The potential combinations were examined in detail clerically to inform the threshold that should be set to ensure all matches assigned automatically by the software are correct. These were reviewed clerically on a periodic basis, especially when processing areas with different demographic characteristics.

8.2.2.3   Automatic link rates for the 2011 Census

This section summarises the results from the automatic linkage stage for both households and persons.

The ONS (2012b) provides full details of the linkage rates. A total of 198 164 households and 451 736 persons were automatically linked across the CCS sample contained in the 348 LAs in England and Wales. This gave an overall household automatic link rate of 60% and an overall person automatic link rate of 70%.

The household automatic link rates for each LA ranged from 1 to 87% with a median of 68%. The person automatic link rates ranged from 38 to 94% with a median of 73%.

The six LAs with the lowest household automatic link rate were among the first to be linked automatically and were moved into the clerical linkage phase despite low link rates, while the automatic linkage algorithms were optimised for subsequent areas.

8.2.2.4   Overall quality of the 2011 linkage processes

This section outlines the overall quality of the linkage, which includes the later clerical and manual stages. Following the completion of the linkage process, a sample of areas were selected for relinking which involved an independent team repeating the clerical linkage phase in order to assess the quality of the linkage process and the decisions made as described by the ONS (2013a). This information helped to establish the effect that linkage accuracy had on the population estimate. The relinking was performed by experienced linkers, and to ensure independence, no one relinked an area that they had worked on originally.

This process identified decisions that had the same outcome both originally and at relinking and also decisions that had different outcomes. The sample contained a total of 83 356 original link decisions, representing approximately 17% of the original linkage decisions. For sets of decisions that had different outcomes, these were checked to identify which decision was correct.

From the sample, 229 errors in the original linkage were identified (0.27% of total decisions). These errors were classified as 63 incorrect links and 166 missed links. These translate into an overall precision of 99.9% and sensitivity of 99.75%. Further classification and analysis of the error rates by area types and teams were reported by the ONS (2013a). The conclusion was that the quality of the linkage between the 2011 Census and the CCS was very high as was required. Nevertheless, it took a significant amount of clerical resource to achieve this.

8.3   Population-level linkage in countries that operate a population register: register-based censuses

8.3.1   Introduction

A register-based census is a method of producing data on population, households and dwellings by linking together existing administrative and statistical data sources without using large-scale fieldwork enumeration. Many countries are investigating the possibility of using more administrative data for statistical purposes. The United Nations Economic Commission for Europe (2007) outlined three key prerequisites for undertaking such a project:

(a) *Legislation which enables the linkage of data from different sources*

Legislation provides a key foundation for the use of administrative data sources for statistical purposes. National legislation will happen if there is a broadly held view that it makes good sense to take advantage of existing administrative data sources rather than collect data for statistical purposes. For example, all Nordic countries have a national statistics act that gives the NSI the right to access identifiable unit level administrative data and to link them with other administrative registers for statistical purposes. Furthermore, the statistics act provides a detailed definition of data protection.

(b) *Establishment of appropriate administrative and/or statistical sources with a unique identifier (e.g. personal identification number, address)*

One major factor that facilitates the statistical use of administrative data is the use of unified identification systems across different sources. In their absence, it is difficult to link different registers, which is central to register-based statistics production. A minimum requirement is to have a unified identification system for base registers.

(c) *Appropriate topics in the sources which cover all demands of users and legislation*

The first country to undertake a completely register-based census was Denmark in 1981. They used their central population register, established in 1964, as the backbone for the register-based Census. The personal identification number was used to link the population register to other registers and administrative sources. However, this was not the earliest use of a population register within a census. Both Finland and Norway used their central population registers in their 1970 Censuses, having operated their registers since 1969 and 1964, respectively.

A number of countries have adopted such an approach. In the 2010 round of censuses in the UNECE region, a review of approaches by Valente (2012) found that eight countries (Andorra, Austria, Belgium, Denmark, Finland, Norway, Slovenia and Sweden (Statistics Sweden, 2001)) used a register-only-based approach, five used registers combined with surveys (Iceland, Israel, Netherlands, Switzerland and Turkey) and a further eight (Czech Republic, Estonia, Italy, Latvia, Liechtenstein, Lithuania, Poland and Spain) used registers combined with a full enumeration.

In terms of linkage technology, the availability of a unique person level identification number allows highly accurate linkage between sources, and therefore, in many cases, there is no need for probabilistic techniques. However, in some cases, the linkage does require some backup in the form of clerical resolution for cases where a link was not possible.

In Switzerland, a population register and an annual set of surveys are linked using their unique social security number. This approach was adopted in 2010. During introduction and development of the system, they found that it was inevitable that a small number of people were not yet assigned a social security number or that their number had to be subsequently corrected. In such cases, links to register data were attempted using family name, first name, date of birth and address. Processing cases which cannot be linked through identifiers was found to be very time-consuming, but at the end, there were less than 0.5% unmatched records (Swiss Federal Statistical Office, 2012).

The following sections provide brief case studies for four countries, one which uses a register only (Finland), one which combines a population register with surveys (the Netherlands) and one which uses registers and some form of enumeration (Poland). The fourth case study is the only country in Europe that uses a population register but without a unique identification number (Germany).

8.3.2   Case study 1: Finland

In Finland, the central population register was founded in 1969. The establishment of the register and the introduction of the personal identity number into the compilation of statistics was a significant change which enabled the combination of individual-level data. The central population register was used for the first time for pre-filling personal data in the 1970 Population Census, although the distribution and collection of questionnaire forms were still completed with the help of the population registration organisation. Income data for the Census were derived from the taxation register. In this Census, data from two nationwide registers were combined with the help of personal identity numbers for the first time in Finland.

Over the 1970s, several administrative registers were set up in the country, and their coverage and quality level were judged to be reliable enough to utilise as source data for population censuses. In the 1980 population Census, the majority of the demographic and qualification data were for the first time drawn from registers, again using the personal identity number for linkage. The census questionnaires collected missing information, such as place of work and occupation.

In 1990, the population Census was conducted totally on the basis of register data. Finland was the second country after Denmark to compile the population and housing census using only data collected from registers and administrative records. Since 1990, data from over 30 registers have been used for population censuses, making it possible to produce all population census data yearly.

However, as Statistics Finland (2004) notes, there are some items in the Finnish register system where data linking has caused difficulty. The employment pension data do not use the same business code as the taxation and business registers, and therefore, extra work is needed to link individuals to the company where they are employed. Likewise, the linking of enterprises to the building where they are based is not always straightforward since the company address data are not necessarily fully accurate, or they may differ from the information in the buildings register. However, no information on linkage accuracy is published.

8.3.3   Case study 2: The Netherlands Virtual Census

The Dutch system is based upon their central population register, which is a combination of municipal population registers. The last Dutch census was in 1971, after which public objection to the burden of the census resulted in its cancellation (Schulte-Nordholt, Hartgers and Gircour, 2004). As an alternative, the Netherlands linked available administrative data to the population register using their unique social security and fiscal (SoFi) number, a personal identifier for every registered Dutch inhabitant. The use of the SoFi number is widespread and is considered normal for all citizens. However, there are some issues with a limited amount of SoFi numbers being abused, for example, by illegal workers. This results in false matches. For example, when the jobs register and the population register are linked, a worker might turn out to be an infant or show an unusually high income, which is actually the total income of all people using the same SoFi number (Schulte-Nordholt, Hartgers and Gircour, 2004).

The approach to producing detailed attribute statistics here is different to that in other Nordic countries such as Sweden, as there are not as many variables available in the registers. Survey data are used to supplement administrative data for those topics not available. However, in household sample surveys, like the Labour Force Survey, records do not have a SoFi number. For those surveys, an alternative linkage key is used, which is often built up by a combination of sex, date of birth and address. In its linkage strategy, Statistics Netherlands tries to maximise the number of links and to minimise the number of false links. So, in order to achieve a higher linkage rate, more efforts are made to link the remaining unlinked records by means of different variants of the linkage key, for example, leaving out the house number and tolerating variations in the numeric characters of the postal code. Overall, around 97% of Labour Force Survey records can be linked to the population register (Schulte-Nordholt, Hartgers and Gircour, 2004). From 2004, the population register was used as a sampling frame for the Labour Force Survey, thus removing the need for this linkage for the 2011 Virtual Census.

To produce census statistics, Statistics Netherlands developed a repeated weighting procedure (Schulte-Nordholt, Hartgers and Gircour, 2004) which allows the production of a set of consistent population-level tables from combined data together with estimates of their quality.

8.3.4   Case study 3: Poland

Poland adopted a unique approach in their 2011 Census as described by Dygaszewicz (2012). Prior to the 2011 Census, they combined 28 administrative sources from government, local government and administrators outside public administration such as real estate administrators and telecommunication operators. These combined data provided values of most census variables, both at the stage of creating a specification of census units (population and housing census) and for qualitative comparisons. Due to a stable system of identifiers (personal identification number and also a dwellings register), it was possible to merge data from different registers and from statistical surveys, including sample surveys. The Polish statistics office has the right to access all unit data stored in information sources of the public and commercial sectors, through specific legislation. The obtained data included necessary identifiers and personal data supporting the linkage of data from different sources. The Census was then carried out completely electronically by initially asking the population to log into a secure web service and then check and update the details from the linked administrative sources and complete questions related to topics that could not be obtained through administrative data. Follow-up computer-assisted personal interviews (CAPI) were available for those with no web access. A 2% survey was also used to check the quality of resulting data.

8.3.5   Case study 4: Germany

Germany has a series of population registers which are maintained in a decentralised way by approximately 12 500 municipalities in about 5 400 computing centres, but there is no unique identifier which would allow them to be combined easily to create a national register or allow easy linkage with other sources. In addition, there is no central register of buildings and addresses.

Federal Statistical Office (2012b) describes how a temporary statistical register of addresses and buildings (Anschriften- und Gebäuderegister – AGR) was set up specifically for purposes of the 2011 Census. To set up the AGR, geo-referenced address data of the land surveying administration, data from the population registers and the registers of persons of the Federal Employment Agency were used. Setting up the AGR required combining data sources by linking text (street names). It is used, first, as the statistical population underlying the census of buildings and housing and, second, as a sampling frame for the 10% census household survey was drawn.

Federal Statistical Office (2012a) outlines the linkage of the municipal population registers to obtain population counts. They are combined into an overall national dataset, linking each record to the temporary address register outlined earlier. However, as an individual is legally allowed to be registered in more than one location, the registers are inflated. In addition, the lack of a unique personal identifier does not provide an easy way to solve this. Therefore, duplicates are identified through a set of variables suited to identify persons (including names, date of birth, gender and place of birth). However, this requires much more effort than data combination by means of numerical identifiers. For duplicate cases which were defined to be incorrect (a person with a main residence and a secondary residence), a questionnaire was used to collect data to determine the correct place of residence. These combined register data are then used as core data to ascertain both the number of inhabitants and information on the demographic structure of the population living in private households.

Lastly, a sample survey conducted among less than 10% of the population assures quality of the population register data by ascertaining, for every municipality, the rates of outdated entries and missing entries and taking these rates into account when determining the number of inhabitants of the municipalities. The survey also collects additional data that cannot be obtained from registers. Thus, the census is closer to a 10% sample census, with a large coverage survey providing coverage adjustments for the combined population register.

8.3.6   Summary

This section has demonstrated that in most countries which do not operate a traditional census, the use of a population register with a unique personal identifier means that statistical data linkage technology is generally not required. Instead, any effort is focussed on clerical resolution for a small proportion of records for which the unique identifier is not available. However, in cases where a unique identifier is not available, such as in Germany, standard techniques are used to de-duplicate and link sources.

While the availability of large registers facilitates this, one issue not always addressed is that of hard to count or hard to register populations such as temporary workers or illegal immigrants. These can be important and moreover there may be incentives to falsify any IDs they may be given or for certain groups to remain anonymous. This results in either coverage or linkage problems (as noted in the Netherlands case study). Organisations using a population register find it hard to deal with these, as it is not desirable to publicly acknowledge the existence of these populations. There are only a few cases where there have been attempts to specifically include such populations, measure coverage or linkage accuracy, and these are generally internal unpublished reviews. In contrast, the issue of hard-to-count populations is a well-known problem for traditional censuses. Efforts to improve data collection and measure coverage errors have developed significantly since the 1970s (see, e.g. Abbott and Compton, 2014, US Government Accountability Office, 2010 and the case study in Section 8.2.2). It is clear that while a population register-based approach has advantages over a traditional census, the quality of the linkage, and resulting statistics, is harder to quantify.

The next section outlines the exploration of administrative data in England and Wales as an alternative to a census. In this particular case, many standard linkage techniques cannot be used as data is anonymised prior to linkage.

8.4   New challenges in record linkage: the Beyond 2011 Programme

8.4.1   Introduction

In May 2010, the UK Statistics Authority asked the ONS to begin a review of the future provision of population statistics in England and Wales in order to inform government and parliament about the options for the next census. In response, the ONS set up the Beyond 2011 Programme to undertake this work. The programme has since undertaken extensive research and consultation into new approaches to counting the population and reviewed practices in other countries, culminating in the National Statistician making her recommendation in March 2014 (ONS, 2014a).

A key focus of this work has been the research into making better reuse of administrative data. The ONS has taken a decision to anonymise administrative data prior to linkage to ensure that high levels of anonymity and privacy are maintained. Several strands of work under the Beyond 2011 research programme involve working with large quantities of personal information relating to everyone in England and Wales, obtained from a range of administrative sources. It is recognised that the planned approach of linking multiple administrative sources might elevate the associated risks relating to the privacy of data about people and households. Further information on the policy for safeguarding data during the research phase of the Beyond 2011 Programme can be found in the ONS (2013b).

To inform the discussion as to whether anonymised data can be used for producing population-level official statistics, this section outlines the methodological challenges of developing a linking process that gives suitably low levels of linking error. The ONS research into development of administrative data models will continue, with the expectation that they will be run in parallel with the next Census in 2021.

8.4.2   Beyond 2011 linkage methodology

Data linkage has a vital role in options being researched. One of the major challenges for administrative data options is to exclude individuals listed on administrative data but who are no longer resident in the population. Data linkage will identify individuals that appear on multiple administrative sources and therefore have a higher likelihood of being in the *usually resident* population.[2] The linkage process is crucial in determining rules to construct a 'statistical population dataset' (SPD) that can be used in a process for estimating the population. An SPD is essentially a count of the population from administrative data, as an alternative to undertaking a census enumeration nationally. More information about the construction of SPDs and the rules that have been formulated from administrative data linkage are reported in the ONS (2013c; 2014b).

Additionally, data linkage is likely to play a significant role in estimating the population. In order to make accurate adjustments for under-coverage and over-coverage on administrative data, current thinking is that it will be necessary to link the SPD to a population coverage survey to a very high standard. Further information about the population coverage survey design is reported in the ONS (2013d). Linkage error is of particular concern when linking the SPD to a population coverage survey. Errors will inflate or deflate population estimates under a dual system estimation model as explained in Section 8.2.2. The linkage strategy in the 2011 Census used a combination of exact and score-based linking and clerical searching. Using clerical resources ensured false positives and negatives were minimised, enabling accurate Census population estimates.

Table 8.2 illustrates links that can be made using conventional score-based approaches or clerical resolution using full identifiers. The first pair of candidate records differs on surname only. A string comparison algorithm can provide a similarity score between the two surnames. The overall link score can be calculated as an un-weighted mean. The decision to accept a link can be automated by the score exceeding a specified threshold, for example, 0.95. This threshold may have been established from previous linkage exercises or by inspecting samples of candidate records at various points of the score distribution, for example, around 0.95. The

Table 8.2   Examples of score-based auto-linking and clerical linking.

Source 1				Source 2			
Forename	Surname	DOB	Postcode	Forename	Surname	DOB	Postcode
Sarah	Johnston	22/10/1982	PO15 1HS	Sarah	Johnson	22/10/1982	PO15 1HS
Michael	Smyth	13/02/1970	PO15 1HR	Mike	Smith	13/02/1970	PO11 4FF

Agreement scores				
Forename	Surname	DOB	Postcode	Link score
1	0.87	1	1	0.97
0.32	0.91	1	0.65	0.72

[2] The UN definition of *usually resident* has been adopted – that is, the place at which the person has lived continuously for at least the last 12 months, not including temporary absences for holidays or work assignments, or intends to live for at least 12 months (United Nations, 2008).

second pair of records, which have a lower link score due to a number of inconsistencies, might fail automatic linkage and would be passed for clerical investigation.

The anonymisation referred to in 8.4.1 'transforms' data in such a way that the use of clerical resolution is not possible, as well as restricting the viability of conventional score-based linking. Research at the ONS has concentrated on developing algorithms which attempt to replicate clerical processes, evaluating the linkage quality of these methods against standard methods that include clerical and score-based linkage.

8.4.3   The anonymisation process in Beyond 2011

In order to ensure a high level of privacy, all datasets with person identifiable information are held in an environment with strong physical and electronic security safeguards. Each dataset is loaded separately onto a reception server which only processes a single dataset at a time. It firstly runs a series of data preprocessing steps including geo-referencing, variable standardisation and link-key creation. Following preprocessing, data are anonymised and then moved onto the environment main servers.

A cryptographic hash function[3] is used to anonymise person identifying information including names, dates of birth and addresses. The hash function, which converts a field into a condensed representation of fixed value, is a one-way process that is not easily reversible – once the hashing algorithm is applied, it takes significant effort and the use of tools that are not available in the research environment to recover the original information. The Information Commissioner's Office (ICO's) code of practice (ICO, 2012) describes the difference between 'anonymisation' and 'pseudonymisation'. In record linkage, 'anonymisation' refers to the removal of elements from a linked dataset that would allow identification of individual persons. It is often applied after the linking process before supplying to users of the linked dataset. 'Pseudonymisation' refers to the replacement of field values in a dataset with a reference or pseudonym that is unique for each value and allows linkage between values that are in exact agreement. The hashing technique used by the ONS in this context is more strictly described as pseudonymisation, and for the remainder of the chapter, the word 'pseudonymisation' will be used.

The same hashing algorithm is used on all of the datasets to be linked together, so the same outcome values are generated for values in exact agreement. Therefore, only cases where two records are identical, that is, where names, dates of birth and addresses are recorded in precisely the same string, will an automatic exact link be possible on the hashed values. Table 8.3 shows an example of what different strings may look like after hashing and illustrates that single character differences result in different hash codes.

Once the information has been hashed, it is not possible to compare likenesses with other similar words. Examples of circumstances where this might occur include the following:

- Use of abbreviations or nicknames

- Data capture errors (resulting from discrepancies in spelling, handwriting and typing)

- Recall errors, for example, inaccurate reporting of postcodes[4] or dates of birth

---

[3] SHA-256 hash function used in combination with a secret cryptographic key (National Institute of Standards and Technology, 2012).
[4] Alphanumeric postal codes used by Royal Mail corresponding to a limited number of addresses or a single large delivery point.

Table 8.3   Examples of name and date strings transformed into hash values.

String/value to hash	Hashed value
John	8C 17 A3 BB 4C AF 71 9D 16 50 97 90 0B 39 01 61
Smith	39 E9 3E D6 6E 50 A7 EC 6B F9 4F 9B 9F CF 81 F6
Jon	86 1A 42 1C 1A 05 E0 E8 FA 24 A1 53 41 59 69 1F
John	8C 17 A3 BB 4C AF 71 9D 16 50 97 90 0B 39 01 61
Smyth	CB 36 9F C9 0A 3B A0 2E E9 9C A0 5E E0 69 84 FB
Jonathan	F4 5C C5 B7 A6 59 23 79 B8 5B 81 81 AA AD 38 50
Jonny	ED ED 5C 0E 56 00 83 84 AA 03 8F E7 02 AA AB E3
27/01/1965	4F 6E B0 E4 55 84 BC 0A 8B A3 89 B5 16 F4 49 9A
26/01/1965	2C 5A 2C 3D 80 D1 48 35 70 24 6A D8 E5 2C 94 17
27/02/1965	EC 67 CC 6D C7 23 40 84 09 E7 B5 7C DE 79 6B D4
27/01/1966	90 BF F8 D3 C5 DD 3F DB 3C 6D DC 39 AD EE E6 46
1965	10 B2 57 F8 08 7E 72 F1 2A E6 96 E4 A1 E4 26 DE
1966	5C C9 4A 4C CA E8 48 75 B5 52 68 E0 B0 C5 F3 CA

8.4.4   Beyond 2011 linkage strategy using pseudonymised data

One of the major limitations of hash encoded data is that it cannot be compared for similarity once the transformation has taken place. Consequently, some of the well-established methods for linkage are unavailable. For instance, string comparison algorithms which identify text strings that are similar are ineffectual, as are decisions that are made clerically by directly comparing candidate pairs of records side by side. Therefore, the focus has been to explore alternative approaches that can automate the linkage of pseudonymised records that do not exactly linkage. This is also a major goal in the wider field of record linkage. Methods that have been developed to tackle the issue include trusted third-party methods where a third party carries out the linkage process (Lyons et al., 2009), Bloom filter encryption where multiple hashing algorithms are applied to *n*-grams and stored in large binary arrays (Schnell, Bachteler and Reiher, 2009; 2010) and *n*-gram comparators of encrypted values where bigrams are created prior to hashing allowing the calculation of bigram similarity scores (Churches and Christen, 2004). However, these methods, at least in the short term, are not appropriate for the existing data environment. Costs and logistic complexity of setting up a third-party arrangement was not practical during initial exploratory research. Techniques such as Bloom filter encryption require further consideration of computation and communication complexity for large databases (Christen, 2012a).

The research focus has been methods that identify links that are similar but not in exact agreement when using a secure hashing algorithm. The idea is to carry out standardised intelligent preprocessing steps which allow likely differences of variables to be captured and carried through the hashing process in a non-disclosive way. A number of alternative preprocessing techniques have been explored. These alternative methods can be categorised as either:

- Deterministic or 'rule-based' linkage using link-keys or

- Score-based linkage using logistic regression

An outline of the link-key process is in Section 8.4.4.1. In order to initiate a score-based method, similarity tables for names and dates of birth are also constructed during

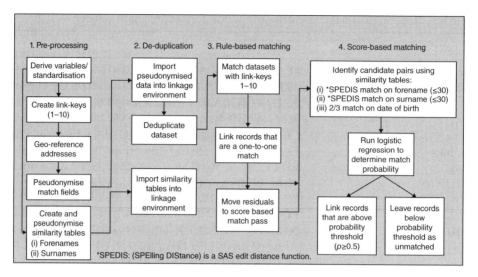

Figure 8.1   Beyond 2011 linkage strategy.

preprocessing, and this is explained in detail in Section 8.4.4.2. The modelling of decision-making through logistic regression is then outlined.

Other preprocessing methods, including the use of name clustering and Soundex algorithms, have been tested (ONS, 2013e). These methods were rejected, either because they performed poorly or because they had limited capacity to improve the algorithm. In the case of name clustering, the goal was to convert and group names into a standardised form using lookup tables prior to hash encoding. This can be achieved with the use of name dictionaries or by comparing similarities with names in public reference tables. However, this approach risks an increase in false links between names that are only marginally similar that have been grouped within the same cluster.

The Soundex algorithm encodes name strings by keeping the first letter in a string and converting remaining non-vowel characters into numbers. The Soundex codes are then hash encoded for use in name linking. This approach has been found to have the opposite effect, with names that are very similar being mapped to different Soundex codes, resulting in an increased risk of missed links. Figure 8.1 shows a flow diagram of the linking strategy. The key components of this are discussed in the subsequent sections.

8.4.4.1   Link-keys

Link-keys are concatenating variables which provide unique keys. These can be hashed and used for automated exact linkage, with the intention of eliminating discrepancies that prevent an exact link. For example, a link-key is a concatenation of the first character of forename and surname, date of birth, sex and postcode district. Figure 8.2 shows this link-key. The link-key is hashed and used to link records between data which have the same link-keys.

The strategy was to define a hierarchical series of link-keys, each designed to take account of common inconsistencies between records belonging to the same individual. These link-keys are the linking fields in a stepwise linkage process, each being a sequential 'link pass' of the deterministic phase of the linkage strategy (Gomatam et al., 2002; Karmel et al., 2011).

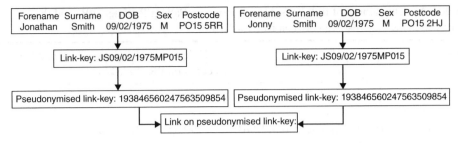

Figure 8.2   Example of link-key creation for linking records.

Such hierarchical deterministic approaches are prevalent in linkage studies across epidemiology (e.g. Li et al., 2006; Pacheco et al., 2008).

To minimise the chances of false positive links, the link-keys were designed to exhibit a high degree of uniqueness across the data. This was important in the context of population-level linkage, as simple combinations such as surname and date of birth will not be unique. For example, a concatenation of forename initial, surname initial, sex, date of birth and post-code district[5] is unique for 99.55% of NHS Patient Register (PR)[6] records in England and Wales. This limits potential false positive links, provided the postcode district and first letters of forename and surname have been correctly recorded.

Inconsistency between linking variables can occur in a number of different forms. A single link-key cannot take account of all inconsistencies that can occur between data sources. Frequency analysis of the PR for a range of variable concatenations resulted in a series of link-keys designed to take account of the most common inconsistencies. Table 8.4 presents these link-keys, their uniqueness on the PR and the type of inconsistency that each was designed to overcome. Section 8.4.5.2 evaluates the performance of this linkage strategy.

To reduce the risk of false positive links, records are only linked on a link-key if it is unique on both datasets (i.e. one-to-one link). If multiple records link on a particular link-key, then a link is not made and those candidates are passed on as a residual to the next link-key pass. This hierarchical linking process means that links made at each stage of the process are linked and removed, and the residuals are passed to the next stage. The ordering of the link-keys is important. Once two records are linked, there is no process to review the link even if the true link pair is identified at a later stage in the process. Future methodological refinements will explore whether this can be improved.

8.4.4.2   Score-based linkage

Following the exact linkage as described previously, the next stage is to pass the residuals through an algorithm that generates scores indicating strength of agreement between candidate pairs. For pseudonymised data, there are two challenges with implementing score-based methods. The first is obtaining string comparison scores for pseudonymised names and dates of birth. The second is how to combine and use similarity scores to make linkage decisions. Both issues are explored in the following.

---

[5] Postcode district is the inward part of a postcode, for example, SW19.
[6] The NHS Patient Register is a dataset containing all current GP registrations in England and Wales.

Table 8.4   Uniqueness of link-keys derived from the Patient Register (PR) and the inconsistencies they resolve between true link pairs.

Link-key		% Unique records on PR	Inconsistencies resolved by link-key
(1)	Forename, surname, DOB, sex, postcode	99.99	None – exact agreement
(2)	Forename initial, surname initial, DOB, sex, postcode district	99.55	Name/postcode discrepancies
(3)	Forename bigram,[a] surname bigram, DOB, sex, postcode area	99.44	Name discrepancies/movers in area
(4)	Forename initial, DOB, sex, postcode	99.84	Surname discrepancy
(5)	Surname initial, DOB, sex, postcode	99.44	Forename discrepancy
(6)	Forename, surname, age, sex, postcode area	99.46	DOB discrepancy/movers in area
(7)	Forename, surname, sex, postcode	99.19	DOB missing/incorrect
(8)	Forename, surname, DOB, sex	98.87	Movers out of area
(9)	Forename, surname, DOB, postcode	99.52	Sex missing/incorrect
(10)	Surname, forename, DOB, sex, postcode (linked on key 1)[b]	99.99	Forename/surname transpositions
(11)	Middle name, surname, DOB, sex, postcode	99.90[c]	Forename/middle name transpositions

[a] In this context, the bigram comprises the first two characters of the name.
[b] Key 10 has a transposition between forename and surname. A link is searched for on key 1 of the other dataset to link individuals that may have used their forename and surname interchangeably.
[c] Key 11 is not produced if middle name is not provided. This is an estimate of uniqueness for the key from records that include middle name. Linking key 11 on key 1 from the other dataset can also be used to link individuals that may have used their forename and middle name interchangeably.

String comparison scores using similarity tables

Similarity tables are an alternative to standard string comparison algorithms. The idea is to derive a lookup table of similar values for a variable, without making direct comparisons across data sources. A standard string comparison algorithm was used to provide scores between similar values for each variable. Using single variables individually (prior to hashing) was non-disclosive on the grounds that individuals were not identifiable from a forename (or surname) alone. A similar technique, utilising a public reference table of names, was proposed by Pang and Hansen (2006), although their method has been shown to perform poorly against other approximate string linking methods (Bachteler, Schnell and Reiher, 2010). However, there was a clear need to develop an approach which allowed score-based linking between candidate records. The string comparison algorithm used was the SAS[7] proprietary SPEDIS (SPElling DIStance) function, an edit distance function similar to Levenshtein distance (Yancey, 2005). This method was chosen over standard Levenshtein

---

[7] Statistical Analysis System (SAS), SAS Institute Inc.

distance and the string comparison metric Jaro–Winkler (Cohen et al., 2003a; Yancey, 2005) due to its ease of use.

Figures 8.3, 8.4 and 8.5 show how a similarity table for forenames is generated:

(a) **Dataset 1 import**: A complete list of all unique forenames is extracted from dataset 1.

(b) **Dataset 2 import**: Any forenames on the second dataset that are not already on the list are added to create a complete list of forenames between two datasets.

(c) **Create similarity table**: A copy of the list of forenames is created, and the SAS SPEDIS string comparison algorithm generates similarity scores between all possible pairings of

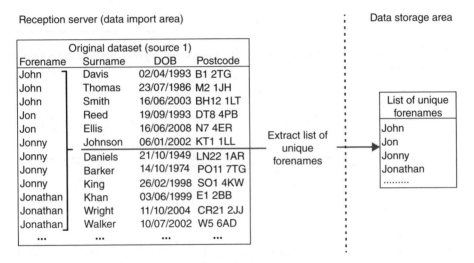

Figure 8.3   Forename extraction from dataset 1.

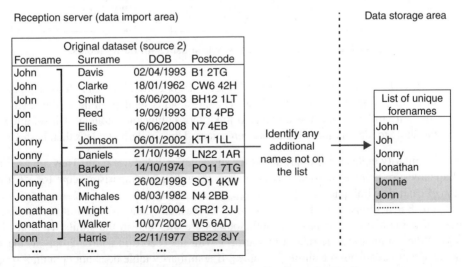

Figure 8.4   Forename extraction from dataset 2.

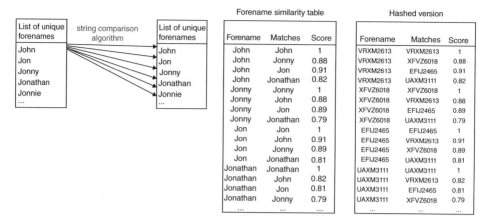

Figure 8.5   String comparison and hashing. The hash values in this example are for illustrative purposes only.

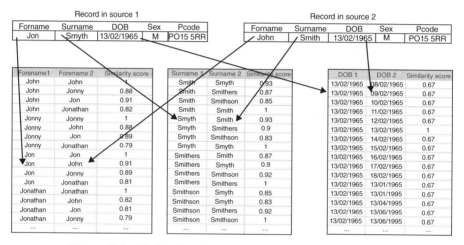

Figure 8.6   Undertake three-way join using similarity tables.

names. Name pairs above a specified threshold are retained in the table (this step purely saves space and later processing time). The threshold is set depending on the degree of similarity to be accepted as a potential link; a loose blocking strategy will set a lower threshold to identify more links between names. This similarity table is then hashed.

Hashed similarity tables are also produced for surnames and dates of birth. They are used as lookup tables for comparing pseudonymous data, providing a comparison score for identification of candidate link pairs.

Figure 8.6 demonstrates the process with 'un-hashed' data for illustrative purposes. Values of name and date of birth on both sources are included in the similarity tables by design. When comparing the record in source 1 with the record in source 2, any available scores are extracted from the similarity tables. If a similarity table does not contain a score for a particular variable comparison, it is assumed the score is zero. Note that since exact

Table 8.5   Agreement scores to be used in score-based linking.

Candidate pair ID	Forename	Surname	DOB
Candidate pair_1	0.91	0.93	0.67

comparisons are included in the similarity tables, this allows for records that are very similar, as well as records where all three variables are similar. The similarity table for forenames can also be supported with a name thesaurus that identifies links on nicknames and established abbreviations. When this information is combined, the following scores can be derived as demonstrated in Table 8.5.

The advantage of this approach is that candidate pairs that have multiple inconsistencies can be identified as potential links based on the level of agreement between forename, surname and date of birth. Having agreement scores for these variables, as well as a measure of name commonality as a percentage frequency of the name distribution, provides opportunities for score-based linkage. To support the decision-making capacity of the algorithm, additional information is also derived between link candidates. Euclidean geographic distances between candidate records are calculated using Lower Layer Super Output Area (LSOA)[8] centroid longitude and latitude coordinates. Sex agreement is also recorded as a binary classification for agreement and disagreement. A postcode agreement score has also been created with four levels representing exact, sector, district and area level agreement. All of these agreement and commonality measures can be stored alongside pseudonymised data as shown in Table 8.6.

The following section considers how decision-making regarding the match statuses of candidate pairs can be modelled with supervised training methods.

Combining similarity scores using logistic regression

Where two records have been identified as a potential match from the similarity tables, a method is required to automate the decision whether or not to declare the two records as a match (i.e. to link them). The use of regression models was tested to develop a prediction function to estimate the predicted probability of a pair of records being a match. The use of prediction functions based on statistical models can be found in many areas of research, including finance and biomedical sciences. However, these are based on the ability to validate the model through a clerical process. Both the Copas–Hilton and the Fellegi–Sunter methods make provision for estimating a score that is indicative of the probability that two records match. However, these methods have traditionally relied upon the reservation of a 'clerical region' comprising of more difficult cases that are manually determined by trained clerical resources. For a more detailed discussion, see Chapter 2.

Typically, existing linkage models depend on the identification of two threshold points in the score distribution. These points are identified by incrementally sampling n records at each point of the distribution and clerically checking the link statuses of candidate pairs. Working downwards from the top of the score distribution, the point where the sample candidates start to include non-links is set as the upper threshold, and all candidates

---

[8]LSOA – Lower Layer Super Output Area – total population between 1000 and 3000 people, average 1600 people. For an introduction to the different types of geography, see http://www.ons.gov.uk/ons/guide-method/geography/beginner-s-guide/index.html.

Table 8.6 Example of score data for link candidates derived from similarity tables.

Candidate pair ID	Forename agreement score	Surname agreement score	Forename % frequency	Surname % frequency	Postcode agreement score	Sex agreement	DOB agreement score	Distance between LSOA centroids
Candidate pair_1	0.91	0.93	0.0025	0.0014	4	1	0.67	2.1
Candidate pair_2	0.78	0.93	0.0025	0.0001	2	1	0.33	6.1
Candidate pair_3	0.69	1.00	0.0025	0.0110	3	1	0.33	31.2

with scores exceeding this point are automatically linked. The same approach is taken working upwards from the bottom end of the score distribution, with the point where sample candidates start to include true links set as the lower threshold. This incremental approach to sampling is problematic with pseudonymised data as only a small number of un-hashed candidate records will be available to researchers for clerical review. An incremental sampling approach based on a small overall sample is likely to result in less than optimal estimates for the location of the upper and lower thresholds. Furthermore, the remaining candidates that have scores lying between the two thresholds would ideally be sent for clerical resolution. Even if identifiable data were being used, this would entail a clerical linkage exercise on a very large scale and would be extremely resource intensive. Automated linkage was instead refined by introducing a single score threshold for identifying whether pairs link or not. Existing linkage models sometimes do this[9] but still clerically check the link statuses of candidate pairs. An automated approach increases the risk of both false positives and false negatives. For more difficult cases, the absence of human judgement in the decision-making requires that data for identifying the single threshold point has good coverage of the types of inconsistencies occurring between true link candidates.

In order to use a single score threshold, an overall agreement score is required. The agreement scores between the linking variables need to be appropriately weighted to generate an overall score. As an initial method, logistic regression was used to combine the agreement scores and yield a probability indicating the likelihood that candidate pairs are matches. The primary objective of logistic regression models in this context is to develop a supervised technique that can effectively be 'trained' to determine whether a particular candidate is a match or not (Köpcke and Rahm, 2008). However, the calculation of match probabilities between candidates has further benefits. They can be used in the design of stratified samples for quantifying errors in the linking algorithm, as well as informing users of linked data about the uncertainty of links made.

The predictor variables for the model consisted of the following:

- Forename similarity score

- Surname similarity score

- Date of birth agreement code (4=full, 3=M/Y, 2=D/Y, 1=D/M, 0=none)

- Sex agreement code (1=yes, 2=no)

- Postcode agreement code (4=full, 3=postcode sector, 2=postcode district, 1=postcode area, 0=none)

- Forename weight (% frequency)

- Surname weight (% frequency)

- Name count (forename and surname combined)

- Distance between LSOA centroids

---

[9] For instance, the linking methodology used by Statistics New Zealand (2006) in the Integrated Data Infrastructure Project.

In practice, a sample of un-hashed candidate records will be made available without compromising data protection policy and security safeguards. The sampling strategy is still under development; however, it is likely that stratification by age, sex and area-based characteristics (e.g. urban/rural[10]) will feature in the sample design. The sample candidates are subject to a clerical decision (match or non-match) which is used as the logistic regression response variable. The fitted model can serve as training data for the remaining candidate pairs. Logistic regression is used because it is a simple way of developing a binary classification model based on a single score threshold. Firstly, the model coefficients serve as weights for each linking variable, to generate an overall predicted probability of a link. Secondly, the regression equation can be used as a prediction function to automatically classify the remaining candidates as a match or not, depending on whether they are above or below the single threshold score. For logistic regression, a common default threshold for classifying a binary outcome is $p = 0.5$. However, when the proportions of matches and non-matches are not equal within the sample, the logistic regression output within the functions domain is not symmetrical, but deviates towards the extreme that has a greater number of cases (Rojas et al., 2001 cited Real, Barbosa and Vargas, 2005). Further analysis of the optimum threshold point can be undertaken with data used to fit the model.

This technique has been applied to a number of test datasets (after the removal of exact matches) with consistent results achieved. On training datasets, the model is able to predict the link status in concordance with the clerical decision in approximately 97% of cases. When the model equations are used on an independent sample of pairs, which are clerically linked for comparison, the agreement level is usually higher than 95%. Some initial sensitivity analysis has been undertaken to identify whether the optimum threshold for classifying links or non-links is located somewhere other than at 0.5 in the score distribution. The early indications are that the optimum threshold can vary depending on the sample that has been selected as training data. The blocking strategies used have tended to result in a fairly even split between the number of links and non-links identified as potential candidates. Under these conditions, the optimum threshold score has always been located between 0.45 and 0.55, resulting in a small increase in the percentage of correct decisions being made. However, sensitivity analysis will be crucial for identifying the optimum classification threshold in circumstances where a more relaxed blocking strategy is used.

A number of issues arise in the application of logistic regression with clerically matched training data. The first relates to the size of the samples drawn for clerical review and the confidence intervals associated with the parameter estimates used to calculate match probabilities. Larger sample sizes ensure that a more complete range of linking scenarios are captured in training data, thus reducing the risk of over-fitting models that are biased towards the particular characteristics of the records sampled. Decisions need to be made based on empirical evidence whether to increase overall sample size to account for other effects, for example, if it is expected the true parameters are likely to vary depending on ethnic group. Tackling this problem could involve stratified sampling or including such characteristics as effects in the logistic regression model. However, these approaches will need larger sample sizes. Decisions about the acceptable number of records that can be used for clerical review need to be balanced with risks associated with data privacy. In circumstances where sample sizes are limited, it may be viable to provide confidence intervals around the match probability itself.

---

[10] For example, see Bibby and Brindley (2013).

A second issue is that the procedure assumes independence between the parameters esti-mated for each matching variable. The joint probability of similarity across different varia-bles is computed as the product of the separate probabilities. In truth, independence may not be present across matching fields, particularly with Census data where the prevalence of typographical error in one field is often indicative of an increased likelihood of typographical error in another. Violation of the conditional independence assumption is a well-known prob-lem in probabilistic record linkage, with varying consequences depending on data being linked. Herzog, Scheuren and Winkler (2007) discuss possible solutions with the use of gen-eral interaction models, the principles of which could possibly be incorporated within the framework outlined earlier.

Alternative methods for modelling decision-making
While logistic regression models derived from training data appear to be viable based on the evidence of research to date, there are a number of classification techniques that could be used in its place. It is intended that research will continue to identify the optimum method for classifying pairs into links and non-links. Alternative methods include decision trees (Cochinwala et al., 2001; Elfeky, Verykios and Elmagarmid, 2002), random forests (Criminisi, Shotton and Konukoglu, 2012) and support vector machines (Bilenko, Basu and Sahami, 2005). There is also scope to consider the Fellegi–Sunter method if a suitable approach for identifying a single classification threshold can be developed. This would have the advantage of not requiring training data when the EM algorithm is incorporated into the method.

8.4.5   Linkage quality

One of the essential requirements of this linkage research was to measure the quality loss due to pseudonymisation. It was expected that the use of suboptimal string comparison algo-rithms and the unavailability of clerical resolution would result in higher false positives and false negative error rates compared to the quality levels achieved by the 2011 Census to CCS linking presented in Section 8.2.2.4.

8.4.5.1   Comparison study

One of the early assessments of quality used a clerical exercise to link 10 000 HESA student records[11] to the Patient Register (PR), based on a random sample of 20 dates of birth (ONS, 2013e). The aim was to confirm the feasibility of linking pseudonymised data by measuring the error rates of a simple pseudonymised linkage approach, using un-hashed data. A small number of link-keys and an early version of the scoring algorithm outlined in Section 8.4.4.2 were used.

Estimation of the number of false positives and false negatives requires 'gold standard' linked data. This comprises a set of perfectly linked records between two datasets, where all of the true links have been identified and all of the true non-links are left unlinked. For this study, the limited size and the restriction to agreement on date of birth made this practi-cally possible. The creation of the gold standard link used standard rule-based and score-based linking, followed by clerical resolution of all pairs in a widely drawn range of scores deemed not high enough for certain links and not low enough to be certain non-links. The

---

[11] Higher Education Statistics Agency list of all students registered with higher education institutions in England and Wales (see https://www.hesa.ac.uk/overview).

links identified from the gold standard exercise were then compared with the links made by the pseudonymised linkage algorithm described in the preceding text.

The link rate was 88.1%, compared with 89.9% achieved by the gold standard. False positives were 1% (89 errors out of 8708 linkages), and false negatives were 2.5% (224 missed links out of 8932 available). However, the conditions under which the comparison was made may have generated some bias. Firstly, it is certainly not the case that for all true link pairs, date of birth agrees and so the restriction to use a sample of data with particular dates of birth will underestimate error rates. Secondly, the clerical exercise undertaken as part of the gold standard was not conducted by an independent team and was therefore not a fully independent comparison.

Nevertheless, while there were some limitations with the study design, the results were encouraging and suggested that the linking of two pseudonymised administrative data sources was viable.

8.4.5.2   Comparison with 2011 Census quality assurance linkage

A key part of the 2011 Census quality assurance (QA) process was the comparison of Census population estimates by age and sex with administrative data (ONS, 2012c). This included a large-scale linking exercise for a selected subset of 58 LAs. The linkage used a combination of exact, probabilistic (Fellegi–Sunter) and clerical methods to combine the Census data with the PR. These studies provided the opportunity to examine the performance of the pseudonymised linkage algorithm when applied to linkage of administrative and survey data. As discussed in the ONS (2013c), the framework for producing population estimates being researched for Beyond 2011 uses administrative data linked to a survey, the population coverage survey. In the comparison study reported here, the PR was a proxy for an SPD, and the Census, limited to the postcodes that formed part of the CCS sample, was a proxy for the population coverage survey. This linkage will be a vital part of the population estimation process, requiring high accuracy assuming linkage at individual level for application in a capture–recapture estimation process (ONS, 2013d).

For this evaluation, the Census QA links were viewed as a lower bound for, but reasonably close to, the true gold standard. False positives are unlikely, and overall, there will be a very small number of missed true links.

The Census QA links were compared with links identified by the pseudonymised linkage algorithm, including the score-based linkage process. Table 8.7 shows the link rates (as a percentage of PR records) for the Census QA links and the links using the pseudonymised linkage algorithm. It also shows the false positive rate (as a percentage of all the links that were made) and false negative rate (as a percentage of all Census QA links made).

The comparison exercise showed that the pseudonymised linkage algorithm has the capacity to link administrative and survey data despite the challenges imposed by hashing data. Considering the simplifications imposed for the comparison described in Section 8.4.5.1, performance when linking to survey data was rather better.

The closeness of the Census QA links to the gold standard means the false positive and false negative rates are indicative of the quality loss associated with hashing data. However, these error levels are considerably higher than the 2011 Census to CCS linking, which achieved estimated rates of less than 0.1% false positives and 0.25% false negatives as reported in Section 8.2.2.4. However, it should be noted that the 2011 Census was designed to be linked to the CCS and that expecting such accuracy when linking administrative sources to a coverage survey is unrealistic.

Table 8.7   Table of link results: Census QA comparison.

LA	Census QA link rate (%)	Pseudonymous data link rate (%)	Pseudonymous data false positives (%)	Pseudonymous data false negatives (%)
Birmingham	82.0	80.2	0.4	2.5
Westminster	65.1	63.6	0.4	2.7
Lambeth	64.0	62.9	0.5	2.2
Newham	68.3	66.5	0.5	3.0
Southwark	66.3	64.3	0.4	3.3
Powys	94.3	92.9	0.2	1.7
Aylesbury Vale	89.9	89.1	0.2	1.1
Mid Devon	88.6	88.3	0.6	0.9

Table 8.7 shows linkage error was higher in areas of high population churn, such as Birmingham and the London Boroughs of Westminster, Lambeth, Newham and Southwark. The pseudonymised linkage algorithm misses approximately two to three per cent of true links in these areas.

8.4.5.3   Linkage errors and population estimates

Following on from the studies in Sections 8.4.5.1 and 8.4.5.2, research is ongoing to reduce linkage errors through improvements to linkage methods and data capture and cleaning processes. The impact of linkage error on the population estimates is dependent on the estimation method that is used. As noted previously, if a capture–recapture method is used, the rate of false positive links will result in an equivalent negative bias in the population estimate. Similarly, the rate of false negative links will result in an equivalent positive bias in the estimates. Given the challenges associated with automating linkage of pseudonymised data, it might not be possible to reduce linkage errors to an acceptable level to produce robust population estimates using capture–recapture methods. While alternatives to capture–recapture are being explored, one possible solution is to develop a robust sampling strategy to quality assure linkages and obtain estimates for the rate of false positives and false negatives. In theory, these estimated error rates could be used to adjust for linkage biases in the capture–recapture method. This area of research continues in parallel with the development of existing methods to improve the accuracy of the linkage algorithm.

8.4.6   Next steps

There are a number of avenues for further research. As outlined in Section 8.4.5.3, the focus will be on attempting to reduce false negatives to a level that is compatible with the estimation approach, which is still under development. In the Census QA linkage exercise, it became apparent that previous addresses collected on the 2011 Census questionnaire were useful pieces of information to draw upon when making clerical decisions. As a result, a small test examined the impact of using previous addresses to improve linkage rates, showing some small improvements in reducing linkage error (~0.6 percentage point reduction of false negatives), and this research will continue.

The ONS (2014b) describes research to develop linkage procedures which use the concept of associative linkage. While this has not been fully developed, initial indications are that a number of additional links might be possible by drawing upon the strength of another individual who has already been linked within the same address, for example, a spouse, partner, child or parent. This is useful for individuals that have recently moved addresses, allowing for a relaxation of linkage criteria at the individual level. In particular, it enables accurate links to be made for individuals that have very common names or discrepancies in the recording of linking variable information.

8.4.7   Conclusion

The comparison exercises that have been undertaken so far have provided the ONS with a robust framework to develop and quality assure data linkage in Beyond 2011. Having access to a comparison from Census QA linking has been invaluable and will continue to provide an ongoing basis for improving the algorithm. The development of the algorithm will continue as attempts are made to reduce the number of false positives and false negatives that are generated.

Based on the evidence currently available, the proposed approach to linking pseudonymised data shows that linking population scale administrative data can be achieved, although with higher error levels than would be achieved with the original data. While it is crucial to understand how the reported increase in linking error will impact on the accuracy of population estimates, the computational efficiency of the approach means it is suitable for implementation. The scale of record linkage proposed in Beyond 2011 is considerably larger than the linking exercises that were undertaken for the 2011 Census. In practice, it would be very resource intensive to run similar clerical exercises between all of the potential administrative sources.

The population estimation framework is being developed in parallel with linkage research, and the tolerance for error in the linking process has not yet been fully understood. For SPD creation, which requires the linking of administrative sources, linkage errors of the order reported in this paper may be acceptable. Census non-response results in under-coverage, as will a result of failure to link administrative records when constructing an SPD. For Census estimation, non-response is adjusted for by linking Census records to the CCS and using the results to apply a dual system estimation. In principle, the same method can be used with administrative data which has under-coverage; however, this will require a very high standard of linkage between the SPD and population coverage survey, where tolerance for error is much lower. For the 2011 Census, the error rate for false positives was estimated to be less than 0.1% and less than 0.25% for false negatives.

It is recognised that Census and CCS linkage is very different from linking administrative sources to a coverage survey. Firstly, Census and CCS data are collected over a 6–8-week period, thereby increasing the likelihood that respondents will be recorded correctly at the same place on both sources. This cannot be controlled with administrative data, where lags in people's interaction will result in them being recorded in different places. For example, health system registrations are generally updated when an appointment is needed, not when a move occurs. Secondly, data collected from Census and CCS field exercises were designed to be linked. Administrative data are collected for operational purposes. There is no consideration for record linkage in their design. Considering these factors, it is likely that error rates for false positives and false negatives will be larger when linking the SPD to population coverage survey. While further research might improve the error rates so they are closer to those achieved with Census and CCS linkage, a realistic target for false positive and false negative errors in the Beyond 2011 context has yet to be developed. This target will need to be compatible with the estimation approach, which itself is still being developed as described by the ONS (2013d).

Reducing false negatives is the priority for future development. Use of previous address data and associative linking are promising in this regard, with linkage error for some trials achieving below 1%. It is also important to look beyond the linking algorithm as the only basis for reducing errors. Improving survey data quality by redesigning forms and collection mode could improve linking accuracy, for example, online data collection and use of hand-held field devices which have inbuilt validation checks for misspellings, inconsistencies and address entries.

Understanding bias will be a major focus of future research. The error rates reported in this chapter are likely to be more prominent for particular subgroups of the population (see Chapter 4), and this could have an adverse affect on small area estimates or age/sex estimates at the LA level. There is also a need to evaluate the capacity to accurately link records where the location of the individual is recorded in different LAs. The Census QA comparison reported in this chapter was limited to linking records within the same LA, and a comparison of records linked nationally is being planned.

Measuring the quality of linking is fundamental to success. The linking exercises undertaken by the Census QA team serve as an initial basis for measuring the precision and recall of the algorithm. However, as it was used to develop the algorithm, there is a risk of understating error rates. Work to identify or acquire an independent gold standard linked dataset is ongoing.

A process is being developed for obtaining access to a sample of un-hashed records in a way that does not compromise the ONS policy to protect data by appropriate privacy and security safeguards, and this sample may be used to train the models in the score-based linking and could be used to quality assure the methods that have been described.

Research into the implications of linking pseudonymised data will continue, and new methods may emerge from research being undertaken outside of the ONS and from the literature available. Of particular interest in the emerging field of privacy-preserving record linkage is the development of new encryption techniques for identifying string similarities (Schnell, Bachteler and Reiher, 2009) and research into alternative methods for automatically classifying links between records (summarised by Christen, 2012b). All future research will be subject to methodological review and will continue to be shared with wider public interest groups.

8.5 Summary

This chapter has discussed the application of record linkage methods in the context of large-scale data collection activities undertaken by NSIs to enumerate and measure the characteristics of resident populations.

The resource-intensive survey data collection processes which have underpinned population censuses for many decades are being subject to increasing scrutiny and re-evaluation from both users and producers of official statistics across the world. This has been driven by a range of common factors including increased diversity of respondent households, falling response rates (with corresponding increasing data collection costs) and rising user expectations about more timely statistics.

The existence of high quality population registers has already led to the replacement of survey-based censuses with register-based alternatives in jurisdictions where such data infrastructure is established. More recently, rises in the quality and coverage of computerised administrative datasets, the availability of powerful technologies for storing, manipulating and bringing together massive datasets and the financial pressures generated by a challenging economic climate have enabled others to begin exploring new possibilities. For instance, the ONS has invested substantial resources in research to assess the viability of an administrative data-based census without a population register.

These new approaches to the delivery of census-type statistics are underpinned fundamentally by record linkage techniques, both in the derivation of population data and – equally importantly – in the evaluation of their quality. The second of these raises significant new challenges given the common scenario of linked administrative data without common identification numbers that is faced by NSIs in countries without population registers. The accurate linking of coverage surveys to census enumeration responses has been a key component of census quality evaluation since the 1990s. However, this was primarily achieved through large-scale clerical exercises that were economically viable only in the context of one-off decennial enumeration and permissible because of specific census legislation enabling the use of personal identifiers for that purpose.

At the time of writing, linking administrative and survey data in the context of the ONS Beyond 2011 Programme are predicated on pseudonymisation of administrative sources to ensure confidentiality is preserved, especially where multiple sources are brought together. This chapter has presented initial findings from the work of the programme. These indicate that the use of careful preprocessing and combinations of key variables deliver reasonable performance compared to clerical linking of the same source data, albeit far from achieving the low error levels in the Census to CCS linkage. A key issue going forward remains how to robustly estimate the error associated with this process in the absence of an empirical 'truth'. There is clearly more work to be done, especially on the proposal for a sample-based approach to this issue. Finally, there is evidence from academic research (e.g. Schnell, Bachteler and Reiher, 2010) suggesting that encryption methods themselves might be adjusted to reduce the impact of confidentiality protection on the performance of linking algorithms, but the practical implementation of such techniques in the context of official statistics is some way off.

9

Privacy-preserving record linkage

Rainer Schnell
Research Methodology Group, University Duisburg-Essen, Duisburg, Germany

9.1 Introduction

Record linkage is an increasing popular research strategy in medicine, the social sciences, commercial data mining and official statistics. Most often, the purpose of the linkage operation is the production of a dataset containing information on individual persons or organisations. With such *microdata*, two different kinds of privacy concerns arise.

The first problem is that datasets containing more information on the same unit can be re-identified more easily. This problem is the central topic of *statistical disclosure control* (Hundepool et al., 2012). Since this problem is not specific to record linkage, it will not be discussed here.

The second problem concerns the attributes that can be used to identify an individual entity. In most modern societies, protecting such identifiers in administrative databases is required by law. Furthermore, releasing these identifiers for research is usually limited to a few, highly regulated special cases. Therefore, linking records of different databases by identifiers even within the same public administration may be prohibited by law. If such linkages are allowed, usually special techniques protecting the identifiers have to be used. The set of techniques for record linkage without revealing identifiers is called *privacy-preserving record linkage* (PPRL).

Privacy-preserving analysis techniques in general and specifically PPRL have become active fields of research in computer science, statistics and some application fields such as epidemiology, health service research and survey methodology. As a result of this intensive research, the list of available privacy-preserving techniques is growing fast.[1] In total, the list

---

[1] The keyword 'privacy preserving' currently (2014) yield about 4070 citations in CiteSeerX, in Google Scholar about 31 800, in Pubmed about 90 and ScienceDirect about 1 200 publications.

Methodological Developments in Data Linkage, First Edition. Edited by Katie Harron, Harvey Goldstein and Chris Dibben.
© 2016 John Wiley & Sons, Ltd. Published 2016 by John Wiley & Sons, Ltd.

of available privacy-preserving analysis and linkage techniques is impressive. To limit the scope of the chapter, the focus here will be privacy-preserving techniques, which have been used on databases covering national populations to generate general purpose statistical microdata.

9.2   Chapter outline

The number of PPRL techniques actually used for data production of research microdata is small. This chapter will shortly describe the current available techniques which are suitable for large population databases such as census datasets, social security administration data or cancer registries.

Section 9.3 begins with a description of the most basic and widely used standard scenario for PPRL: the use of a trusted third party with error-free identification numbers. Some refinements are described, and finally, the application scenario for many medical research settings is introduced: linking decentralised databases using PPRL by a trustee for the generation of microdata files (Section 9.3.4). The chapter focusses on methods most appropriate for such applications.

A short description of most widely discussed PPRL techniques is given in Section 9.4. The remaining chapter concentrates on one of the most frequently used techniques: Bloom filter-based PPRL.

Files beyond about 50 000 records need special techniques (*blocking*) since not all possible pairs in a record linkage process can be computed. The set of available techniques is described, a new technique introduced and some comparisons to older techniques reported (Section 9.5).

The central problem of PPRL is privacy protection (Section 9.6). Therefore, currently known attacks on PPRL protocols are summarised (Section 9.6.3). Based on this research, countermeasures against these attacks are described (Section 9.7). Finally, research needs in PPRL are delineated (Section 9.8) and policy implementation issues mentioned (Section 9.9).

Although some sections contain standard material covered in reviews previously published, some of the techniques and results are presented here for the first time. This new material is contained in Sections 9.5.2, 9.6.3 and 9.7.

9.3   Linking with and without personal identification numbers

A distinction between *(direct) identifiers* (e.g. personal identification numbers (PIDs)) and *quasi-identifiers* (e.g. names and dates of birth) is useful in practice. If a one-to-one mapping of individuals and personal identification codes is possible, we call this code a direct identifier.[2]

If a unique direct identifier is available, it is most often a national identification number (or *PID*). In such settings, record linkage is in principle a technically trivial file merge

---

[2] Of course, the definition is neither clear-cut nor universally accepted. For example, the American *HIPAA/HITECH* act defines as direct identifiers of an individual 18 items, such as names, geographic subdivisions smaller than a state, including zip codes beyond the third digit, all elements of dates (except year), phone numbers, electronic addresses, social security numbers, account data, fingerprints, face images and more. For details, see Trinckes (2013).

operation.[3] However, few countries have universal national PIDs (e.g. Denmark, Finland, Norway and Sweden). In most other countries, *quasi-identifiers* such as names, dates of birth and addresses must be used. These characteristics are neither unique nor stable over time and often recorded with errors. Record linkage only using exact matching quasi-identifiers will therefore miss many matches. The amount of errors in quasi-identifiers is often remarkably high, if the data quality of the identifier is not important for the organisational purposes for which the data were collected. Therefore, identifiers concerning financial transactions such as bank account numbers usually have lower error rates than quasi-identifiers, where error rates often exceed 10–15% per field. In accordance with this, Winkler (2009) reports that 25% of matches in a census would have been missed if only exact matching identifiers had been used. In many applications, the remaining matching subset is not a random sample of all true matches in the databases. Here, the resulting missing information cannot statistically be considered as missing at random.[4] An example is neonatal databases: children of mothers with changes in their names might be different from children of mothers with no change in their names or different from mothers whose names are missing. In such applications, additional techniques have to be used. Some of the available options will be discussed later.

9.3.1 Linking using a trusted third party

The basic model for PPRL is the use of a trusted third party (Figure 9.1). Database holders A and B submit the personal identifiers and the corresponding identification codes of the persons in their database to the trustee. The trustee identifies identical persons in both databases and delivers the list of corresponding identification codes to the research group, who then links the separate databases A and B (no longer containing personal identifiers) based on the linkage list of the trustee. Therefore, only the trustee sees the identification codes and personal identifiers, whereas the research group sees only the identification code. However, the trustee also learns who is a member of which database.

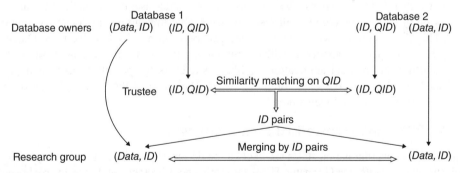

Figure 9.1 Standard model for linking two databases with a trusted third party. Adapted from Schnell, Hill and Esser (2013).

---

[3] In practice, PIDs do contain errors (Grannis, Overhage and McDonald, 2002; Newman and Brown 1997). Most but not all PID systems have checksums, so that most simple data processing errors can be identified easily. The main problems in practice are missing identifiers and multiple PIDs for the same person. Despite this, linking with PIDs is much easier than without.

[4] Identifiers seem to be missing or erroneous more often for vulnerable populations; therefore, mortality may be underestimated in such linkages (Ford, Roberts and Taylor, 2006; Zingmond et al., 2004).

9.3.2   Linking with encrypted PIDs

Knowledge gain of the trustee can be prevented by using encrypted identifiers. Encryption is usually done with cryptographic hash functions (*hash message authentication codes* (*HMACs*)). These are one-way functions, so that two different inputs will be mapped to two different outcomes, but there is no way of finding the input given only the outcome. In practice, HMACs with a password are used (*keyed HMACs*). Currently, *MD-5* or *SHA-1* is most often used as HMAC (Martin, 2012; Stallings, 2011). In countries with PID covering the whole population, usually an ID is generated by hashing the PID with a keyed HMAC: the resulting linkage ID is specific to this linkage project and cannot be used for other linkages.

9.3.3   Linking with encrypted quasi-identifiers

If no universal and unique PID is available, PPRL with a trusted third party uses encrypted quasi-identifiers. These are always prone to errors, for example, by typing or optical character recognition errors or by changes in values such as name changes after marriage or changes of addresses. Slightly different ways of spelling names, for example, the inclusion or exclusion of academic or generational titles or other name suffixes, usually do not strongly affect record linkage procedures with unencrypted identifiers (e.g. see Randall et al., 2014). However, if the identifiers are encrypted with HMACs, even small variations will result in completely different encodings after encryption. Therefore, standardisation (Christen, 2012a) of quasi-identifiers before encryption is highly recommended. The standard technique to make HMAC-encrypted quasi-identifiers resilient to small variations in spelling is the use of phonetic encodings for names. A phonetic code maps similarly pronounced strings to the same key, so that very similar variants of a name form a common group. For almost 100 years, the most popular phonetic function has been *Soundex* (Christen, 2012a), initially developed for census operations. For example, the names Engel, Engall, Engehl, Ehngel, Ehngehl, Enngeel, Ehnkiehl and Ehenekiehl all produce the same code (in this example: E524).

For record linkage, phonetic codes are normally additionally encrypted with a cryptographic function such as SHA-1. Using such a combination of standardisation, phonetic encoding and encryption of the phonetic code will result in acceptable linkage results for many applications. This combination is widely used in medical applications (Borst, Allaert and Quantin, 2001). However, persons appearing with entirely different names in the two databases will be lost; therefore, in practical applications, fallback strategies for potential record pairs with non-matching phonetic codes are commonly used. The effect of these strategies on overall linkage performance is not well studied.

9.3.4   PPRL in decentralised organisations

Organisations covering nation states are likely to be decentralised. An extreme example might be the healthcare system in Germany. There, currently about 2000 hospitals use diverse hospital information systems without a PID or SSN. Individual financial transactions between more than 170 healthcare insurance companies and hospitals are based on company-specific identifiers and names. Information exchange on individual patients between hospitals is usually based on name, sex, date of birth and insurance company. Only statistical information exchange is based on encrypted quasi-identifiers. For such statistical data collection processes, PPRL procedures are legally required. For example, the cancer registries use encrypted phonetic codes for PPRL.[5]

---

[5] The actual organisation of German cancer registries is quite complex. For the technical details, see Hentschel and Katalinic (2008).

In large decentralised organisations as this, legal requirements severely restrict the number of usable PPRL approaches. Most protocols with strong privacy guarantees seem to require repeated interactions between database owners (e.g. see Atallah, Kerschbaum and Du, 2003). Although often technically simple and even in some protocols requiring only few interactions or little network traffic, such protocols are not suited for linkage operations across different organisations. For example, medical data, crime or tax records are distributed among many different agencies for different purposes in most European countries. It is unlikely that such agencies will allow any external internet connection for their databases. Protocols requiring repeated access to external servers are no option for such secure environments.

The standard scenario in settings like these is shown in Figure 9.2. Here, a federal agency (*FA*) will set all required parameters for a linkage operation and send them to the data holding organisations, for example, hospitals. The hospitals split their databases in two sets: {IDs, data} and {IDs, quasi-identifiers. They send the datasets to a federal data warehouse (*DW*). The hospitals encrypt the identifiers according to the parameters specified by the *FA*. The resulting encrypted identifiers (here denoted as *bf*) and the corresponding IDs are sent to a linkage unit which acts as a trustee. The trustee links all records by using the *bf* alone. The list of all linked pairs of IDs is sent to the DW which merges all datasets according to the list of matching IDs.

In such setting, the *FA* does not receive any data and therefore cannot gain knowledge on any sensitive data. The database holders have their own data and do not receive anything new. Therefore, they don't learn anything by the execution of such protocols. The *DW* has access to all non-sensitive data but to no identifiers at all. Nevertheless, in such settings, the non-sensitive data could be linked to external information containing identifiers. Since this kind of attack

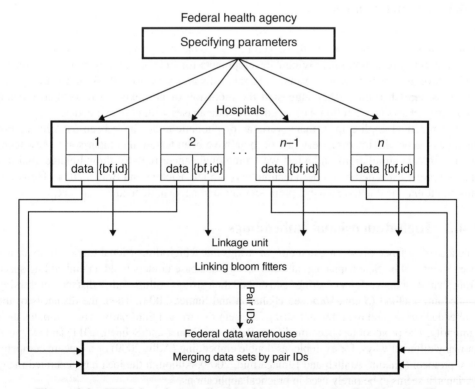

Figure 9.2   PPRL in a decentralised healthcare system [pprlhealthorg2.pdf].

is always possible if microdata are available, such attacks can only be limited by statistical disclosure protection measures (Hundepool et al., 2012).

All technical interesting things happen within the linkage unit. In most security analysis in PPRL, the linkage unit acting as trustee is the attacker. Since the unit receives only encrypted identifiers, the trustee might try to re-identify the encrypted keys. Most of the relevant literature in PPRL discusses ways to prevent re-identification by the trustee. It should be noted that nearly all protocols intended for applications in PPRL assume *semi-honest* or *honest-but-curious* parties. Semi-honest parties act according to the protocol but try to learn secret information of the other parties. They may use additional information or use information they gain during the execution of the protocol. For the scenario described in Figure 9.2, this is widely regarded as a realistic assumption.

9.4   PPRL approaches

The literature on PPRL approaches is widely scattered across academic fields between statistics, computer science and cryptography. A number of reviews, tutorials and taxonomies on available techniques have been published since 2010, for example, Hall and Fienberg (2010); Navarro-Arribas and Torra (2012); Christen, Verykios and Vatsalan (2013); Vatsalan, Christen and Verykios (2013a) and Verykios and Christen (2013). Therefore, the basic approaches will be described here only briefly. A large part of the recent literature on PPRL consists of combinations and extensions of these basic approaches.

9.4.1   Phonetic codes

The idea of using phonetic codes for PPRL has been described in Section 9.3.3. For most real-world settings, variations of these techniques are the standard method for PPRL. After a long neglect in research, recently new developments for linkage techniques using phonetic codes have been reported. For example, Karakasidis and Verykios (2009) and Karakasidis, Verykios and Christen (2012) suggested the inclusion of non-existing records to prevent frequency attacks (see Section 9.6) on encrypted databases with phonetic codes.

For practical applications, many variants of phonetic codes have been used for record linkage in general. However, very few of them have been tested in comparison to new techniques. Recent simulations and a test with a regional cancer registry show linkage qualities that are rarely exceeded by modern techniques (Schnell, Richter and Borgs, 2014). However, this result may be due to extensive preprocessing and needs independent replication.

9.4.2   High-dimensional embeddings

The idea of distance-preserving mapping of strings into a high-dimensional Euclidean space has been suggested by Scannapieco et al. (2007). Two database holders build an embedding space from shared random reference strings and embed their strings within using a distance-preserving embedding method (*SparseMap*; see Hjaltason and Samet, 2003). Then, the distances of the embedded strings and the reference strings are sent to a trusted third party, who computes their similarity. The protocol has been modified (Bachteler, Reiher and Schnell, 2011) and extended in many different ways, for example, as double embedding (Adly, 2009) or as secure computation protocol (Yakout, Atallah and Elmagarmid, 2009). Although the idea has generated many variants, it seems to be rarely used in practical applications.

9.4.3   Reference tables

A protocol based on a public list of reference strings was suggested by Pang and Hansen (2006) and Pang et al. (2009). For a given identifier, both database holders compute a distance between the identifier string and all reference strings in the set. For distances lower than a threshold, the reference string is encrypted using a key known to the database holders. For each identifier string, the resulting set of encrypted reference strings and the computed distances are sent to a third party. This party computes an approximation to the distances between the plain text identifiers.

In a simulation study, Bachteler et al. (2010) compared the reference string method (Pang et al., 2009) with the high-dimensional embedding (Scannapieco et al., 2007) and the Bloom filter approach (see Section 9.4.5). The reference string method performs inferior to the other approaches. However, due to privacy considerations, the reference string method has generated a series of variants and combinations, for example, the protocol suggested by Vatsalan, Christen and Verykios (2011).

9.4.4   Secure multiparty computations for PPRL

The field of *secure multiparty computation (SMC)* protocols is concerned with joint computations of a function by a set of parties with private inputs. The parties should learn only the intended output of the protocol. Even if some of the parties collude, it should be impossible to obtain more information (Lindell and Pinkas, 2009). Data mining is an obvious application for such protocols. Hence, a large number of SMC protocols to solve specific data mining problems have been suggested, for example, SMC k-means clustering (Vaidya and Clifton, 2003).[6] Naturally, the idea can be applied to the secure computation of similarities of quasi-identifiers. Since this is the core of a PPRL problem, there are suggestions for SMC protocols in PPRL. For example, Atallah, Kerschbaum and Du (2003) proposed an SMC protocol for the computation of *edit distances*, the number of edit operations such as inserting, deleting, substituting characters to transform one string into another string. Another SMC protocol for the computation of other string distances has been suggested by Ravikumar, Cohen and Fienberg (2004). However, all currently known SMC protocols in PPRL can hardly be applied for large datasets, since the required computing time is infeasible. Furthermore, SMC protocols require network-based interactions between database holders. In highly secure environments such as Social Security Administrations or medical registries, this is rarely an acceptable proposal. Therefore, in real-world decentralised PPRL applications, SMC protocols are currently not used.

9.4.5   Bloom filter-based PPRL

The idea of Bloom filter-based PPRL was suggested by Schnell, Bachteler and Reiher (2009). The method is based on the idea of splitting an identifier into substrings of length 2 (*bigrams*) and mapping the bigrams by HMACs to a binary vector. Only these vectors are used for linkage.

---

[6] It should be noted that SMC protocols are not suitable for exploratory work during the initial development of a statistical model. Since diagnostics based on residuals are essential for the development of a statistical model, SMCs are of limited use in such applications.

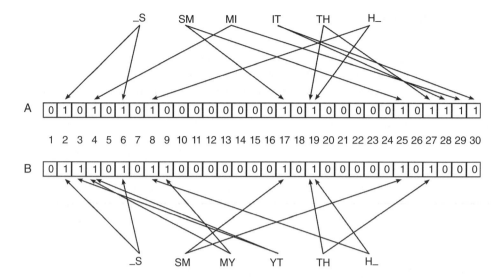

Figure 9.3 Example of the encoding of SMITH and SMYTH with two different cryptographic functions into 30-bit Bloom filters A and B. Taken from Schnell, Bachteler and Reiher (2009).

For example, the set of bigrams of the name *SMITH* is the set[7]

$$\{\_S, SM, MI, IT, TH, H\_\}$$

This set of bigrams is mapped with a hash function to a binary vector (see Figure 9.3). For the mapping of each bigram, Schnell, Bachteler and Reiher (2009) proposed the use of several different HMACs for each bigram. The combination of a bit vector with hash functions is called Bloom filters in computer science (Bloom, 1970). Hereby, the similarity of two strings can be computed by using the Bloom filters only.

The procedure is best explained using an example. If we want to compare the similarity of the names 'Smyth' and 'Smith' using bigrams, we can use a standard string similarity measure like the *Dice coefficient*:

$$D_{a,b} = \frac{2h}{(|a|+|b|)}$$

where h is the number of shared bigrams and $|a|$, $|b|$ is the number of bigrams in the strings a, b. For example, the bigram similarity of 'Smith' and 'Smyth' can be computed by splitting the names into two sets of six bigrams each ($\{\_s, sm, mi, it, th, h\_\}$ and $\{\_s, sm, my, yt, th, h\_\}$) counting the shared bigrams $\{\_s, sm, th, h\_\}$ and computing the Dice coefficient as $(2\times4)/(6+6)\approx0.67$.

If we want to compare the two strings with a Bloom filter encoding, we could, for example, use bigrams and Bloom filters with 30 bits and two HMACs only (in practice, Bloom filters with 500 or 1000 bits and 15–50 hash functions are used). Figure 9.3 shows the encoding for this example. In both Bloom filters, 8 identical bits are set to 1. Overall, $1+10$

---

[7] The bigrams _S and H_ are due to padding: start and end of a string are marked by adding a blank on the left, respectively, on the right end of the string.

bits are set to 1. Using the Dice coefficient, the similarity of the two Bloom filters is computed as $(2 \times 8)/(11 + 10) \approx 0.76$. In general, the similarity of two Bloom filters approximates the similarity of the unencrypted strings. Since numerical identifiers such as date of birth can be represented as strings, numerical data can also be encoded in Bloom filters. Therefore, all available information on quasi-identifiers can be used for PPRL with Bloom filters.

In the initial proposal, each quasi-identifier is mapped to one Bloom filter. Therefore, this approach can be used with little or no modification with most record linkage programmes. However, in some legal environments, record linkage has to be done with exactly one identifier, for example, a PID may be required by law. For such settings, Schnell, Hill and Esser (2013) suggested the use of the encoding described previously but with one common Bloom filter (called a *cryptographic long-term key* (*CLK*)) for all identifiers. So first name, last name, addresses, sex, date of birth, etc. are all mapped to the same Bloom filter (but with different hash functions and different passwords for each identifier). The authors suggested varying the number of hash functions k between identifiers i, for example, to reflect the assumed discriminating power of identifiers for possible pairs. This can be approximated by selecting k_i proportional to the entropy H_i of the identifier.

Simulations and real-world applications consistently show acceptable performance of CLKs. For example, in an application of a German cancer registry (Richter, 2013), a CLK based on first name, last name, date of birth, zip code and place of residence was used to link two files with 138 142 and 198 475 records. Considering only exact matches on the CLK, 18 pairs were found which had been not matched before using the procedures of German cancer registries (for details, see Hentschel and Katalinic, 2008) and clerical editing on unencrypted names. In general, record linkage based on separately encoded Bloom filters should perform slightly better than linkages based on CLKs of the same identifiers. However, CLKs have an obvious advantage over separate identifiers: An attack on CLKs seems to be more difficult than an attack on separate Bloom filters (for details, see Section 9.6.3). Since strings encoded in binary vectors are a flexible data structure for PPRL string similarity computations, several modifications of the basic idea have been suggested (see Section 9.7).

Bloom filter-based record linkage has been used in real-world medical applications, such as in Brazil (Napoleão Rocha, 2013), Germany (Schnell, 2014) and Switzerland (Kuehni et al., 2011). The largest application so far has been an Australian study (Randall et al., 2014). Here, healthcare data with more than 26 million records have been used. PPRL with Bloom filters showed no difference in linkage quality compared with traditional probabilistic methods using fully unencrypted personal identifiers.

9.5   PPRL for very large databases: blocking

Comparing each record of a file with each record of a second file requires $n \times m$ comparisons. With a national database holding millions of records, computing the similarity between all pairs is inconceivable. In practice, record linkage is therefore usually based on comparisons within small subsets of all possible pairs. Techniques for selecting these subsets are called *blocking* or *indexing* methods (Christen, 2012a; 2012b). In most PPRL projects, blocking also has to be done in a privacy-preserving way (*privacy-preserving blocking*). Privacy-preserving blocking has become a field of research on its own. Recent proposals include Karakasidis and Verykios (2011; 2012a; 2012b); Vatsalan, Christen and Verykios (2013b) and Karapiperis and Verykios (2014). However, only a subset of the proposed blocking methods can be used with Bloom filter-based PPRL.

9.5.1   Blocking for PPRL with Bloom filters

Linking two databases consisting of Bloom filters implies the search for pairs of similar binary vectors. This may be seen as a problem of finding nearest neighbours in a high-dimensional binary space. In the case of population databases, a nearest neighbour among more than 100 million candidates has to be found. With regard to Bloom filter-based PPRL, the number of suitable candidates for blocking is quite limited. Five promising methods will be described here.

The first obvious method is the use of external blocks. External blocks are formed by encrypting a quasi-identifier with an HMAC and using the hash value as a block. In practice, very often, regional identifiers or birth cohorts are used as blocks. This kind of blocking (called *standard blocking*, Herzog, Scheuren and Winkler, 2007) relies on blocking variables without errors. Errors in block identifiers of two records for the same person will usually result in a missed link for this pair. Therefore, in practice, most often, different blocking variables (e.g. postcodes, sex, date of birth, phonetic codes of names) are used sequentially.[8]

The second obvious method is sorting. The approach introduced by Hernández and Stolfo (1998) as *sorted neighbourhood* (*SN*) *method* has become the standard for handling large files with encrypted identifiers. Both input files are pooled and sorted according to a blocking key. For binary vectors, this can, for example, be the number of bits set to one (the *Hamming weight*). A window of a fixed size is then slid over the records. Two records from different input files form a candidate pair if they are covered by the window at the same time.

Canopy clustering (*CC*) (McCallum, Nigam and Ungar, 2000) forms candidate pairs from records placed in the same *canopy*. All records from both input files are pooled. The first canopy is created by choosing a record at random from this pool. This randomly chosen record constitutes the central point of the first canopy. All records within a certain loosely defined distance *l* from the central point are added to the canopy. Then, the central point and any records in the canopy within a certain more closely defined distance *t* from the former are removed from the record pool. Additional canopies are built in the same way as the first until there are no more remaining records. The result is a set of potentially overlapping canopies. Pairs which can be formed from the records of the same canopy constitute the set of candidate pairs.

LSH-blocking is based on *locality-sensitive hashing* (*LSH*) (Indyk and Motwani, 1998), a general technique for the search of approximate nearest neighbours. For the search on binary data, very often, *MinHash* (Broder, 1997) has been used as hash function for LSH (for details, see Leskovec, Rajaraman and Ullman, 2014). However, LSH for Bloom filters simply samples bits from the binary vectors and uses similar patterns of samples as blocks (Durham, 2012). Many variations of the LSH-blocking have been suggested recently (Karapiperis and Verykios, 2014; Steorts et al., 2014). For the setting described in Section 9.3.4, multiparty protocols or protocols requiring many iterations between database owners cannot be used. However, in general, the performance of simple LSH-blocking with very large datasets seems to be disappointing (Bachteler, Reiher and Schnell, 2013).

---

[8] This practice is common in cancer registries or during census operations. Given the ease of re-identification by unique combinations of encrypted demographic information, this is a questionable routine.

Finally, the use of *Multibit trees* (*MBT*) (Kristensen, Nielsen and Pedersen, 2010) for blocking in general record linkage, without reference to PPRL, was suggested recently as *q-gram blocking* by Bachteler, Reiher and Schnell (2013). However, the method can also be used for blocking binary vectors such as Bloom filters in PPRL (Schnell, 2013; 2014). With de-duplicated datasets, after blocking Bloom filters with MBT, no further processing is needed, since the search already yields the nearest neighbour. Since the technique is new, it will be explained in more detail.

9.5.2   Blocking Bloom filters with MBT

MBT were introduced to search huge databases of structural information about chemical molecules (Kristensen, Nielsen and Pedersen, 2010). If the query vectors are all binary, a query A is searched in a database of binary vectors B. All records in the database with a similarity to A above a certain threshold t should be retrieved. In chemoinformatics, very often, the *Tanimoto coefficient* $A \cap B / A \cup B$ is used for measuring similarity of binary vectors.[9] The coefficient is simply the ratio of the number of 1s the vectors have in common to the number of 1s where either vector has a 1. The algorithm uses the fact stated by Swamidass and Baldi (2007) that given the number of 1s in A and B (denoted by $|A|$ and $|B|$), the upper bound of the Tanimoto coefficient is $T_{max} = \min(|A|,|B|) / \max(|A|,|B|)$. If all vectors are stored in database indexed by $|B|$, searching for the vector A can be limited to those entries for which $|B| \leq t|A|$ or $|B| \geq |A| / t$. The increased speed of the algorithm is primarily due to those eliminations and the use of some special data structures.[10]

For the application of MBT on Bloom filters, the tree structure is built for the first file, and the records of the other file are queried sequentially. Therefore, the time required for querying the records of the second file is more important for the overall running time than the time needed to build the tree. In general, the average query time in MBT shows a linear increase with the number of records in the second file. This is an attractive scaling property of the method.

9.5.3   Empirical comparison of blocking techniques for Bloom filters

In the initial publication of q-gram blocking by Bachteler, Reiher and Schnell (2013), comparisons inter alia between MBT, CC, SN and standard blocking were reported. In most situations, MBT outperformed the other methods, even those that had performed best in other comparison studies (Christen, 2012b). After the promising results of the initial simulations, the original Java implementation of the Multibit tree algorithm was implemented as an R-library using C++. With this version, computing time was further decreased by a factor of more than five.

The performance of that implementation of MBT was studied in a series of simulations (Schnell, 2014). For the simulation reported here, files were generated with Febrl (Christen, 2008). Files with 1 000, 5 000, 10 000, 50 000, 100 000, 500 000 and 1 million records were prepared. CLKs with 1000 bits based on name, surname, sex and day/month/year of birth as identifiers and $k = 20$ hash functions for each of the six fields were generated with an additional Python script. The second file was a copy of the first file but with 0, 5, 10, 15 and 20% records containing errors.

---

[9] Both Dice and Tanimoto coefficients have a range of 0–1; they are monotone related.

[10] Details on the Multibit tree algorithm and an implementation in Java can be found in Kristensen et al. (2010).

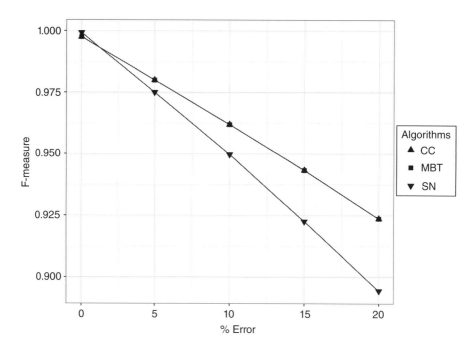

Figure 9.4   F-measure for canopy clustering (CC), sorted neighbourhood (SN) and Multibit trees (MBT). Errors in 5, 10, 15 and 20% of the records. Results for CC and MBT are nearly identical. Taken from Schnell (2014).

Figure 9.4 shows the F-measure for CC, SN and MBT. The performance of all blocking methods decreases with increasing error rates but more sharply for the SN technique. The results for CC and MBT are nearly identical. In general, the precision achieved by MBT is independent of error and independent of file size. The observed recall for MBT decreases linearly with error but is independent of file size. Overall, MBT performs as well as the best known traditional technique.

It must be kept in mind that all blocking methods need careful specification of parameters, for example, the window size in SN or the thresholds l and t in CC. For the use of MBT, this parameter is the Tanimoto threshold as described in Section 9.5.2. If this threshold is selected too high, the algorithm will be very fast but will miss many possible pairs. Selecting the threshold too low will increase the computing time. Hence, the threshold has to be selected carefully. The optimal threshold depends among other parameters on the number of errors in the quasi-identifiers.

Therefore, to achieve sufficient recall, the Tanimoto threshold must be lowered with increasing number of errors. In the simulations reported in Schnell (2014), a threshold of 0.85 gives a minimum recall of 0.85 even with 20% errors. This threshold shows a minimum precision of 0.95. For most applications, the 0.85 threshold therefore seems to be a reasonable start value. If the application has higher demands on precision and recall, using a threshold of 0.8 with blocks of at most 100 000 records will increase recall beyond 0.93 despite 20% errors.

For MBT, the computing time will increase with decreasing similarity thresholds, since the number of pairwise comparisons will increase. However, even with a low similarity threshold

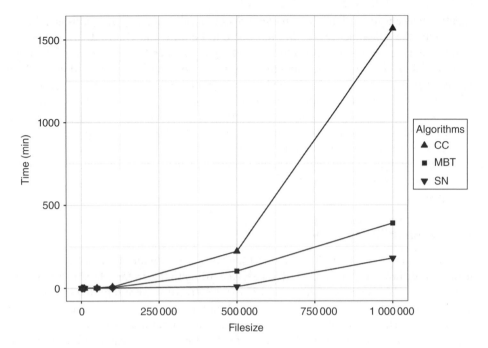

Figure 9.5 Time in minutes for finding best matching pairs (1 000–1 000 000 records) for canopy clustering (CC), sorted neighbourhood (SN) and Multibit trees (MBT), 10% errors. Taken from Schnell (2014).

of 0.85, two files of 500 000 records with 10% errors could be matched in 5902 seconds. For this combination of parameters, a recall of 0.931 and a precision of 0.977 were observed: exactly the same performance as CC in about 40% of the time (see Figure 9.5).

9.5.4   Current recommendations for linking very large datasets with Bloom filters

Given current hardware and currently available algorithms for very large datasets such as a population census, very few techniques are suitable for Bloom filter-based PPRL. The simplest option would be external blocking, for example, by encrypted year of birth. This key would form a block, and within each block, other techniques could be used. SN is a robust option in such settings. MBT would be another option. Both techniques seem to perform well. Restricting the blocks to about 1 million records, PPRL based on Bloom filters could be done with a small cluster of servers within 24 hours. Given other restrictions of PPRL, this is already an acceptable time for most research applications.

9.6   Privacy considerations

Currently, from a mathematical point of view, it seems impossible to achieve the goal of a dataset that cannot be re-identified at all. This is attributed by Dwork and Pottenger (2013) to '...the fact that the privacy-preserving database is useful'. Therefore, the current focus in computer science is the notion of *differential privacy*, usually targeting the quasi- identifiers.[11] Interestingly, the consequences for lawyers seem to be different. Ohm (2010) argues (in a chapter called 'From Math to Sociology') that regulators need to ask questions that help reveal the risk of re-identification and threat of harm: 'because easy reidentification [sic!, RS] has taken away purely technological solutions that worked irrespective of these messier, human considerations, it follows that new solutions must explore, at least in part, the messiness'. Correspondingly, German jurisdiction defines *de facto anonymity* as modification of identifiers such as only a disproportionate investment of time, cost and labour would lead to re-identification. Therefore, the analysis of a cryptosystem for an epidemiological cancer registry might depend on the assumed motives of an attacker. Some facts on reported privacy breaches will be summarised, before the technical details on preventing attacks will be given.

9.6.1   Probability of attacks

The American ITRC (www.idtheftcenter.org), a non-profit organisation, collects information on privacy breaches in the United States. According to their yearly breach report 2013 (ITRC, 2014), 614 breaches with 91 982 172 exposed records were reported in the United States. About 269 breaches with about 8.8 million records concerned medical or healthcare databases. Hence, more than 40% of all breaches pertain to medical or healthcare databases. In 2014, one incident alone concerned 4.5 million records in a hospital information system (BBC-News, 2014). In the United States, medical databases seem to be attractive targets for attacks. However, it must be considered that American medical and healthcare databases very often contain financial information, such as credit card information. Furthermore, there may be a market for social security numbers or healthcare identification numbers with the aim to access medical services. For countries with national health services or differing health insurance systems, this is not necessarily true. Therefore, medical or health databases might be of lesser interest to external attacks outside the United States. For example, the reports of the Federal German Data Protection Agencies for 2012 and 2013 do list a couple of incidents concerning medical databases (e.g. loss of backup tapes) but not a single case of an outsider attack. In accordance with that, US data also show that most privacy breaches are due to human error. In a study of 1046 total privacy breach incidents in the United States between 2005 and 2008, Liginlal, Sim and Khansa (2009) reported that human error caused 67% of the incidents and malicious acts 33%. Finally, it must be kept in mind that from the attacker's point of view, a social engineering attack on a human is usually easier than a mathematical attack on an encryption scheme.

Finally, the overall success probability of an attack on a medical database should be considered. De-anonymisation attacks on databases for research purposes have been rarely reported in the international literature. In a systematic review, Emam et al. (2011) reported that only 14 attacks could be found in the literature. About 26% of the records could be re-identified in all studies. Only one of the attacks was aimed at a medical database anonymised according to current standards. In this study, 2 of 15 000 records could be correctly re-identified. Therefore, the overall probability of an attack on a research database and the success probability of such an attack seem to be entirely different from the 'proof-of-concept'

---

[11] However, Dwork and Pottenger (2013) clearly state that '…preventing re-identification does not ensure privacy…'.

attacks considered in computer science and statistics. For actual real implementations, this difference should be kept in mind (see Section 9.9).

9.6.2   Kind of attacks

Recently, Vatsalan et al. (2014) classified the attacks most frequently discussed in the PPRL literature in five groups:

1. Dictionary attack: If the encryption function is known, an attacker can encrypt a large dictionary of possible quasi-identifiers to find matching encrypted identifiers.

2. Frequency attack: If a suitable population distribution of quasi-identifiers is available, the frequency distribution of encrypted quasi-identifiers can be used for assigning records to quasi-identifiers even if the encryption function is not known.

3. Cryptanalysis: Some encoding techniques, for example, Bloom filters, are prone to cryptanalysis. Using the bit patterns of frequent names or frequent q-grams, some records might be correctly re-identified.

4. Composition attack: Using auxiliary information on the databases or at least some records, information might be combined to learn sensitive values of certain records.

5. Collusion: In multiparty protocols, a subset of database owners and the third party violate the protocol and try to learn the other database owner's data.

Since either keyed HMACs or seeded random number generators are used for encryption, dictionary attacks on PPRL procedures don't seem promising. It should be noted that collusion is not excluded by the honest-but-curious assumption. Most of the PPRL schemes in practical use today seem to be susceptible to collusion.[12] Therefore, in practice, the implementation of a PPRL protocol has to rely on the enforcement of the corresponding jurisdiction. Composition attacks have been defined by Ganta, Kasiviswanathan and Smith (2008) as attacks, in which an adversary uses independent anonymised releases to breach privacy (for a textbook example with hospital data, see Chen et al., 2009). These kinds of attacks have received little attention in the PPRL literature, since most protocols minimise the amount of information available for an attacker. In accordance with this reasoning, the published attacks on Bloom filter-based PPRL approaches concentrate on frequency attacks and cryptanalysis.

9.6.3   Attacks on Bloom filters

So far, three studies by two research groups have been published on attacking PPRL Bloom filters. Furthermore, there is a recent unpublished report by one of the groups. All attacks will be described shortly.

Kuzu et al. (2011) sampled 20 000 records from a voter registration list and encrypted the bigrams of forenames (with $k=15$ and $l=500$). The authors formulated their attack as a *constraint satisfaction problem* (*CSP*) which defines a set of variables, which have to

---

[12] Dalenius in 1977 cited Hansen as early as 1971: 'The US Bureau of the Census accepts the view that "(…) it is not feasible to protect against disclosure by collusion" '.

satisfy certain constraints. CSP problems can be solved by the application of constraint programming (Marriott and Stuckey, 1999). Usually, special programmes called CSP solvers are used for this. To limit the problem size given to the CSP solver, Kuzu et al. (2011) used a frequency analysis of the identifiers from the voter registration list and of the Bloom filters encodings. For assigning possible names to the Bloom filters, generated frequency intervals for the forenames in the voting list and for the Bloom filters were applied. To restrict the number of alternative names that could correspond to a Bloom filter, two assumptions were used: the encrypted records are a random sample of a known resource, and the attacker has access to the resource from which the sample is drawn. Given the described setting, the CSP solver assigned the 400 most frequent names of approximately 3500 different forenames correctly.

However, the assumptions used by the authors are rarely found in practical applications. In their second paper, Kuzu et al. (2013) evaluated the practical use of their own attack more criti-cally. Personal identifiers in a given application database such as a medical registry are unlikely to be a random sample of an available population list. Thus, Kuzu et al. (2013) investigated whether voter registration records could be used to identify encrypted personal identifiers from a medical centre. In this more realistic scenario, the attacked database is not a random sample of the available population list. After several modifications of the attack and restricting the problem to a set of just 42 names, the CSP solver failed even after a week of runtime. Restricting the problem further to the set of only the 20 most frequent names, the CSP assigned 4 of those 20 names correctly. Nevertheless, Kuzu et al. (2013) concluded that the attack remains feasible in practice. This remains to be demonstrated with an independently encrypted database. No replication of a CSP attack on Bloom filters from other research groups has been reported in the literature.

A different and highly successful attack on simple Bloom filters has been published by Niedermeyer et al. (2014). Very little computational effort is needed, and only publicly available name frequency lists are used for this form of attack. The attack concentrates on the frequency of bigrams as the building blocks of Bloom filters instead of the frequency of entire names.

In the standard Bloom filters used for PPRL (Schnell, Bachteler and Reiher, 2009), the k hash functions are based on the *double hashing scheme*:

$$h_i = (f + i \times g) \bmod L \text{ for } i = 0, \ldots, k - 1$$

where L is the length of the Bloom filter and f and g are the cryptographic hash functions such as MD-5 or SHA-1. This was originally proposed in Kirsch and Mitzenmacher (2006) as a fast and simple hashing method for Bloom filters yielding satisfactory performance results. Using this scheme, each bigram will set at most k bits to one, since k hash functions are used. Niedermeyer et al. (2014) denote the Bloom filter generated by one bigram as an *atom*. Then, the Bloom filter of a name is the bitwise OR operation of the atoms corresponding to the bigrams of the name.[13]

For the demonstration of the attack, the authors used 10 000 Bloom filters with stand-ard settings ($m = 1000$, $k = 15$). The Bloom filters were sorted and de-duplicated, yielding 7580 unique Bloom filters. For analysis, they used only those 934 Bloom filters, which occurred at least twice. Because they did not know the hash functions used, they generated

---

[13] The bitwise OR of two bits gives 1 if either or both bits are 1, otherwise it returns 0.

every possible atom. The pairwise combination of two vectors with 1 000 bits resulted in 1 000 000 possible atoms. The next step was testing which atoms actually occurred in the 934 most frequent Bloom filters. They matched the bit positions set to one in the possible atoms with the bit positions set to one in the given Bloom filters, which resulted in 3952 atoms.

By excluding possible atoms that do not encrypt a bigram (these atoms have a high probability to have less than k bits set to one), they only used atoms with k bits for further analyses.

After that, they determined which of the remaining 805 possible atoms are contained in each Bloom filter. Finally, they assigned the three most frequent bigrams to the most frequent atoms by hand. For that, 934 Bloom filters as well as the 805 atoms were sorted according to their frequencies. By manually assigning further atoms to bigrams, they deciphered all 934 Bloom filters. In total, they found 338 bigrams (of all possible 729 bigrams) through deciphering the 934 most frequent Bloom filters. With more manual effort, nearly all bigrams could have been deciphered. Given the knowledge of nearly all bigrams, every name and even unique names could be deciphered. Therefore, the attack described in that paper can be used for the deciphering of a whole database instead of only a small subset of the most frequent names, as in reported previous research. The authors clearly state that this kind of filtering atoms is only due to the double hashing scheme used. If other hash functions would have been used, this method is not suitable for attacking Bloom filters.

Finally, in a yet unpublished paper, Steinmetzer and Kroll (2014) present a fully automated attack on an encrypted database containing Bloom filters, encrypting forenames, surnames and place of birth. They suppose that the attacker only knows some publicly available lists of the most common forenames, surnames and locations. The attack is based on analysing the frequencies and the combined occurrence of bigrams from the identifiers of these lists.

The authors generated Bloom filters with quasi-identifiers according to the distribution in the population. The identifiers were truncated after the tenth letter and padded with blanks. The bigrams of each record were hashed with $k=20$ hash functions into one Bloom filter of length 1000. It is important to note that they used the double hashing scheme for the generation of k hash functions. They modified an automatic cryptanalysis of substitution ciphers as described by Jakobsen (1995). In addition to the general approach of Niedermeyer et al. (2014) to identify *atoms*, Steinmetzer and Kroll (2014) used additional information about the joint frequency distribution of bigrams in the target language. After this modification, the algorithm was able to reconstruct 59.6% of the forenames, 73.9% of the surnames and 99.7% of the locations correctly. For 44% of the 10 000 records, all identifier values were reconstructed successfully. However, the authors note that the attack is specific to the use of double hashing scheme. Furthermore, the attack described avoided encoded numerical data. Although the attack seems to be highly successful, the authors doubt that this way of attack will still be a viable option if some of the methods described in the following section are applied.

9.7   Hardening Bloom filters

To counteract the attacks described previously, the construction of Bloom filters for PPRL can be modified. Most of the currently available options will be described here.

9.7.1   Randomly selected hash values

The attack described by Niedermeyer et al. (2014) was conceived for the construction scheme of the hash functions as used by Schnell, Bachteler and Reiher (2009). Therefore, this vector of attack can be eliminated by modifying the hash function. This could be done by randomly selecting hash values. If the k hash functions $h_0, \dots, h_{k-1}$ are randomly sampled from the set of all functions that map the bigram set Σ^2 to $\{0, \dots, 999\}$, the number of possible atoms increases. For example, given the parameters $l = 1000$ and $k = 15$, the number of candidate atoms increases from $493\,975$ (when using the double hashing scheme) to approximately 6.9876×10^{32} when permitting arbitrary hash functions. Therefore, Niedermeyer et al. (2014) strongly suggested the use of random independent hash functions for applications. By the use of randomly selected hash values, filtering phantom atoms by selecting atoms with maximal Hamming weight would result in a smaller reduction of remaining atoms, making this way of attack unusable in practice.

9.7.2   Random bits

An attack on a Bloom filter-encrypted quasi-identifier might use the fact that the same q-gram will be mapped to identical positions in all Bloom filters. The frequency distribution of such bit patterns might be used in different ways for an attack. For example, some patterns frequently occur together. By using information on the joint distribution of q-grams in unencrypted quasi-identifiers in combination with the joint frequency distribution of bit patterns, assignments of q-grams to bit patterns can be checked with an automated procedure. Many different ways of setting up such a system are possible. Obvious candidates are generic algorithms (Haupt and Haupt, 2004, for a cryptographic application, see Morelli and Walde, 2003) or constrained satisfaction problems solvers (Marriott and Stuckey, 1999, for an application to Bloom filters see Kuzu et al., 2011). If the constraints or optimisation criteria of such automatic assignment systems depend on deterministic rules, such attacks can be made much harder if random noise is added to the bit patterns. Adding random noise to encrypted information is common in computer science – see, for example, Rivest (1998). In PPRL, the idea of adding random bits has been mentioned by Schnell, Bachteler and Reiher (2009). The simplest option is adding noise randomly to a Bloom filter. Here, bit positions are sampled randomly and set to one (*srs-1*). Alternatively, the complement of the bit is used. The random noise can be made dependent on the q-gram, so that for different q-grams, different noise is added. For example, frequent q-grams can be encoded with more bits set randomly. To our knowledge, the effects of these variations on linkage quality and privacy measures have not been studied systematically.[14] As an illustration, the effect of *srs-1* on F- Scores will be described in the following.

Adding random bits will affect precision and recall of PPRL procedures. Since PPRL should be resistant to errors, adding small amounts of random bits will affect performance only slightly. However, very high rates of random error will reduce recall and precision. The amount of loss will depend on error rates in the identifiers themselves. For example, given perfect identifiers, adding even 100 random bits to a Bloom

---

[14] Note that this is different from differential privacy (for an introduction, see Dwork and Pottenger, 2013) for the items encoded in a Bloom filter. This problem has been studied by Alaggan et al. (2012). They show that differential privacy can be satisfied if each bit of a Bloom filter is flipped with a probability $p = 1/(1 + e\varepsilon/k)$, where k is the number of hash functions and ε is the privacy parameter.

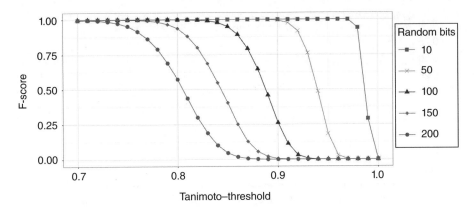

Figure 9.6   The effect of adding random bits to files with 10000 Bloom filters each on the F-score depending on the similarity threshold. Initial identifiers have no errors.

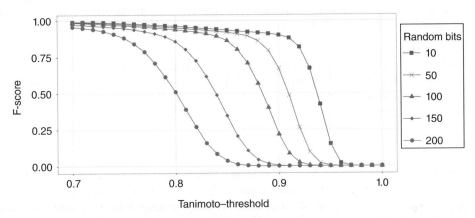

Figure 9.7   The effect of adding random bits to files with 10000 Bloom filters each on the F-score depending on the similarity threshold. Twenty per cent errors in the identifiers.

filter ($l = 1000$) shows small effects on the performance for a CLK using first name, second name, sex, date of birth and city with $k = 20$ (see Figure 9.6, $n = 10\,000$ records). Choosing a similarity threshold of 0.85 would have reduced the F-score to 0.95 with 100 random bits.

However, if identifiers with errors have to be used, the number of random bits that can be added without loss in precision and recall will be lower. Repeating the experiment described previously with 20% errors per identifier gives the result shown in Figure 9.7: 100 random bits would have reduced the F-score to about 0.25 given a similarity threshold of 0.85. Therefore, at most 50 random bits should have been used, giving an F-score of about 0.93.

In contrast to our expectation, the amount of overlap between the two files to be linked does not show an effect on the amount of random noise which could be added (see Figure 9.8). Even files with little overlap of records (50%) and high error rates in identifiers (20% per identifier), a similarity threshold of 0.85 yields a precision of 1.0 and recall of 0.8706.

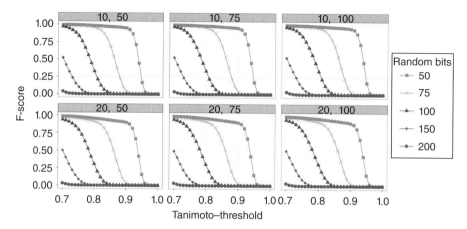

Figure 9.8 The effect of adding random bits to files with 10 000 Bloom filters each on the F-score depending on the similarity threshold, errors in identifiers and different overlap. First row: 10% errors in the identifiers, second row: 20% errors in the identifiers. First column: 50% overlap, second column 75% overlap, third column 100% overlap.

Adding 5% random bits to Bloom filters seems to affect PPRL performance only slightly. Given the fact that deterministic attacks are likely to fail with noisy Bloom filters, adding up to 5% random bits will enhance security of Bloom filter PPRL without serious losses in precision and recall.

9.7.3   Avoiding padding

In record linkage applications based on q-grams, adding blanks at the beginning and end of an identifier is common practice. This *padding* allows the identification of q-grams at the beginning or end of an identifier in a q-gram set. Usually, padding at least increases precision in a record linkage process. However, padded q-grams are usually among the most frequent q-grams in identifiers. For example, among the 50 most frequent bigrams in German surnames, 18 are padded bigrams. Since frequent padded q-grams can be identified easily even after encryption, padding identifiers is not recommended for PPRL.

9.7.4   Standardising the length of identifiers

The distributions of quasi-identifiers such as names are usually not uniform, but show high variations and skewness. For example, in a large German administrative database covering about 40% of the population, the length of first names varies between 2 and 24 with a mean of 9.7 (and a skewness of 0.52); the length of last names varies between 2 and 46 with a mean of 7.2 (skewness 1.9). Very long or very short names can be easily identified in a Bloom filter, since the number of bits set to one is exceptionally large or small. Therefore, to protect against this way of re-identification, the length of identifiers should be standardised. Long names could be shortened by deletion or sampling of q-grams. Shortening the identifiers will prevent the identification of longer names. Furthermore, the distribution of bigram frequencies will change. Short identifiers may be extended by *key stretching* (Kelsey et al., 1998). The basic idea of key stretching is the extension of a g-bit key to

$g + t$ bits. Key stretching is a standard technique in cryptography, but so far has not been used in PPRL. Key stretching for PPRL can, for example, be implemented by random sampling q-grams of an extended alphabet and concatenating these with the short name. Of course, key stretching will also modify the frequency distribution of q-grams. Standardising the length of identifiers will make re-identification of rare short or long names more difficult; furthermore, attacks based on q-gram frequencies will need additional information. However, no empirical studies on the cryptographic and PPRL properties of these techniques seem to be currently available.

9.7.5   Sampling bits for composite Bloom filters

Sampling from identifiers can be seen as a special case of deleting characters. Therefore, instead of deleting characters, sampling can be used. Durham (2012) published a variation of CLKs, denoted by Durham et al. (2013) as *composite Bloom filters*. Bit positions from separate Bloom filters for each identifier are sampled. The initial Bloom filters are built either statically (constant values for the length of the Bloom filters and the number of hash functions) or dynamically (such that an approximately equal number of bit positions is set to one in each Bloom filter). Next, bits are sampled from these separate Bloom filters, either the same number of bits from each or proportional to the discriminatory power of each Bloom filter. Finally, the sampled bits are concatenated and permuted. Applying the attack described previously on these kinds of Bloom filters would not be promising, because composite Bloom filters consist of multiple identifiers, like CLKs, and their bit positions are sampled from the initial Bloom filters.

9.7.6   Rehashing

To impede attacks on q-gram-encodings, the resulting bit arrays can be transformed. Obvious ideas for the transformation of bit arrays such as rotating (Schnell, Bachteler and Reiher, 2011) or permutation (Durham, 2012) offer no protection against attacks as described previously. Therefore, other techniques are needed. As an example, a new technique will be described here. The method is based on a second hashing of the already hashed q-grams.

Consider a database of CLKs or other Bloom filters of length m equal to 1000 bits, built from multiple identifiers. For rehashing a CLK, we define a window of w bit positions, which slides along the CLK. The number of bit positions the window slides forward is denoted with s. The bits covered by the window are used as the binary representation of an integer. This integer serves as a seed for a random sample of k_{re} integers, which are drawn with replacement from the set $\{0, \ldots, m-1\}$. Next, a new second stage bit array is initialised with zeros. The bit positions that correspond to the random numbers are set to one. Finally, the window will shift s positions to the right, and the rehashing procedure is repeated.

The procedure will be explained using an example: assume a CLK of length $m = 1000$ and a window of size $w = 8$ with step size $s = 6$ (see Figure 9.9). Then, the binary vector $v = (0,1,0,1,0,0,1,1)$ of length 8, which is defined by the window, serves as pattern for the binary representation of an integer:

$$1 \cdot 2^0 + 1 \cdot 2^1 + 0 \cdot 2^2 + 0 \cdot 2^3 + 1 \cdot 2^4 + 0 \cdot 2^5 + 1 \cdot 2^6 + 0 \cdot 2^7$$
$$= 1 + 2 + 16 + 64$$
$$= 83.$$

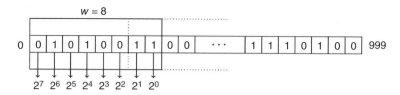

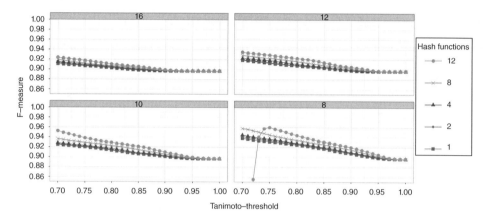

Figure 9.9 Rehashing a CLK $l = 1000$ with a window of size $w = 8$. The bits covered by the window are used as integer seed for the generation of a set of k_{re} random numbers.

Figure 9.10 F-scores for PPRL of two files with 10 000 records after rehashing of CLKs with $k = 1, 2, 4, 8, 12$ hash functions, window size $w = 8, 10, 12, 16$ and step size s equal to window size ($s = w$).

Next, using 83 as the seed for a random generator, a random sample of $k_{re} = 3$ numbers from the set $\{0, \ldots, 999\}$ is drawn and assigned to 83. Thus, for each binary representation which produces the integer 83, the same positions in the new bit array are set to one. Finally, the window is shifted 6 bits to the right. The bits that are now covered by the window are used as binary representation of another integer. Finally, a new random sample of three numbers is assigned to this integer, and the bit positions corresponding to the new sample are also set to one in the new bit array. This new second stage CLK is used like a traditional Bloom filter for PPRL.

The results of a small simulation of PPRL using two files with 10 000 records are shown in Figure 9.10. Larger window sizes decrease the performance (at least for step sizes equal to the window size). Larger number of hash functions increase performance for rehashing. For the parameter settings used here (no additional errors, overlap of 100%), lower similarity thresholds show better results for all but one experiment. The lower right figure ($w = 8$) demonstrates a decrease in linkage quality below a similarity threshold of 0.75. Below this threshold, the number of false positives increases sharply; therefore, the precision and accordingly the F-score become unacceptable. However, high values of precision and recall can be achieved with moderate ($8 < w < 12$) window sizes, high numbers of hash functions ($k \geq 12$) and moderate similarity thresholds ($0.75 \leq t \leq 0.8$). Therefore, the idea of rehashing CLKs or other Bloom filters seems to deserve further study. Since the choice of these parameters depends on m and k and the number of q-grams per identifier, the choice of optimal parameters for rehashing is subject to ongoing research.

9.7.7   Salting keys with record-specific data

In computer science, salt is an additional random string that is concatenated with passwords before a one-way function for hashing is used (Morris and Thompson, 1979; Schneier, 1996). In this application, salts are a defence against dictionary attacks. The idea can be used for Bloom filter-based PPRL as suggested by the author in Niedermeyer et al. (2014). *Salting* describes the process of generating hash values that depend on record-specific keys. Short identifiers such as date or year of birth are obvious candidates for such a key. Then, for a single bigram *b* appearing in two names, the same bit positions will be set to one in the corresponding Bloom filters only if the keys coincide. If the keys are not equal, it is very unlikely that all hash values for the bigram *b* are the same. If the keys are erroneous in one file, the records will not match, since the bit pattern is different for the same records. Therefore, the key values for salting should contain no errors at all. In practice, very few identifiers beyond date of birth are suitable candidates. If such keys can be used, salting in PPRL increases precision and does not reduce recall. The effect of salting is similar to blocking. However, the use of salting increases the entropy of encrypted identifiers. For example, the bigrams resulting from the name FELLEGI would be hashed completely different if the year of birth is used as a key and two persons with this name were born in 1959 and 1972. Therefore, filtering phantom atoms as described previously would be much harder with salting. Hence, if suitable blocking variables with very low error rates are available, the values of the blocking variables should be used within each block as a salt for hashing.

9.7.8   Fake injections

All proposed attacks on Bloom filters strongly depend on comparing observed frequencies of bit patterns and expected frequencies of encoded entities. Names and *q*-grams of names show highly skewed distributions.[15] Hence, the success of these attacks can be reduced if the frequency distribution of the input is modified artificially. This could be achieved, for example, by inserting random strings which contain rare *q*-grams. Thus, the overall frequency distribution of hashed *q*-grams will be closer to a uniform distribution, which makes re-identification more difficult. Karakasidis, Verykios and Christen (2012) described three such fake injection methods in the context of phonetic codes. These approaches could be adapted to Bloom filters. However, all these methods have serious drawbacks.

9.7.9   Evaluation of Bloom filter hardening procedures

Most of the methods described here have been proposed quite recently. This is also true for the criteria used for evaluating these methods. The most elaborated contribution here by Vatsalan et al. (2014) suggested a series of standardised measures of disclosure risk *DR* based on $P_s(a^M)$ as *probability of suspicion*. Given n_g as the number of values in the dataset G^M matching a value a^M in the anonymised dataset D^M, the probability of suspicion is $1/n_g$. Normalising this to $0 \le P_s(a^M) \le 1$ and denoting with N the number of records in G^M yield

$$P_s(a^M) = \frac{(a/n_g) - (1/N)}{1 - (1/N)}$$

---

[15] Fox and Lasker (1983) showed that the distribution of English surnames is highly skewed and obeys Zipf's law by a discrete Pareto distribution. The same phenomenon is observed for the *q*-gram frequencies.

This probability is primarily used for the definition of:

Maximum risk, DR_{max}, as the maximum $P_s(a^M)$ over all values in $\boldsymbol{D}^M$

Marketer risk, DR_{Mark}, as the number of records in $\boldsymbol{D}^M$, which can be re-identified with $P_s(a^M)=1.0$

Mean risk, DR_{Mean}, as the mean of all $P_s(a^M)$

Although Vatsalan et al. (2014) presented first results for some PPRL techniques, their proposal must still be proven to be useful in practice. However, systematically testing the privacy properties of the procedures discussed previously is currently the most urgent research problem within Bloom filter-based PPRL. It must be kept in mind that a cryptanalytic attack on a building block of a PPRL (such as a cryptographic hash function) can invalidate the results of computing privacy metrics. Since it is impossible to prove that information protection designs are unbreakable (Pieprzyk, Hardjono and Seberry, 2003), privacy metrics are just a necessary first step for the evaluation of PPRL procedures.

9.8   Future research

Progress in PPRL has been remarkable during the last 5 years. PPRL is now a very active research field in statistics, computer science and application areas such as medicine and official statistics. However, for practical applications using real-world population size databases, some problems deserve further study.

Most PPRL approaches are currently based on encrypted string data. However, in some situations, either geographical proximities or temporal distances are among the set of available quasi-identifiers. Despite some recent progress (Farrow, 2014), using the ordinal or metric information as quasi-identifiers in PPRL is an unresolved topic up to now.

One of the most urgent problems is due to missing identifiers or quasi-identifiers. This problem has received very little attention (Ong et al., 2014). Regarding encrypted identifiers in PPRL, currently very little is known. Therefore, for this important practical problem, systematic research is lacking.

Privacy-preserving blocking for datasets with about 100 million records on current hardware needs about a day of computing time. Using the most promising approaches from PPRL blocking, massive parallel or GPU implementations should be easy by comparison, since the results of blocks are independent in many applications. Although, parallel implementations of SN (Kolb, Thor and Rahm, 2012) and CC (https://mahout.apache.org) have been published, practical parallel implementations of PPRL blocking for secure environments are currently not readily available.

Instead of using functions of identifiers to compute similarities, Wong and Kim (2013) suggested a protocol to compute similarity coefficients of binary vectors by exchanging only some temporary summation variables with the help of a homomorphic encryption. The authors did not intend this approach to be used in PPRL, but these building blocks can be used as part of a PPRL protocol. Although Zhang and Zhang (2012) showed that the approach of Wong and Kim (2013) has security problems, the idea of using summation variables for comparing Bloom filters is new to PPRL. A different approach for cryptographic secure Bloom filter similarity computations was introduced by Beck and Kerschbaum (2013). They encrypt every bit of a Bloom filter in a two-party protocol to compute an approximation to the similarity of two Bloom filters. However, although none of these protocols meets the requirements for applications in real-world settings of medical research, they open new areas of research in PPRL.

9.9   PPRL research and implementation with national databases

Finally, it must be emphasised that the most important obstacles against the widespread use of PPRL techniques are not technical problems or the availability of easy to use software. More important than precision, recall and runtime performance is the acceptance of the protocols by the data protection agencies supervising the data custodians according to the relevant jurisdiction. Even if trusted and tested standard techniques such as anonymous linking codes are used, getting the legal permission for a national linkage project seems to require about 2 years in most jurisdictions. If new techniques have to be approved, longer delays should be expected. A recent example is given by a report for the British Office for National Statistics. They considered several methods for linking administrative data within the *Beyond 2011 Programme* but refrained from all '(…) recent innovations, such as Bloom filter encryption (…)' since they '(…) have not been fully explored from an accreditation perspective' (Office for National Statistics, 2013e; see Chapter 8). Therefore, if new PPRL techniques are to be widely used, systematic research on cryptographic properties according to European and other international legal standards has to be done. This will require the joint effort of lawyers, computer scientists, statisticians and cryptographic experts. Coordinated efforts across disciplines and across national borders within existing research structures usually require many years. Therefore, the actual implementation of new PPRL procedures may require at least as much political action as additional research efforts.

Acknowledgements

For computational assistance, I am indebted to Christian Borgs. For the clarification of some mathematical details, I have to thank Simone Steinmetzer. This research has been partly supported by the grant SCHN 586/17-1 of the German Research Foundation (DFG) awarded to author.

10

Summary

Katie Harron[1], Chris Dibben[2] and Harvey Goldstein[3,4]
[1] *London School of Hygiene and Tropical Medicine, London, UK*
[2] *University of Edinburgh, Edinburgh, UK*
[3] *Institute of Child Health, University College London, London, UK*
[4] *Graduate School of Education, University of Bristol, Bristol, UK*

10.1   Introduction

Methodological developments in data linkage brings together a collection of chapters that present the current state, immediate future, and potential future of data linkage methodology. The contributions from expert members of the international data linkage community fill a niche in the data linkage literature, focussing on up-to-date, cutting-edge methodology with applications to data systems internationally.

This concluding chapter summarises the issues with data linkage methodologies as they exist today, discusses how new developments will address these issues and highlights future areas of research.

10.2   Part 1: Data linkage as it exists today

The current state of data linkage methodology was summarised by Winkler with an overview of well-established probabilistic methods and parameter estimation techniques that have been in use for over 40 years (Chapter 2). Winkler also introduces the problem of linkage error and discusses methods for estimating false-match rates and adjusting for linkage error.

Chapter 3, contributed by authors within the UK Administrative Data Research Network, introduces the data linkage environment and models for data access and linkage. This chapter highlights the importance of well-organised, consistent and secure data linkage environments for sharing and linking data while minimising the risk of security breaches and protecting confidential information. In this context, practitioners have a responsibility to ensure that

Methodological Developments in Data Linkage, First Edition. Edited by Katie Harron, Harvey Goldstein and Chris Dibben.
© 2016 John Wiley & Sons, Ltd. Published 2016 by John Wiley & Sons, Ltd.

data is being shared and linked in such a way that it is also fit for purpose and that the quality of linked data can be evaluated. This makes close communication and collaboration between data custodians, data linkers and data users of vital importance.

The importance of evaluating linkage quality cannot be overemphasised. Data security requirements often mean that data linkers are separated from those who analyse the data so that any implications of linkage error for the efficiency or quality of the data analysis may not inform linkage procedures. Likewise, data users are separated from in-depth information on linkage methods so that uncertainties resulting from the linkage may not be apparent and hence not incorporated into the data analysis (Bohensky et al., 2010). High match rates alone may be sufficient for some purposes, but the examples presented by Bohensky in Chapter 4 demonstrate the dramatic effects that linkage error can have on results based on linked data, even when high match rates have been achieved. Bohensky explores common issues affecting linkage quality, provides a comprehensive review of the ways in which linkage error impacts on the quality of research findings and suggests recommendations for improving the quality of linkage through quality control procedures, transparent reporting and validation studies.

The chapters forming the first section of the book highlight several challenges for data linkage as it exists today, relating to different aspects of the data linkage process: quality of identifiers, quality of methods, quality of evaluation and quality of data security.

10.3   Part 2: Analysis of linked data

The middle section of the book attempts to present the immediate future of data linkage methodologies and focusses on the impact of the quality of identifier variables, linkage methods and non-random errors on the analysis of linked data.

10.3.1   Quality of identifiers

The issue of incomplete and imperfect identifiers is central to the problem of linkage error. This is particularly relevant when linkage is required between administrative datasets that were not necessarily collected with linkage in mind. If well-completed, unique identifiers were available in administrative datasets, linkage of data between sources would be straightforward, linkage error would be non-existent, and bias due to linkage error would not be present.

However, the dynamic and error-prone nature of administrative data means that identifiers are subject to recording error, missing values and changes over time. For cross-sectoral linkage (e.g. between health and educational data), the use of unique identifiers such as the NHS number in the United Kingdom or similar health system identifiers is not feasible, and key variables such as name, date of birth and place of residence have to be used. In practice, whatever data capture methods are used, recording errors will occur. Additionally, for longitudinal linkage, time-dependent identifiers (such as postal codes and surnames) can be unreliable and subject to change even when the actual recording is accurate, and other identifiers such as surname, sex and date of birth may not provide sufficient discrimination within large datasets (where different people share common identifiers).

Given these issues, linkage using incomplete and imperfect identifiers is likely to remain a significant problem for analyses based on linked data. Chapter 4 highlights the limitations of commonly used approaches for linkage of imperfect identifiers.

10.3.2   Quality of linkage methods

Probabilistic linkage is perhaps the most widely recommended approach for satisfactory linkage of data with imperfect or incomplete identifiers but has some outstanding issues, in particular the choice of appropriate thresholds. Typically, thresholds are selected subjectively by ordering potentially matching record pairs by match weight and (where feasible) performing clerical review. Ideally, the thresholds are chosen to minimise the total number of errors (i.e. false matches plus missed matches) or so that the errors cancel out (i.e. to minimise the absolute difference between the number of false matches and missed matches). However, without knowledge of the expected number of linkage errors for a particular match weight, choice of optimal thresholds is difficult. Manual review may also be unfeasible for the large numbers of records included in linkage systems for total populations.

A further issue with probabilistic linkage is the assumptions underlying match weight calculations and, in particular, the requirement for independence between identifiers (Daggy et al., 2013). There is relatively limited evidence in the literature on the impact of the failure of these assumptions on linkage. However, Tromp et al. (2008) found that dependence between highly correlated variables (such as expected birth date and actual date of birth) had a negative impact on match weights assigned to non-dependent variables and that this resulted in an incorrect ranking of record pairs ordered by match weight (Tromp et al., 2008). Similarly, Herzog, Scheuren and Winkler (2010) found that match weights assigned to non-dependent identifiers were too low in the presence of dependent identifiers (Herzog, Scheuren and Winkler, 2010). It is, however, commonly believed that the impact of dependence between identifiers is small and that the failure of the independence assumption can be ignored (Herzog, Scheuren and Winkler, 2007; Winkler, 1999). Chapter 6 suggests one approach that would, in principle, avoid the need for dependence between identifiers would be to directly calculate match probabilities jointly over a set of identifiers. It suggests that a set of match probabilities could be based, for example, on a log-linear model estimating the probability of a match given agreement and disagreement over a joint set of identifiers. Such a model would be able to take into account associations between the probability of agreement or disagreement and other variables (e.g. age, ethnicity, etc.) that might occur when particular groups of records are more prone to linkage error than others. Work in this area is currently ongoing.

The limitations of current methods highlight the need for continued development of methods to handle linkage error within analysis. These methods should take into account the fact that analysts may not have access to the original data (including identifiers). Two such methods are described in Chapters 5 and 6. In Chapter 5, Chambers and Kim focus on regression analyses, describing an approach for modelling bias due to incorrect linkage and for developing methods to correct it. Chapter 6 concentrates instead on a missing data imputation framework for handling uncertainty in linkage due to poor quality identifiers. The method proposed in Chapter 6 – prior-informed imputation – aims to produce efficient and unbiased results from a linked dataset derived using imperfect identifiers.

10.3.3   Quality of evaluation

Although measures of linkage error (e.g. sensitivity, specificity, match rate, etc.) are reported in the data linkage literature, there is no single universal method used for evaluating linkage quality (Pinto da Silveira and Artmann, 2009). This is likely to be because different methods of evaluation are appropriate in different situations.

One method for evaluating linkage quality was demonstrated by Lariscy (2011), where sensitivity analyses based on a range of linkage criteria were used for identifying 'differential' linkage, where particular groups of records are more likely to link than others (Lariscy, 2011). Such structured sensitivity analyses can provide a range of plausible results and reflect inherent uncertainty in the linkage process. To allow data users to perform sensitivity analyses, data linkers would need to provide the linkage quality data associated with each record pair being linked. In the case of probabilistic linkage, for example, this implies that match weights should be provided for all 'candidate' record pairs (not just the record with the highest match weight).

Comparing the characteristics of linked and unlinked data has also been shown to be useful in identifying potential sources of bias due to linkage error. For example, Ford, Roberts and Taylor (2006) compared the characteristics of linked and unlinked maternal and birth records and found that particular groups of records were under-represented in the linked pairs (Ford, Roberts and Taylor, 2006). These records were less likely to link, demonstrating non-random linkage error. To allow data users to compare the characteristics of linked and unlinked data, data linkers should also provide information on the unlinked records, so that these can be compared with the linked records to identify any potential sources of bias.

Gold-standard (or reference) data are also particularly useful for estimating linkage error and for evaluating the quality of linkage. Such datasets can be obtained through detailed manual review, the use of additional identifiers not available in all records, or external datasets (Fonseca et al., 2010; Monga and Patrick, 2001; Newgard, 2006; Wiklund and Eklund, 1986; Zingmond et al., 2004).

10.4   Part 3: Data linkage in practice: new developments

The final section of the book addresses the future of data linkage.

As described previously, many of the algorithms underpinning data linkage date back over four decades. The same applies to the approach taken to manage linked data, which has traditionally been done through relational databases. As the number of records we wish to link increases, the practicalities of storing multiple candidate links and associated match weights or probabilities need to be further explored. Chapter 7 presents a graph database approach, which provides much more flexibility, scalability and efficiency than traditional methods by storing records and links in the form of edges and nodes.

Chapter 8, contributed by authors from the UK Office for National Statistics, discusses how data linkage might be used as an alternative approach to more traditional methods of providing official statistics for total populations, in the context of recent drives to make increased use of administrative data and for transparency, open data and data sharing. One of the major challenges presented in this chapter is the requirement for linkage of identifiers that have been encrypted or 'pseudonymised' by each data provider. The chapter discusses a method of deriving the probability of a correct match based upon computing distance or similarity measures for each identifier. Where there is no perfect agreement, for example, on names, a thesaurus-based similarity measure between all possible congruences or candidate records can be computed and carried through the encryption process. Training data, based upon a subset of non-encrypted records, is developed through a process of manual review where match status is then assumed known. This training data is then used in a generalised linear model where the predictors are the similarity scores. The advantage of this approach is that dependencies among the error distributions across identifiers are implicitly taken into account. However, this method does rely upon the quality of the training set and the relevance of any chosen thesaurus to the data being linked. This is a similar motivation to the use of Bloom filters discussed in Chapter 10 although in principle is more general since it can define 'similarity' in a broader sense, rather than just based upon matching string sequences.

The theme of encryption and privacy protection is continued in Chapter 10, where Schnell addresses the situation where pseudonymisation of identifiers takes place at source or at least before files are linked. This approach increases privacy, since the transmission and possession of data are under enhanced protection through the removal of identifiers. Using encryption methods based upon Bloom filters, measures of similarity are estimated for all pairs of records. Thus, where an identifier agrees in both files, this will be detected, and a measure of similarity of agreement is derived in all other cases. These similarity measures can then be used to derive the weights for probabilistic linkage or as with thesaurus-based methods a predicted match probability based on training data. The chapter presents examples where this technique performs well and is an area of active research (Smith and Shlomo, 2014). An area for further research would be the study of procedures that in some way combine those discussed in Chapters 9 and 10.

An alternative approach based upon encryption methods that has had little use and that is not discussed in the present volume is a privacy-preserving method based upon commutative encryption (see Adam et al., 2007), which works as follows. Suppose, for simplicity, we have two data providers and a trusted third party (TTP). Data provider 1 securely encrypts all their data with an encryption and decryption key known only to themselves and which is never released to anyone else. They also randomly permute the columns (variables) in their dataset and retain this information securely. The data are securely passed to provider 2 who proceed to encrypt the data received from provider 1 with their own secret key which is also not revealed to anyone else. They use the same key to encrypt their own data file and also permute the columns and encrypt the permutation key using a private/public key system. This permutation adds a further layer of security against dictionary attack. The two resulting files are then sent securely to the TTP who encrypts both files with their own secret key. At this point, the data package is totally secure in the sense that none of the providers nor the TTP can decrypt the data, neither can any outside attacker. Within the data package, the identification of the provider is available, although this too can be encrypted using a private/public key system in order to add a further level of security.

When there is a requirement to link the two datasets, the decryption proceeds as follows. The data package is sent by the TTP to one of the providers (say, provider 1) who decrypts each dataset within the package with their own secret decryption key. The data remain secure and are sent to the next provider who does the same with their key. The resulting data which is still secured by the TTP encryption is sent to the TTP who at this stage is able to recover the clear data using their own decryption key together with the key to decrypt the permutation information.

The security advantages of such a scheme (which can be extended to any number of providers) are that only the TTP is ever able to see the clear data and can only do this with the permission of every data provider. Also, if at any future time the TTP wishes to add data from a further provider or to update the data from an existing provider, they need to only send the dataset, encrypted by the TTP alone or jointly with the original providers, call it dataset 1

(DS1), to the provider for them to encrypt DS1 and add another encrypted dataset. The provider has no access to the clear data since this remains encrypted within DS1. This package will be returned and lodged with the TTP. When linking is required, the new provider is added to the list of providers who need to decrypt the data. Thus, security is maintained with only the TTP ever able to see clear data. Governance arrangements within the TTP will be needed to ensure that clear data is only available for linkage purposes after which the identifiers are pseudonymised to ensure security within the TTP when they are further anonymised prior to release.

From the viewpoint of privacy-preserving data linkage, such a scheme would appear to be less secure than pseudonymisation at source (PAS) since at the data linkage stage, the clear identifiers are available. However, it actually has a stronger element of security in that, unlike PAS the encryption, no keys (except the permutation keys which are securely encoded) are transferred among a possibly large number of providers as pointed out previously. Each provider retains their own secret key and this will allow a greater ownership of the data. The important advantage, however, is that it allows fully efficient probabilistic linkage using established algorithms.

A further method is one based upon widely used public key cryptography methods used in commercial and other transactions. In this case, the linkage agency makes available its 'public' encryption key to every provider who then uses it to encrypt its file. Because this form of encryption is asymmetric, the decryption key is separate and held only by the linking agency. Transmission is secure, and when the linking agency has received all the files, it applies its secret decryption key to obtain the unencrypted data. Since this method is widely used (Zimmerman, 2014), it would seem to be an obvious candidate for general adoption. It does rely upon the linkage agency acting as a TTP, as pointed out previously, and thus could be viewed as less secure than other pseudonymisation procedures. However, since the linking agency will also typically be charged with the responsibility for anonymisation of any linked data that it makes available, this implies that it is formally trusted to safeguard the pre-release linked data *before* anonymisation. In both this case and in the case of commutative encryption methods, it seems to us that it would be somewhat bizarre if an agency were to be trusted with anonymising a linked (and hence potentially disclosive) dataset prior to distribution, but not trusted to manage the original unencrypted data before linking so as to preserve privacy.

10.5   Concluding remarks

The value of data linkage is well accepted, as it promises considerable time and cost advantages over new data collection for large numbers of individuals (Holman et al., 2008). The rich, informative datasets created through linkage of administrative data and administrative data with research survey data allow new insights into questions that could not otherwise have been addressed (Holman et al., 2008; Kelman et al., 2003; Merrall, Bird and Hutchinson, 2012). The opportunity to link data between institutional processes, technology in everyday use and commercial transactions means that linked data is playing an increasingly dominant role in social, economic and medical science. Nevertheless, the process required for linking, analysing, evaluating and managing these data sources is complex. Where current linkage approaches fail to provide reasonable solutions, new methodologies, as set out in the chapters of this book, are crucial for fully exploiting the opportunities presented by data linkage. Traditional forms of analysis may also need to be refined. Looking forward, it may be that advances in data linkage methodologies, as outlined in this book, require and lead to equally innovative developments in the field of statistical methodology. We finally very briefly speculate on some of the key issues that arise from a future increasingly dominated by linked administrative and transactional data.

In the context of linked data analysis, the uncritical application of statistical techniques that were developed in the context of experiments and survey methodologies may be inappropriate. Techniques designed to incorporate the uncertainty emerging from traditional sampling designs may be much less helpful in providing information on estimates derived from very large datasets. With very large data, the (mis)use of confidence intervals or significance tests as a heuristic for indicating an 'important' finding, for example, needs to be treated with even more caution than in traditional data environments. Data covering large real populations will not necessarily provide adequate study numbers. If there is only a small 'exposed' group within a population, then the power of any study to detect effects may be limited despite every individual being in the study. Traditional power calculations may not have the same relevance. This further emphasises both the importance of linkage to increase power and of utilising data from several populations.

New data infrastructures may be very rich in terms of certain important dimensions of research interest, but can be very sparse in others. For example, linked administrative and transactional data typically contain exact times for events, allowing sophisticated analysis of time to or between events. On the other hand, they rarely contain information on an individual's attitudes, beliefs or intentions. In contrast, more traditional survey and interview based tools have almost the opposite strengths and weaknesses. It is therefore unlikely that either of these broad approaches will replace the other. However, development in techniques for analysing unstructured text such as Natural Language Processing may allow the use of unsolicited expressions derived from online sources such as Facebook or Twitter for capturing sentiment in linked data. Effective methods for jointly analysing the two types of data structures are required (e.g. graphical models for combining mismatched data (Molitor et al., 2009)).

Finally, even linked datasets based on universal systems (i.e. total coverage of a real population) will be affected by missing data for a complex set of reasons. Importantly, these reasons are likely to vary between different datasets. The process of data linkage itself can also produce missing data, as discussed in Chapter 6. As well as dealing with main sources of missing data (e.g. non-response, follow up attrition, etc.), as is common with traditional study data, researchers may also need to consider systematic (institutional) as well as personal (individual) reasons for missingness. These reasons will vary between variables in the same dataset. For example, a dataset that combines data from welfare and hospital systems may have missingness within the welfare system because a particular regional office has not been promoting eligibility for a specific grant, certain population groups may be unwilling to apply for a grant or data may be missing in the hospital system because of the urgency of treatment. Missingness may also be related to the priority staff place on recording certain data and whether the individual concerned needs to be asked for the information. Patterns of missingness will be complex, and any assessment of whether they will bias results is difficult. Understanding how missing data arise is an important component of both the production and analysis of linked data so that existing procedures for handling missing data (Carpenter and Kenward, 2012) can be utilised.

We have aimed to provide a stimulating set of contributions in this volume, which we hope will motivate further methodological developments in data linkage.

References

3M Health Information Systems, 2013. 3M™ Healthcare Data Dictionary, USA. Available at: http://solutions.3m.com/ [accessed 28 November 2014].

Abbott, O., 2009. 2011 UK Census coverage assessment and adjustment methodology. Population Trends, 137(Autumn), 25–32.

Abbott, O. and Compton, G., 2014. Counting and estimating hard-to-survey populations in the 2011 Census. In: Tourangeau, R., Edwards, B., Johnson, T. P., Wolter, K. M. and Bates, N. A., editors. Hard-to-Survey Populations. Cambridge: Cambridge University Press, p 58–81.

Abrahams, C. and Davy, K., 2002. Linking HES maternity records with ONS birth records. Health Statistics Quarterly, 13, 22–30.

Acheson, E., 1967. Medical Record Linkage. London: Oxford University Press.

Adam, N., White, T., Shafiq, B., Vaidya, J. and He, X., 2007. Privacy preserving integration of health care data. AMIA Annual Symposium Proceedings, 2007, p 1–5.

Adly, N., 2009. Efficient record linkage using a double embedding scheme. In: Proceedings of the International Conference on Data Mining, 13–16 July 2009, Las Vegas, NV. Athens, GA: CSREA Press, p 274–281.

Agichstein, E. and Ganti, V., 2004. Mining reference tables for automatic text segmentation. In: ACM Knowledge Discovery and Data Mining Conference, 22–25 August 2004, Seattle, WA. New York: ACM, p 20–29.

Agresti, A., 2007. An Introduction to Categorical Data Analysis (2nd Edition). Hoboken, NJ: John Wiley & Sons, Inc.

Alaggan, M., Gambs, S. and Kermarrec, A.-M., 2012. BLIP: Non-interactive differentially-private similarity computation on bloom filters. In: Richa, A. W. and Scheideler, C., editors. Stabilization, Safety, and Security of Distributed Systems: Proceedings of the 14th International Symposium, 1–4 October 2012, Toronto, ON. Berlin/New York: Springer, p 202–216.

Atallah, M. J., Kerschbaum, F. and Du, W., 2003. Secure and private sequence comparisons. In: Samarati, P. and Syverson, P., editors. Proceedings of the ACM Workshop on Privacy in the Electronic Society, 30 October 2003, Washington, DC. New York: Association for Computing Machinery, p 39–44.

Aurelius, 2012–2014. Titan Distributed Graph Database. Available at: http://thinkaurelius.github.io/titan/ [accessed 26 June 2015].

Australian Bureau of Statistics, 2013. Wage and salary earner statistics for small areas. Available at: www.abs.gov.au/ausstats/abs@.nsf/mf/5673.0.55.003 [accessed 28 November 2014].

Aylin, P., Lees, T., Baker, S., Prytherch, D. and Ashley, S., 2007. Descriptive study comparing routine hospital administrative data with the Vascular Society of Great Britain and Ireland's National Vascular Database. European Journal of Vascular and Endovascular Surgery, 33(4), 461–465.

Bachteler, T., Schnell, S. and Reiher, J., 2010. An empirical comparison of approaches to approximate string matching in private record linkage. In: Proceedings of Statistics Canada Symposium 2010:

Social Statistics: The Interplay among Censuses, Surveys and Administrative Data. Ottawa: Statistics Canada, p 290–295.

Bachteler, T., Reiher, J. and Schnell, S., 2011. A simplified variant of a protocol for privacy-preserving string comparison. Technical Report 2011-01, Nuremberg: German Record Linkage Center.

Bachteler, T., Reiher, J. and Schnell, R., 2013. Similarity Filtering with Multibit Trees for Record Linkage. Working Paper WP-GRLC-2013-02. Nuremberg: German Record Linkage Center.

Baldi, I., Ponti, A., Zanetti, R., Ciccone, G., Merletti, F. and Gregori, D., 2010. The impact of record linkage bias in the Cox model. Journal of Evaluation in Clinical Practice, 16(1), 92–96.

Baxter, J., 1998. One number census matching. One Number Census Steering Committee Paper 98/14. Office for National Statistics. Available at: www.ons.gov.uk/ons/guide-method/census/census-2001/design-and-conduct/the-one-number-census/methodology/steering-committee/key-papers/matching-strategy.pdf [accessed 28 November 2014].

BBC-News, 2014. Community health systems data hack hits 4.5 million. Available at: http://www.bbc.com/news/technology-28838661 [accessed 28 November 2014].

Beck, M. and Kerschbaum, F., 2013. Approximate Two-Party Privacy-Preserving String Matching with Linear Complexity. IEEE International Congress on Big Data, BigData Congress, 2013 June 27–July 2.

Belin, T. and Rubin, D., 1995. A method for calibrating false-match rates in record linkage. JAMA, 90(430), 694–707.

Bentley, J. P., Ford, J. B., Taylor, L. K., Irvine, K. A. and Roberts, C. L., 2012. Investigating linkage rates among probabilistically linked birth and hospitalization records. BMC Medical Research Methodology, 12, 149.

Bhattacharya, I. and Getoor, L., 2006. A latent Dirichlet allocation model for entity resolution. In: Proceedings of the 6th SIAM Conference on Data Mining (SDM '06), 20–22 April 2006, Maryland. New York: Society for Industrial & Applied Mathematics, p 47–58.

Bibby, P. and Brindley, P., 2013. Urban and rural area definitions for policy purposes in England and Wales: Methodology. Available at: www.gov.uk/government/uploads/system/uploads/attachment_data/file/239477/RUC11methodologypaperaug_28_Aug.pdf [accessed 28 November 2014].

Bilenko, M., Basu, S. and Sahami, M., 2005. Adaptive product normalization: Using online learning for record linkage in comparison shopping. In: Proceedings of the International Conference on Data Mining, 27–30 November 2005, Houston, TX. Washington, DC: IEEE Computer Society, p 58–65.

Bilenko, M., Kamath, B. and Mooney, R. J., 2006. Adaptive blocking: Learning to scale up record linkage. In: Proceedings of the 6th IEEE International Conference on Data Mining, 18–22 December 2006, Hong Kong. Los Alamitos, CA: IEEE Computer Society.

Bilmes, J. A., 1998. A Gentle Tutorial of the EM Algorithm and Its Application for Parameter Estimation for Gaussian Mixture and Hidden Markov Models. Berkeley, CA: International Computer Science Institute. Available at: http://ssli.ee.washington.edu/people/bilmes/mypapers/em.pdf [accessed 28 November 2014].

Bishop, Y. M. M., Fienberg, S. E. and Holland, P. W., 1975. Discrete Multivariate Analysis. Cambridge, MA: MIT Press.

Bishop, G. and Khoo, J., 2007. Methodology of evaluating the quality of probabilistic linking. Technical Report 1351.0.55.018, Canberra, ACT: Australian Bureau of Statistics.

Black, N., Barker, M. and Payne, M., 2004. Cross sectional survey of multicentre clinical databases in the United Kingdom. BMJ, 328(7454), 1478.

Blakely, T., Woodward, A. and Salmond, C., 2000. Anonymous linkage of New Zealand mortality and Census data. Australian & New Zealand Journal of Public Health, 24(1), 92–95.

Bloom, B. H., 1970. Space/time trade-offs in hash coding with allowable errors. Communications of the ACM, 13(7), 422–426.

Bohensky, M. A., Jolley, D., Sundararajan, V., Evans, S., Pilcher, D., Scott, I. and Brand, C., 2010. Data linkage: A powerful research tool with potential problems. BMC Health Services Research, 10(1), 346–352.

Bohensky, M. A., Jolley, D., Sundararajan, V., Evans, S., Ibrahim, J. and Brand, C., 2011a. Development and validation of reporting guidelines for studies involving data linkage. Australian & New Zealand Journal of Public Health, 35(5), 486–489.

Bohensky, M. A., Jolley, D., Sundararajan, V., Pilcher, D. V., Evans, S. and Brand, C. A., 2011b. Empirical aspects of linking intensive care registry data to hospital discharge data without the use of direct patient identifiers. Anaesthesia and Intensive Care, 39(2), 202–208.

Bopp, M., Braun, J., Faeh, D. and Gutzwiller, F., 2010. Establishing a follow-up of the Swiss MONICA participants (1984–1993): Record linkage with census and mortality data. BMC Public Health, 10, 562.

Borkar, V., Deshmukh, K. and Sarawagi, S., 2001. Automatic segmentation of text into structured records. In: Association of Computing Machinery SIGMOD 2001, 17–19 March 2010, Hong Kong. New York: ACM, p 175–186.

Borst, F., Allaert, F. A. and Quantin, C., 2001. The Swiss solution for anonymous chaining patient files. In: Patel, V., Rogers, R. and Haux, R., editors. Proceedings of the 10th World Congress on Medical Informatics. Amsterdam: IOS Press, p 1239–1241.

Boyd, J. H., Ferrante, A. M., O'Keefe, C. M., Bass, A. J., Randall, S. M. and Semmens, J. B., 2012. Data linkage infrastructure for cross-jurisdictional health-related research in Australia. BMC Health Services Research, 12, 480.

Boyd, J. H., Randall, S., Ferrante, A., Bauer, J., Brown, A. and Semmens, J., 2014. Technical challenges of providing record linkage services for research. BMC Medical Informatics and Decision Making, 14(1), 23.

Brenner, H., Stegmaier, C. and Ziegler, H., 1995. Estimating completeness of cancer registration: an empirical evaluation of the two source capture-recapture approach in Germany. Journal of Epidemiology and Community Health, 49(4), 426–430.

Brenner, H., Schmidtmann, I. and Stegmaier, C., 1997. Effects of record linkage errors on registry-based follow-up studies. Statistics in Medicine, 16(23), 2633–2643.

Broder, A. Z., 1997. On the resemblance and containment of documents. In: Proceedings of Compression and Complexity of Sequences, Positano, Italy. Washington, DC: Institute of Electrical and Electronics Engineers, p 21–29.

Brown, J. J., 2000. Design of a Census Coverage Survey and Its Use in the Estimation and Adjustment of Census Underenumeration [unpublished PhD thesis]. Southampton: University of Southampton.

Budzinsky, C. D., 1991. Automated spelling correction. Statistics Canada Technical Report, Ottawa: Statistics Canada.

Buerli, M., 2012. The current state of graph databases. Available at: http://www.cs.utexas.edu/~cannata/dbms/Class%20Notes/09%20Graph_Databases_Survey.pdf [accessed 28 November 2014].

Campbell, K. M., Deck, D. and Krupski, A., 2008. Record linkage software in the public domain: A comparison of Link Plus, The Link King, and a 'basic' deterministic algorithm. Health Informatics Journal, 14(1), 5–15.

Campbell, K. M., 2009. Impact of record-linkage methodology on performance indicators and multivariate relationships. Journal of Substance Abuse Treatment, 36(1), 110–117.

Carpenter, J. and Kenward, M., 2012. Multiple Imputation and Its Application. Chichester: John Wiley & Sons, Ltd.

Chambers, R., 2009. Regression analysis of probability-linked data. Research Series, Official Statistics. Available at: www.statisphere.govt.nz/~/media/statisphere/Files/official-statistics-research-series/osr-series-v4-2009-regression-analysis-probability-linked-data.pdf [accessed 28 November 2014].

Chambers, R., Chipperfield, J., Davis, W. and Kovacevic, M., 2009. Inference based on estimating equations and probability-linked data. In: Centre for Statistical & Survey Methodology, Working Paper Series. Wollongong: University of Wollongong, p 38.

Chambers, R. L., Steel, D. G., Wang, S. and Welsh, A., 2012. Maximum Likelihood Estimation for Sample Surveys, Chapman and Hall/CRC Monographs on Statistics and Applied Probability. Hoboken, NJ: CRC Press.

Charlton, C., Michaelides, D., Cameron, B., Szmaragd, C., Parker, R., Yang, H., Zhang, Z. and Browne, W., 2012. Stat-JR Software. Center for Multilevel Modelling, University of Bristol and Electronics and Computer Science, University of Southampton.

Chattopadhyay, A. and Bindman, A. B., 2005. Accuracy of medicaid payer coding in hospital patient discharge data: Implications for medicaid policy evaluation. Medical Care, 43(6), 586–591.

Chen, B.-C., Kifer, D., LeFevre, K. and Machanavajjhala, A., 2009. Privacy-Preserving Data Publishing, Foundations and Trends in Databases, Vol. 2. Boston, MA: Now.

Chipperfield, J. O., Bishop, G. R. and Campbell, P., 2011. Maximum likelihood estimation for contingency tables and logistic regression with incorrectly linked data. Survey Methodology, 37(1), 13–24.

Chipperfield, J. O. and Chambers, R., 2015. Using the bootstrap to analyse binary data obtained via probabilistic linkage. Journal of Official Statistics (in press).

Christen, P., Churches, T. and Zhu, J. X., 2002. Probabilistic name and address cleaning and standardisation. In: The Australian Data Mining Workshop, November. Available at: http://datamining.anu.edu.au/projects/linkage [accessed 28 November 2014].

Christen, P. and Goiser, K., 2005. Assessing deduplication and data linkage quality: What to measure? In: Proceedings of the 4th Australasian Data Mining Conference, 5–6 December 2005, Sydney. Canberra, ACT: Australian National University.

Christen, P. and Goiser, K., 2007. Quality and complexity measures for data linkage and deduplication. Studies in Computational Intelligence, 43, 127–151.

Christen, P., 2008. Febrl: An open source data cleaning, deduplication and record linkage system with a graphical user interface. In: Li, Y., Liu, B. and Sarawagi, S., editors. Proceedings of the 14th ACM SIGKDD International Conference on Knowledge Discovery and Data Mining. New York: ACM, p 1065–1068.

Christen, P., 2012a. Data Matching: Concepts and Techniques for Record Linkage, Entity Resolution and Duplicate Detection. Berlin: Springer.

Christen, P., 2012b. A survey of indexing techniques for scalable record linkage and deduplication. IEEE Transactions on Knowledge and Data Engineering, 24(9), 1537–1555.

Christen, P., Verykios, V. and Vatsalan, D., 2013. A tutorial on techniques for scalable privacy-preserving record linkage. Available at: http://cs.anu.edu.au/~Peter.Christen/cikm2013pprl-tutorial/cikm-2013-pprl-tutorial-slides.pdf [accessed 28 November 2014].

Churches, T., Christen, P., Lu, J. and Zhu, J. X., 2002. Preparation of name and address data for record linkage using hidden Markov models. BMC Medical Informatics and Decision Making, 2, 9.

Churches, T. and Christen, P., 2004. Some methods for blindfolded record linkage. BMC Medical Informatics and Decision Making, 4, 9.

Cochinwala, M., Kurien, V., Lalk, G. and Shasha, D., 2001. Efficient data reconciliation. Information Sciences, 137(1–4), 1–15.

Cohen, W. W., Ravikumar, P. and Fienberg, S. E., 2003a. A comparison of string metrics for matching names and addresses. In: International Joint Conference on Artificial Intelligence, Proceedings of the Workshop on Information Integration on the Web, Acapulco, Mexico, August 2003.

Cohen, W. W., Ravikumar, P. and Fienberg, S. E., 2003b. A comparison of string distance metrics for name-matching tasks. In: Proceedings of the ACM Workshop on Data Cleaning, Record Linkage and Object Identification, Washington, DC, August 2003.

Cohen, W. W. and Sarawagi, S., 2004. Exploiting dictionaries in named entity extraction: Combining semi-Markov extraction processes and data integration methods. In: Proceedings of the ACM Knowledge Discovery and Data Mining Conference 2005, 21–24 August 2005, Chicago, IL. New York: ACM, p 89–98.

Cooper, W. S. and Maron, M. E., 1978. Foundations of probabilistic and utility-theoretic indexing. Journal of the Association for Computing Machinery, 25, 67–80.

Copas, J. B. and Hilton, F. J., 1990. Record linkage: Statistical models for matching computer records. Journal of the Royal Statistical Society, A, 153, 287–320.

Criminisi, A., Shotton, J. and Konukoglu, E., 2012. Decision forests: A unified framework for classification, regression, density estimation, manifold learning and semi-supervised learning. Foundations and Trends in Computer Graphics and Vision, 7(2), 81–227.

Daggy, J., Xu, H., Hui, S., Gamache, R. and Grannis, S., 2013. A practical approach for incorporating dependence among fields in probabilistic record linkage. BMC Medical Research Methodology, 13(1), 97.

Dalenius, T., 1977. Towards a methodology for statistical disclosure control. Statistisk Tidskrift, 15, 429–444.

Deming, W. E. and Gleser, G. J., 1959. On the problem of matching lists by samples. Journal of the American Statistical Association, 54, 403–415.

Dempster, A. P., Laird, N. M. and Rubin, D. B., 1977. Maximum likelihood from incomplete data via the EM algorithm. Journal of the Royal Statistical Society, B, 39, 1–38.

Dickinson, H. O., Salotti, J. A., Birch, P. J., Reid, M. M., Malcolm, A. and Parker, L., 2001. How complete and accurate are cancer registrations notified by the National Health Service Central Register for England and Wales? Journal of Epidemiology and Community Health, 55(6), 414–422.

Dolson, D., 2010. Census coverage studies in Canada: A history with emphasis on the 2011 census. In: Proceedings of the Section on Survey Research Methods JSM 2010, 31 July – 5 August 2010. Alexandria, VA: American Statistical Association, p 441–445.

Doyle, P., Lane, J. I., Theeuwes, J. M. and Zayatz, L. M., 2001. Confidentiality, Disclosure and Data Access. New York: Elsevier.

Duncan, G., Elliot, M. J. and Salazar, J. J., 2011. Statistical Confidentiality. New York: Springer.

Dunn, H., 1946. Record linkage. American Journal of Public Health, 36(12), 1412–1416.

Durham, E. A., 2012. A Framework for Accurate, Efficient Private Record Linkage [PhD thesis]. Nashville: Vanderbilt University.

Durham, E. A., Kantarcioglu, M., Xue, Y., Toth, C., Kuzu, M., and Malin, B., 2013. Composite Bloom filters for secure record linkage. IEEE Transactions on Knowledge and Data Engineering, 99, 1.

Duvall, S. L., Fraser, A. M., Kerber, R. A., Mineau, G. P. and Thomas, A., 2010. The impact of a growing minority population on identification of duplicate records in an enterprise data warehouse. Studies in Health Technology and Informatics, 160(Pt 2), 1122–1126.

Dwork, C. and Pottenger, R., 2013. Toward practicing privacy. Journal of the American Medical Informatics Association, 20(1), 102–108.

Dygaszewicz, J., 2012. Modern census in Poland. Paper presented at United Nations International Seminar on Population and Housing Censuses: Beyond the 2010 Round, 27–29 November 2012, Seoul, Republic of Korea. Available at: unstats.un.org/unsd/demographic/meetings/Conferences/Korea/2012/docs/s07-4-1-Poland.pdf [accessed 2 December 2014].

Elfeky, M. G., Verykios, V. and Elmagarmid, A. K., 2002. TAILOR: A record linkage toolbox. In: International Conference on Data Engineering, 26 February – 1 March 2002, San Jose, CA. Washington, DC: IEEE Computer Society, p 17–28.

Ellenberg, J. H., 1994. Selection bias in observational and experimental studies. Statistics in Medicine, 13(5–7), 557–567.

Elliot, M. J., 2005. Statistical Disclosure Control: Encyclopaedia of Social Measurement, Vol. 3. New York: Elsevier, p 663–670.

Elmagarmid, A., Ipeirotis, P. and Verykios, V., 2007. Duplicate record detection: A survey. IEEE Transactions on Knowledge and Data Engineering, 19(1), 1–16.

Emam, E. K., Jonker, E., Arbuckle, L. and Malin, B., 2011. A systematic review of re-identification attacks on health data. PLoS ONE, 6(12), e28071.

Evans, S. M., Bohensky, M., Cameron, P. A. and McNeil, J., 2011. A survey of Australian clinical registries: Can quality of care be measured? Internal Medicine Journal, 41(1a), 42–48.

Farrow, J. and Churches, T., 2011. A Graph-Based Approach to Managing Linkage Data. Canberra, ACT: PHRN Technical Forum.

Farrow, J., 2012a. A graph-based approach to managing linkage data: Exploiting modern hardware and computing techniques. In: International Data Linkage Conference 'Inside the Black Box' Workshop, 2–4 May 2012, Perth, Western Australia.

Farrow, J., 2012b. NGLS Technical Architecture. Melbourne, VIC: PHRN Technical Forum.

Farrow, J., 2012c. Using graph theory and graph databases to manage record linkage data. In: International Data Linkage Conference, 2–4 May 2012, Perth, Western Australia.

Farrow, J., 2014. Privacy preserving distance-comparable geohashing. Presentation at the International Health Data Linkage Conference 2014, 28–30 April 2014, Vancouver, Canada.

Federal Statistical Office, 2012a. The register of addresses and buildings – a combination of different registers. UNECE-Eurostat Expert Group Meeting on Censuses Using Registers, Geneva, 22–23 May 2012. Available at: www.unece.org/fileadmin/DAM/stats/documents/ece/ces/ge.41/2012/use_of_register/WP_12_Germany.pdf [accessed 2 December 2014].

Federal Statistical Office, 2012b. The population registers in Germany – the main data source in the 2011 Census. UNECE-Eurostat Expert Group Meeting on Censuses Using Registers, Geneva, 22–23 May 2012. Available at: www.unece.org/fileadmin/DAM/stats/documents/ece/ces/ge.41/2012/use_of_register/WP_13_Germany.pdf [accessed 2 December 2014].

Fellegi, I. and Sunter, A., 1969. A theory for record linkage. Journal of the American Statistical Association, 64(328), 1183–1210.

Ferrante, A. and Boyd, J., 2012. A transparent and transportable methodology for evaluating Data Linkage software. Journal of Biomedical Informatics, 45(1), 165–172.

Fett, M. J., 1984. The development of matching criteria for epidemiological studies using record linkage techniques. International Journal of Epidemiology, 13(3), 351–355.

Finney, J. M., Walker, A. S., Peto, T. E. and Wyllie, D. H., 2011. An efficient record linkage scheme using graphical analysis for identifier error detection. BMC Medical Informatics and Decision Making, 11, 7.

Fonseca, M., Coeli, C., Lucena, F., Veloso, V. and Carvalho, M., 2010. Accuracy of a probabilistic record linkage strategy applied to identify deaths among cases reported to the Brazilian AIDS surveillance database. Cadernos de Saúde Pública, 26, 1431–1438.

Ford, J. B., Roberts, C. L. and Taylor, L. K., 2006. Characteristics of unmatched maternal and baby records in linked birth records and hospital discharge data. Paediatric and Perinatal Epidemiology, 20(4), 329–337.

Ford, D. V., Jones, K. H., Verplancke, J. P., Lyons, R. A., John, G., Brown, G., Brooks, C. J., Thompson, S., Bodger, O., Couch, T. and Leake, K., 2009. The SAIL Databank: Building a national architecture for e-health research and evaluation. BMC Health Services Research, 9, 157.

Fournel, I., Schwarzinger, M., Binquet, C., Benzenine, E., Hill, C. and Quantin, C., 2009. Contribution of record linkage to vital status determination in cancer patients. Studies in Health Technology and Informatics, 150, 91–95.

Fox, W. R. and Lasker, G. W., 1983. The distribution of surname frequencies. International Statistical Review, 51(1), 81–87.

Freund, Y. and Schapire, R. E., 1996. Experiments with a new boosting algorithm. In: Machine Learning: Proceedings of the 13th International Conference, 3–6 July 1996, Bari. San Francisco, CA: Morgan Kaufmann, p 148–156.

Gamma, E., Helm, R., Johnson, R. and Vlissides, J., 1994. Design Patterns: Elements of Reusable Object-Oriented Software. Indianapolis, IN: Pearson Education.

Ganta, S. R., Kasiviswanathan, S. P. and Smith, A., 2008. Composition attacks and auxiliary informa-tion in data privacy. In: Proceedings of the 14th ACM SIGKDD International Conference on Knowledge Discovery and Data Mining. New York: ACM, p 265–273.

German, R. R., 2000. Sensitivity and predictive value positive measurements for public health surveil-lance systems. Epidemiology, 11(6), 720–727.

Gill, L., 1997. OX-LINK: The oxford medical record linkage system. In: Alvey, W. and Jamerson, B., edi-tors. Record Linkage Techniques: Proceedings of an International Workshop and Exposition. Washington, DC: Federal Committee on Statistical Methodology, Office of Management and Budget, p 15–33.

Gill, L., 2001. Methods of automatic record matching and linking and their use in national statistics. National Statistics Methodological Series, No. 25. Available at: http://www.ons.gov.uk/ons/guide-method/method-quality/specific/gss-methodology-series/gss-methodology-series--25--methods-for-automatic-record-matching-and-linkage-and-their-use-in-national-statistics.pdf [accessed 17 December 2014].

Goeken, R., Huynh, L., Lynch, T. and Vick, R., 2011. New methods of census record linking. Historical Methods, 44(1), 7–14.

Goldberg, A. and Borthwick, A., 2004. The Choicemaker 2 record matching system. Available at: cs.nyu.edu/artg/publications/goldberg_borthwick_The_ChoiceMaker_2_Record_Matching_System_2007.pdf [accessed 2 December 2014].

Goldstein, H., Carpenter, J., Kenward, M. G. and Levin, K. A., 2009. Multilevel models with multivari-ate mixed response types. Statistical Modelling, 9(3), 173–197.

Goldstein, H. and Kounali, D., 2009. Multilevel multivariate modelling of childhood growth, numbers of growth measurements and adult characteristics. Journal of the Royal Statistical Society: Series A, 172(3), 599–613.

Goldstein, H., Harron, K. and Wade, A., 2012. The analysis of record-linked data using multiple impu-tation with data value priors. Statistics in Medicine, 31(28), 3481–3493.

Goldstein, H., Carpenter, J. and Browne, W., 2014. Fitting multilevel multivariate models with missing data in responses and covariates that may include interactions and nonlinear terms. Journal of the Royal Statistical Society: Series A, 177(2), 553–564.

Gomatam, S., Carter, R., Ariet, M. and Mitchell, G., 2002. An empirical comparison of record linkage procedures. Statistics in Medicine, 21(10), 1485–1496.

Grannis, S. J., Overhage, J. M. and McDonald, C. J., 2002. Analysis of identifier performance using a deterministic linkage algorithm. Proceedings of the AMIA Symposium, 2002, p 305–309.

Grannis, S. J., Overhage, J. M., Hui, S. and McDonald, C. J., 2003. Analysis of a probabilistic record linkage technique without human review. AMIA Annual Symposium Proceedings, 2003, 259–263.

Gutman, R., Afendulis, C. C. and Zaslavsky, A. M., 2013. A Bayesian procedure for file linking to ana-lyze end-of-life medical costs. Journal of the American Statistical Association, 108(501), 34–47.

Hall, P. A. V. and Dowling, G. R., 1980. Approximate string comparison. Association of Computing Machinery, Computing Surveys, 12, 381–402.

Hall, R., Fienberg, S. E., 2010. Privacy-preserving record linkage. In: Domingo-Ferrer, J. and Magkos, E., editors. Privacy in Statistical Databases, Lecture Notes in Computer Science No 6344. Berlin: Springer, p 269–283.

Harron, K., Wade, A., Muller-Pebody, B., Goldstein, H. and Gilbert, R., 2012. Opening the black box of record linkage. Journal of Epidemiology and Community Health, 66(12), 1198.

Harron, K., Wade, A., Muller-Pebody, B., Goldstein, H., Parslow, R., Gray, J., Hartley, J. C., Mok, Q. and Gilbert, R., 2013. Risk-adjusted monitoring of blood-stream infection in paediatric intensive care: A data linkage study. Intensive Care Medicine, 39(6), 1080–1087.

Harron, K., Wade, A., Gilbert, R., Muller-Pebody, B. and Goldstein, H., 2014. Evaluating bias due to data linkage error in electronic healthcare records. BMC Medical Research Methodology, 14, 36.

Hastie, T., Tibshirani, R. and Friedman, J., 2001. The Elements of Statistical Learning: Data Mining, Inference, and Prediction. New York: Springer.

Haupt, R. L. and Haupt, S. E., 2004. Practical Genetic Algorithms (2nd Edition). Hoboken, NJ: John Wiley & Sons, Inc.

Hentschel, S. and Katalinic, A. (Eds), 2008. Das Krebsregister-Manual der Gesellschaft der epidemiologischen Krebsregister in Deutschland e.V. München: Zuckerschwerdt Verlag

Herman, A., McCarthy, B., Bakewell, J., Ward, R., Mueller, B., Maconochie, N., Read, A., Zadka, P. and Skjaerven, R., 1997. Data linkage methods used in maternally-linked birth and infant death surveillance data sets from the United States (Georgia, Missouri, Utah and Washington State), Israel, Norway, Scotland and Western Australia. Paediatric and Perinatal Epidemiology, 11(S1), 5–22.

Hernández, M. A. and Stolfo, S. S., 1998. Real-world data is dirty: Data cleansing and the merge/purge problem. Data Mining and Knowledge Discovery, 2(1), 9–37.

Herzog, T. N., Scheuren, F. J. and Winkler, W. E., 2007. Data Quality and Record Linkage Techniques. New York: Springer.

Herzog, T. N., Scheuren, F. and Winkler, W. E., 2010. Record Linkage. In: Scott, D. W., Said, Y. and Wegman, E., editors. Wiley Interdisciplinary Reviews: Computational Statistics. New York: Wiley, p 535–543.

Hills, B., 2014. Combing through the grey: Use of linkage outcome strings to complement record weights for linkage at Population Data BC. In: 2014 International Health Data Linkage Conference, 28–30 April 2014, Vancouver, Canada.

Hjaltason, G. R. and Samet, H., 2003. Properties of embedding methods for similarity searching in metric spaces. IEEE Transactions on Pattern Analysis and Machine Intelligence, 25(5), 530–549.

Hof, M. H. P. and Zwinderman, A. H., 2012. Methods for analyzing data from probabilistic linkage strategies based on partially identifying variables. Statistics in Medicine, 31(30), 4231–4242.

Hogan, H., 1992. The 1990 post-enumeration survey: An overview. The American Statistician, 46, 261–269.

Holman, C., Bass, A., Rouse, I. and Hobbs, M., 1999. Population based linkage of health records in Western Australia: Development of a health services research linked database. Australian & New Zealand Journal of Public Health, 23(5), 453–459.

Holman, C., Bass, J., Rosman, D., Smith, M., Semmens, J., Glasson, E., Brook, E., Trutwein, B., Rouse, I. and Watson, C., 2008. A decade of data linkage in Western Australia: Strategic design, applications and benefits of the WA data linkage system. Australian Health Review, 32(4), 766–777.

Hundepool, A., Domingo-Ferrer, J., Franconi, L., Giessing, S., Schulte Nordholt, E., Spicer, K. and de Wolf, P.-P., 2012. Statistical Disclosure Control. Chichester: John Wiley & Sons, Ltd.

Huntington, S. E., Bansi, L. K., Thorne, C., Anderson, J., Newell, M. L., Taylor, G. P., Pillay, D., Hill, T., Tookey, P. A. and Sabin, C. A., 2012. Using two on-going HIV studies to obtain clinical data from before, during and after pregnancy for HIV-positive women. BMC Medical Research Methodology, 12, 110.

Identity Theft Resource Centre, 2014. 2013 data breach category summary. Technical Report, San Diego, CA: Identity Theft Resource Center.

Iezzoni, L. I., 1997a. The risks of risk adjustment. JAMA, 278(19), 1600–1607.

Iezzoni, L. I., 1997b. Assessing quality using administrative data. Annals of Internal Medicine, 127(8 Pt 2), 666–674.

Indyk, P. and Motwani, R., 1998. Approximate nearest neighbors: Towards removing the curse of dimensionality. In: Proceedings of the 30th Annual ACM Symposium on the Theory of Computing, Dallas, 23–26 May 1998. New York: ACM.

Information Commissioners Office, 2012. Code of practice. Available at: www.ico.org.uk/for_organisations/data_protection/topic_guides/anonymisation [accessed 2 December 2014].

Jakobsen, T., 1995. A fast method for the cryptanalysis of substitution ciphers. Cryptologia, 19(3), 265–274.

Jamieson, E., Roberts, J. and Browne, G., 1995. The feasibility and accuracy of anonymized record linkage to estimate shared clientele among three health and social service agencies. Methods of Information in Medicine, 34(4), 371–377.

Karakasidis, A. and Verykios, V. S., 2009. Privacy preserving record linkage using phonetic codes. In: Proceedings of the 2009 4th Balkan Conference in Informatics, BCI'09, 17–19 September 2009. Washington, DC: IEEE Computer Society, p 101–106.

Karakasidis, A. and Verykios, V. S., 2011. Secure blocking + secure matching = secure record linkage. Journal of Computing Science and Engineering, 5(3), 223–235.

Karakasidis, A. and Verykios, V. S., 2012a. A sorted neighbourhood approach to multidimensional privacy preserving blocking. In: 2012 IEEE 12th International Conference on Data Mining Workshops (ICDMW), 10 December 2012. Los Alamitos, CA: IEEE Computer Society, p 937–944.

Karakasidis, A. and Verykios, V. S., 2012b. Reference table based k-anonymous private blocking. In: Proceedings of the 27th Annual ACM Symposium on Applied Computing. New York: ACM, p 859–864.

Karakasidis, A., Verykios, V. S. and Christen, P., 2012. Fake injection strategies for private phonetic matching. In: Garcia-Alfaro, J., Navarro-Arribas, G., Cuppens-Boulahia, N., de Capitani di Vimercati, S., editors. Data Privacy Management and Autonomous Spontaneous Security, Lecture Notes in Computer Science, Vol. 7122. Berlin: Springer, p 9–24.

Karapiperis, D. and Verykios, V. S., 2014. A distributed near-optimal LSH-based framework for privacy-preserving record linkage. Computer Science and Information Systems, 11(2), 745–763.

Karmel, R. and Rosman, D., 2008. Linkage of health and aged care service events: Comparing linkage and event selection methods. BMC Health Services Research, 8, 149.

Karmel, R., Anderson, P., Gibson, D., Peut, A., Duckett, S. and Wells, Y., 2011. Empirical aspects of record linkage across multiple data sets using statistical linkage keys: The experience of the PIAC cohort study. BMC Health Services Research, 10, 41.

Karr, A., Lin, X., Sanil, A. and Reiter, J., 2009. Privacy-preserving analysis of vertically partitioned data using secure matrix products. Journal of Official Statistics, 25(1), 125–138.

Kawai, H., Garcia-Molina, H., Benjelloun, O., Menestrina, D., Whang, E. and Gong, H., 2006. P-Swoosh: Parallel algorithm for generic entity resolution. Stanford University CS Technical Report, Stanford, CA: Stanford University.

Kelman, C. W., Bass, A. J. and Holman, C. D. J., 2002. Research use of linked health data—a best practice protocol. Australian & New Zealand Journal of Public Health, 26(3), 251–255.

Kelman, C. W., Kortt, M. A., Becker, N. G., Li, Z., Mathews, J. D., Guest, C. S. and Holman, C. D. J., 2003. Deep vein thrombosis and air travel: Record linkage study. BMJ, 327(7423), 1072–1075.

Kelsey, J., Schneier, B., Hall, C. and Wagner, D., 1998. Secure applications of low-entropy keys. In: Okamoto, E., Davida, G. and Mambo, M., editors. Information Security. Berlin: Springer, p 121–134.

Kendrick, S. and Clarke, J., 1993. The Scottish record linkage system. Health Bulletin, 51(2), 72.

Kenig, B. and Gal, A., 2013. MFI blocks: An effective blocking algorithm entity resolution. Information Systems, 38(6), 908–926.

Kho, M. E., Duffett, M., Willison, D. J., Cook, D. J. and Brouwers, M. C., 2009. Written informed consent and selection bias in observational studies using medical records: Systematic review. BMJ, 338, b866.

Kim, G. and Chambers, R., 2011. Regression analysis under probabilistic multi-linkage. Statistica Neerlandica, 66(1), 64–79.

Kim, G. and Chambers, R., 2012a. Regression analysis under incomplete linkage. Computational Statistics and Data Analysis, 56, 2756–2770.

Kim, G. and Chambers, R., 2012b. Regression analysis under probabilistic multi-linkage. Statistica Neerlandica, 66(1), 64–79.

Kim, G. and Chambers, R., 2013. Bias Reduction for Correlated Linkage Error. Working Paper Series. Wollongong: NIASRA, University of Wollongong.

Kirsch, A. and Mitzenmacher, M., 2006. Less hashing, same performance: Building a better bloom filter. In: Azar, Y. and Erlebach, T., editors. Proceedings of the 14th Annual European Symposium on Algorithms, 11–13 September 2006, Zurich, Switzerland. Heidelberg: Springer, p 456–467.

Kolb, L., Thor, A. and Rahm, E., 2012. Multi-pass sorted neighbourhood blocking with MapReduce. Computer Science - Research and Development, 27(1), 45–63.

Kolb, L. and Rahm, E., 2013. Parallel entity resolution with Dedoop. Datenbank-Spektrum, 13(1), 23–32. Available at: http://dbs.uni-leipzig.de/file/parallel_er_with_dedoop.pdf [accessed 2 December 2014].

Köpcke, H. and Rahm, E., 2008. Training selection for tuning entity matching. In: Proceedings of the Sixth International Workshop on Quality in Databases and Management of Uncertain Data (QDB/MUD '08), 24 August 2008, Auckland, New Zealand. CTIT Workshop Proceedings Series (WP-CTIT-08-02). Centre for Telematics and Information Technology University of Twente, Enschede, The Netherlands. Enschede: CTIT, p 3–12.

Krewski, D., Dewanji, A., Wang, Y., Bartlett, S., Zielinski, J. and Mallick, R., 2005. The effect of record linkage errors on risk estimates in cohort mortality studies. Survey Methodology, 31(1), 13–21.

Kristensen, T. G., Nielsen, J. and Pedersen, C. N. N., 2010. A tree-based method for the rapid screening of chemical fingerprints. Algorithms for Molecular Biology, 5, 9.

Kuehni, C. E., Rueegg, C. S., Michel, G., Rebholz, C. E., Strippoli, M.-P. F., Niggli, F. K., Egger, M. and von der Weid, N. X., 2011. Cohort profile: The Swiss childhood cancer survivor study. International Journal of Epidemiology, 41(6), 1553–1564.

Kuhn, M. and Anderson, R. J., 1998. Soft tempest: Hidden data transmission using electromagnetic emanations. In: Aucsmith, D., editor. Information Hiding, 2nd International Workshop, IH'98, Portland, Oregon, 15–17 April 1998, Proceedings, LNCS 1525. Berlin/New York: Springer-Verlag, p 124–142.

Kuzu, M., Kantarcioglu, M., Durham, E. A. and Malin, B., 2011. A constraint satisfaction cryptanalysis of bloom filters in private record linkage. In: Fischer-Hübner, S. and Hopper, N., editors. The 11th Privacy Enhancing Technologies Symposium. Berlin: Springer, p 226–245.

Kuzu, M., Kantarcioglu, M., Durham, E. A., Toth, C. and Malin, B., 2013. A practical approach to achieve private medical record linkage in light of public resources. Journal of the American Medical Informatics Association, 20(2), 285–292.

Lahiri, P. and Larsen, M. D., 2005. Regression analysis with linked data. Journal of the American Statistical Association, 100, 222–230.

Lain, S. J., Algert, C. S., Tasevski, V., Morris, J. M. and Roberts, C. L., 2009. Record linkage to obtain birth outcomes for the evaluation of screening biomarkers in pregnancy: A feasibility study. BMC Medical Research Methodology, 9, 48.

Langan, S. M., Benchimol, E. I., Guttmann, A., Moher, D., Petersen, I., Smeeth, L., Sorensen, H. T., Stanley, F. and Von Elm, E., 2013. Setting the RECORD straight: Developing a guideline for the REporting of studies Conducted using Observational Routinely collected Data. Clinical Epidemiology, 5, 29–31.

Lariscy, J. T., 2011. Differential record linkage by Hispanic ethnicity and age in linked mortality studies. Journal of Aging and Health, 23(8), 1263–1284.

Larsen, M. D. and Rubin, D. B., 2001. Alterative automated record linkage using mixture models. Journal of the American Statistical Association, 79, 32–41.

Larsen, K., 2005. Generalized naïve Bayes classifiers. SIGKDD Explorations, 7(1), 76–81.

Lauer, M. S. and D'Agostino, R. B. Sr., 2013. The randomized registry trial: The next disruptive technology in clinical research? New England Journal of Medicine, 369(17), 1579–1581.

Lawson, E. H., Ko, C. Y., Louie, R., Han, L., Rapp, M. and Zingmond, D. S., 2013. Linkage of a clinical surgical registry with Medicare inpatient claims data using indirect identifiers. Surgery, 153(3), 423–430.

Legarrete, L. and Ayestaran, M., 2004. Applying methods of record linkage for census validation in the Basque statistics office. Paper presented at European Conference on Quality and Methodology in Official Statistics (Q2004). Available at: www.eustat.es/documentos/datos/pon_19_i.pdf [accessed 2 December 2014].

Leiss, J. K., 2007. A new method for measuring misclassification of maternal sets in maternally linked birth records: True and false linkage proportions. Maternal and Child Health Journal, 11(3), 293–300.

Leskovec, J., Rajaraman, A. and Ullman, J. D., 2014. Mining of Massive Datasets (2nd Edition). Cambridge: Cambridge University Press. Available at: www.mmds.org [accessed 2 December 2014].

Li, B., Quan, H., Fong, A. and Lu, M., 2006. Assessing record linkage between health care and Vital statistics databases using deterministic methods. BMC Health Services Research, 6, 48.

Liginlal, D., Sim, I. and Khansa, L., 2009. How significant is human error as a cause of privacy breaches? An empirical study and a framework for error management. Computers and Security, 28(3), 215–228.

Lindell, Y. and Pinkas, B., 2009. Secure multiparty computation for privacy-preserving data mining. Journal of Privacy and Confidentiality, 1(1), 5.

LingPipe, 2007. Jaro-Winkler distance c++ code. Available at: http://alias-i.com/lingpipe/docs/api/com/aliasi/spell/JaroWinklerDistance.html [accessed 2 December 2014].

Liseo, B. and Tancredi, A., 2011. Bayesian estimation of population size via linkage of multivariate normal datasets. Survey Methodology, 27(3), 491–505.

Lyons, R. A., Jones, K. H., John, G., Brooks, C. J., Verplancke, J. P., Ford, D. V., Brown, G. and Leake, K., 2009. The SAIL databank: Linking multiple health and social care datasets. BMC Medical Informatics and Decision Making, 9, 3.

Mackey, E. and Elliot, M. J., 2013. Understanding the data environment. XRDS, 20(1), 37–39.

Maggi, F., 2008. A survey of probabilistic record matching models, techniques and tools. Scientific Report TR-2008-22, Milano: DEI, Politecnico di Milano.

Marriott, K. and Stuckey, P. J., 1999. Programming with Constraints: An Introduction. Cambridge: The MIT Press.

Martin, K. M., 2012. Everyday Cryptography: Fundamental Principles and Applications. Oxford: Oxford University Press.

Maso, L., Braga, C. and Franceschi, S., 2001. Methodology used for software for automated linkage in Italy (SALI). Journal of Biomedical Informatics, 34(6), 387–395.

McCallum, A., Nigam, K. and Ungar, L. H., 2000. Efficient clustering of high-dimensional data sets with application to reference matching. In: Proceedings of the 6th ACM SIGKDD International Conference on Knowledge Discovery and Data Mining, 20–23 August 2000, Boston, MA. New York: ACM, p 169–178.

McCusker, M. E., Cress, R., Allen, M., Fernandez-Ami, A. and Gandour-Edwards, R., 2012. Feasibility of linking population-based cancer registries and cancer center biorepositories. Biopreservation and Biobanking, 10(5), 416–420.

McGlincy, M., 2004. A Bayesian record linkage methodology for multiple imputation of missing links. In: Proceedings of the Section on Survey Research Methods. Alexandria, VA: American Statistical Association, CD-ROM. Available at: http://www.amstat.org/sections/srms/Proceedings/y2004/files/Jsm2004-000683.pdf [accessed 6 May 2015].

Mears, G. D., Rosamond, W. D., Lohmeier, C., Murphy, C., O'Brien, E., Asimos, A. W. and Brice, J. H., 2010. A link to improve stroke patient care: A successful linkage between a statewide emergency medical services data system and a stroke registry. Academic Emergency Medicine, 17(12), 1398–1404.

Meng, X. and Rubin, D. B., 1993. Maximum likelihood estimation via the ECM algorithm: A general framework. Biometrika, 80, 267–278.

Merrall, E. L., Bird, S. M. and Hutchinson, S. J., 2012. Mortality of those who attended drug services in Scotland 1996–2006: Record-linkage study. The International Journal on Drug Policy, 23(1), 24–32.

Michelson, M. and Knoblock, C. A., 2006. Learning blocking schemes for record linkage. In: Proceedings of the 21st National Conference on Artificial Intelligence (AAAI-06), 16–20 July 2006, Boston, MA.

Moher, D., Hopewell, S., Schulz, K. F., Montori, V., Gotzsche, P. C., Devereaux, P. J., Elbourne, D., Egger, M. and Altman, D. G., 2010. CONSORT 2010 explanation and elaboration: Updated guidelines for reporting parallel group randomised trials. BMJ, 340, c869.

Molitor, N.-T., Best, N., Jackson, C. and Richardson, S., 2009. Using Bayesian graphical models to model biases in observational studies and to combine multiple sources of data: Application to low birth weight and water disinfection by-products. Journal of the Royal Statistical Society: Series A, 172, 615–637.

Monga, H. and Patrick, T., 2001. Error estimation in linking heterogeneous data sources. Health Informatics Journal, 7(3–4), 135–137.

Moore, H. C., de Klerk, N., Keil, A. D., Smith, D. W., Blyth, C. C., Richmond, P. and Lehmann, D., 2012. Use of data linkage to investigate the aetiology of acute lower respiratory infection hospitalisations in children. Journal of Paediatrics and Child Health, 48(6), 520–528.

Morelli, R. and Walde, R., 2003. A word-based genetic algorithm for cryptanalysis of short cryptograms. In: Russell, I. and Haller, S. M., editors. Proceedings of the 16th International Florida Artificial Intelligence Research Society Conference. Menlo Park, CA: AAAI Press, p 229–233.

Morris, R. and Thompson, K., 1979. Password security: A case history. Communications of the ACM, 22(11), 594–597.

Morris, A., Boyle, D., MacAlpine, R., Emslie-Smith, A., Jung, R., Newton, R. and MacDonald, T., 1997. The diabetes audit and research in Tayside Scotland (DARTS) study: Electronic record linkage to create a diabetes register. BMJ, 315(7107), 524–528.

Mortimer, J. and Salathiel, J., 1995. 'Soundex' codes of surnames provide confidentiality and accuracy in a national HIV database. Communicable Disease Report. CDR Review, 5(12), R183–R186.

Napoleão Rocha, M. C., 2013. Vigilância dos óbitos Registrados com Causa Básica Hanseníase [Master thesis]. Brasilia: Universidade de Brasília.

National Health Service, 2013. NHS data model and dictionary, version 3. Available at: www.datadictionary.nhs.uk [accessed 2 December 2014].

National Institute of Standards and Technology, 2005. NedInfo: Jaro-Winkler string comparator c code. Available at: http://nedinfo.nih.gov/docs/Strcmp95.htm [accessed 2 December 2014].

National Institute of Standards and Technology, 2012. FIPS PUB 180-4: Secure Hash Standard (SHS). US Department of Commerce. Available at: http://csrc.nist.gov/publications/fips/fips180-4/fips-180-4.pdf [accessed 2 December 2014].

Navarro, G., 2001. A guided tour of approximate string matching. Association of Computing Machinery, Computing Surveys, 33, 31–88.

Navarro-Arribas, G. and Torra, V., 2012. Information fusion in data privacy: A survey. Information Fusion, 13(4), 235–244.

Neter, J., Maynes, E. and Ramanathan, R., 1965. The effect of mismatching on the measurement of response error. Journal of the American Statistical Association, 60(312), 1005–1027.

Newcombe, H. B., Kennedy, J., Axford, S. and James, A., 1959. Automatic linkage of vital records. Science, 130(3381), 954–959.

Newcombe, H. B. and Kennedy, J. M., 1962. Record linkage: Making maximum use of the discriminating power of identifying information. Communications of the ACM, 5, 563–567.

Newcombe, H. B. and Smith, M. E., 1975. Methods for computer linkage of hospital admission-separation records into cumulative health histories. Methods of Information in Medicine, 14(3), 118–125.

Newcombe, H. B., 1984. Strategy and art in automated death searches. American Journal of Public Health, 74(12), 1302–1303.

Newcombe, H. B., 1988. Handbook of Record Linkage: Methods for Health and Statistical Studies, Administration, and Business. Oxford: Oxford University Press.

Newcombe, H. B., 1995. Age-related bias in probabilistic death searches due to neglect of the 'prior likelihoods'. Computers and Biomedical Research, 28(2), 87–99.

Newgard, C., 2006. Validation of probabilistic linkage to match de-identified ambulance records to a state trauma registry. Academic Emergency Medicine, 13(1), 69–75.

Newgard, C., Malveau, S., Staudenmayer, K., Wang, N. E., Hsia, R. Y., Mann, N. C., Holmes, J. F., Kuppermann, N., Haukoos, J. S., Bulger, E. M., Dai, M. and Cook, L. J., 2012. Evaluating the use of existing data sources, probabilistic linkage, and multiple imputation to build population-based injury databases across phases of trauma care. Academic Emergency Medicine, 19(4), 469–480.

Newman, T. B. and Brown, A. N., 1997. Use of commercial record linkage software and vital statistics to identify patient deaths. Journal of the American Medical Informatics Association, 4(3), 233–237.

Ng, A. and Jordan, M., 2002. On discriminative vs. generative classifiers: A comparison of logistic regression and naïve Bayes. In: Dietterich, T. G., Becker, S. and Ghahramani, Z., editors. Advances in Neural Information Processing Systems 14. Cambridge, MA: MIT Press, p 841–848.

Niedermeyer, F., Steinmetzer, S., Kroll, M. and Schnell, R., 2014. Cryptanalysis of Basic Bloom Filters Used for Privacy Preserving Record Linkage. Working Paper WP-GRLC-2014-4. Nuremberg: German Record Linkage Center.

Nigam, K., McCallum, A. K., Thrun, S. and Mitchell, T., 2000. Text Classification from Labeled and Unlabelled Documents using EM. Machine Learning, 39, 103–134.

Norén, G. N., Orre, R. and Bate, A., 2005. A hit-miss model for duplicate detection in the WHO drug safety database. In: Proceedings of the 11th ACM SIGKDD International Conference on Knowledge Discovery and Data Mining, 21–24 August 2005, Chicago, IL.

Office for National Statistics, 2012a. Building the address register for the 2011 Census. Available at: http://www.ons.gov.uk/ons/guide-method/census/2011/the-2011-census/the-2011-census-project/design-for-the-census/building-the-address-register-for-the-2011-census.pdf [accessed 17 December 2014].

Office for National Statistics, 2012b. Automatic match rates for the 2011 Census to the census coverage survey. Available at: www.ons.gov.uk/ons/guide-method/census/2011/census-data/2011-census-data/2011-first-release/first-release--quality-assurance-and-methodology-papers/automatic-match-rates-for-the-2011-census-to-the-census-coverage-survey.pdf [accessed 2 December 2014].

Office for National Statistics, 2012c. Quality assurance of 2011 Census population estimates – July 2012. Available at: www.ons.gov.uk/ons/guide-method/census/2011/census-data/2011-census-user-guide/quality-and-methods/quality/quality-assurance/index.html [accessed 2 December 2014].

Office for National Statistics, 2013a. An assessment of the quality of the matching between the 2011 Census and the census coverage survey. Available at: www.ons.gov.uk/ons/guide-method/census/2011/census-data/2011-census-user-guide/quality-and-methods/methods/coverage-assessment-and-adjustment-methods/census-coverage-survey--ccs-/matching-quality-report-ns.pdf [accessed 2 December 2014].

Office for National Statistics, 2013b. Beyond 2011: Safeguarding data for research: Our policy. Paper M10, Office for National Statistics. Available at: www.ons.gov.uk/ons/about-ons/who-ons-are/programmes-and-projects/beyond-2011/reports-and-publications/index.html [accessed 2 December 2014].

Office for National Statistics, 2013c. Beyond 2011: Producing population statistics using administrative data. Methods & Policies Report (M6). Available at: www.ons.gov.uk/ons/about-ons/who-ons-are/programmes-and-projects/beyond-2011/reports-and-publications/index.html [accessed 2 December 2014].

Office for National Statistics, 2013d. Beyond 2011: Producing population statistics using administrative data: In theory. Methods & Policies Report (M8). Available at: www.ons.gov.uk/ons/about-ons/who-ons-are/programmes-and-projects/beyond-2011/reports-and-publications/index.html [accessed 2 December 2014].

Office for National Statistics, 2013e. Beyond 2011: Matching anonymous data. Methods & Policies Report (M9). Available at: www.ons.gov.uk/ons/about-ons/who-ons-are/programmes-and-projects/beyond-2011/reports-and-publications/index.html [accessed 2 December 2014].

Office for National Statistics, 2014a. The census and future provision of population statistics in England and Wales: Recommendation from the national statistician and chief executive of the UK statistics authority – March 2014. Available at: www.ons.gov.uk/ons/about-ons/who-ons-are/programmes-and-projects/beyond-2011/reports-and-publications/index.html [accessed 2 December 2014].

Office for National Statistics, 2014b. Beyond 2011: Statistical research update. Methods & Policies Report (M13). Available at: www.ons.gov.uk/ons/about-ons/who-ons-are/programmes-and-projects/beyond-2011/reports-and-publications/index.html [accessed 2 December 2014].

Ohm, P., 2010. Broken promises of privacy: Responding to the surprising failure of anonymization. UCLA Law Review, 57, 1701–1777.

O'Keefe, C. M., Ferrante, A. M. and Boyd, J. H., 2010a. CDL Operational Model Part 1. Curtin University: Population Health Research Network Centre for Data Linkage.

O'Keefe, C. M., Ferrante, A. M. and Boyd, J. H., 2010b. National Linkage Keys and National Linkage Map: Ownership and Governance. Draft Version 0.5. Perth, WA: Population Health Research Network Centre for Data Linkage.

Ong, T. C., Mannino, M. V., Schilling, L. M. and Kahn, M. G., 2014. Improving record linkage performance in the presence of missing linkage data. Journal of Biomedical Informatics, 52, 43–54.

Organisation for Economic Co-operation and Development (OECD), 2006. Glossary of statistical terms. Available at: http://stats.oecd.org/glossary [accessed 2 December 2014].

Pacheco, A. G., Saraceni, V., Tuboi, S. H., Moulton, L. H., Chaisson, R. E., Cavalcante, S. C., Durovni, B., Faulhaber, J. C., Golub, J. E., King, B., Schechter, M. and Harrison, L. H., 2008. Validation of a hierarchical deterministic record-linkage algorithm using data from 2 different cohorts of human immunodeficiency virus-infected persons and mortality databases in Brazil. American Journal of Epidemiology, 168, 1326–1332.

Pang, C. and Hansen, D., 2006. Improved record linkage for encrypted identifying data. In: Westbrook, J., Callen, J., Margelis, G. and Warren, J., editors. Proceedings of HIC 2006 and HINZ 2006. Brunswick, VIC: Health Informatics Society of Australia, p 164–168.

Pang, C., Gu, L., Hansen, D. and Maeder, A., 2009. Privacy-preserving fuzzy matching using a public reference table. In: McClean, S., Millard, P., El-Darzi, E. and Nugent, E., editors. Intelligent Patient Management. Berlin: Springer, p 71–89.

Parry-Langdon, N., 2011. Social survey non-response update. Office for National Statistics. Available at: www.ons.gov.uk/ons/dcp171766_240879.pdf [accessed 2 December 2014].

Petersen, C. G. J., 1896. The yearly immigration of young plaice into the Limfjord from the German Sea. Reports of the Danish Biological Station, 6, 5–84.

Pieprzyk, J., Hardjono, T. and Seberry, J., 2003. Fundamentals of Computer Security. Berlin: Springer.

Pinto da Silveira, D. and Artmann, E., 2009. Accuracy of probabilistic record linkage applied to health databases: Systematic review. Revista de Saúde Pública, 43(5), 875–882.

Population Health Research Network (PHRN), 2013. PHRN overview and achievements 2009–2013. Available at: http://www.phrn.org.au/media/77248/phrn%20overview.pdf [accessed 6 June 2015].

Potz, N., Powell, D., Lamagni, T., Pebody, R., Bridger, D. and Duckworth, G., 2010. Probabilistic record linkage of infection records and death registrations: A tool to strengthen surveillance. Statistical Communications in Infectious Diseases, 2(1), 6.

Qayad, M. and Zhang, H., 2009. Accuracy of public health data linkages. Maternal and Child Health Journal, 13(4), 531–538.

Randall, S. M., Ferrante, A. M., Boyd, J. H., Bauer, J. K. and Semmens, J. B., 2014. Privacy-preserving record linkage on large real world datasets. Journal of Biomedical Informatics, 50, 205–212.

Ravikumar, P. and Cohen, W. W., 2004. A hierarchical graphical model for record linkage. In: Proceedings of the Conference on Uncertainty in Artificial Intelligence, 9–11 July 2004, Banff, Calgary, CA.

Ravikumar, P., Cohen, W. W. and Fienberg, S. E., 2004. A secure protocol for computing string distance metrics. In: Proceedings of the Workshop on Privacy and Security Aspects of Data Mining at the International Conference on Data Mining, 1–4 November 2004, Brighton, UK. Los Alamitos, CA: IEEE Computer Society, p 40–46.

Real, R., Barbosa, B. A. M. and Vargas, J. M., 2005. Obtaining environmental favourability functions from logistic regression. Environmental and Ecological Statistics, 13(2), 237–245.

Richter, A., 2013. Ergebnis des Abgleichs Nr. 2. Unpublished Memo, Cancer Registry Luebeck.

Rivest, R. R., 1998. Chaffing and winnowing: Confidentiality without encryption. Available at: http://people.csail.mit.edu/rivest/Chaffing.txt [accessed 2 December 2014].

Rochon, P. A., Gurwitz, J. H., Sykora, K., Mamdani, M., Streiner, D. L., Garfinkel, S., Normand, S. L. and Anderson, G. M., 2005. Reader's guide to critical appraisal of cohort studies: 1. Role and design. BMJ, 330(7496), 895–897.

Rodgers, S. E., Lyons, R. A., Dsilva, R., Jones, K. H., Brooks, C. J., Ford, D. V., John, G. and Verplancke, J. P., 2009. Residential Anonymous Linking Fields (RALFs): A novel information infrastructure to study the interaction between the environment and individuals' health. Journal of Public Health, 31(4), 582–588.

Rodgers, S. E., Demmler, J. C., D'Silva, R. and Lyons, R. A., 2011. Protecting health data privacy while using residence-based environment and demographic data. Health & Place, 18, 209–217.

Roos, L. L. and Wajda, A., 1991. Record linkage strategies. Part I: Estimating information and evaluating approaches. Methods of Information in Medicine, 30(2), 117–123.

Roos, N. P., Black, C. D., Frohlich, N., Decoster, C., Cohen, M. M., Tataryn, D. J., Mustard, C. A., Toll, F., Carriere, K. C. and Burchill, C. A., 1995. A population-based health information system. Medical Care, 33(12), DS13–DS20.

Roos, L. L., Gupta, S., Soodeen, R. A. and Jebamani, L., 2005. Data quality in an information-rich environment: Canada as an example. Canadian Journal on Aging, 24(Suppl 1), 153–170.

Rothman, K. J., 2002. Epidemiology: An Introduction. New York: Oxford University Press.

Rubin, D., 1987. Multiple Imputation for Nonresponse in Surveys. New York: Wiley.

Sadinle, M. and Fienberg, S. E., 2013. A generalized Fellegi-Sunter framework for multiple record linkage with application to homicide record systems. Journal of the American Statistical Association, 108(502), 385–397.

Samart, K. and Chambers, R., 2014. Linear regression with nested errors using probability-linked data. Australian & New Zealand Journal of Statistics, 56(1), 27–46.

Sariyar, M., Borg, A. and Pommerening, K., 2011. Controlling false match rates in record linkage using extreme value theory. Journal of Biomedical Informatics, 44(4), 648–654.

Sariyar, M., Borg, A. and Pommerening, K., 2012. Missing values in deduplication of electronic patient data. Journal of the American Medical Informatics Association, 19(e1), e76–e82.

Sauleau, E., Paumier, J. and Buemi, A., 2005. Medical record linkage in health information systems by approximate string matching and clustering. BMC Medical Informatics and Decision Making, 5(1), 32.

Scannapieco, M., Figoti, I., Bertino, E. and Elmagarmid, A., 2007. Privacy preserving schema and data matching. In: Proceedings of the SIGMOD Conference. New York: ACM, p 653–664.

Scheuren, F. and Winkler, W. E., 1993. Regression analysis of data files that are computer matched. Survey Methodology, 19, 39–58.

Scheuren, F. and Winkler, W., 1997. Regression analysis of data files that are computer matched – Part II. Survey Methodology, 23(2), 126–138.

Schneier, B., 1996. Applied Cryptography: Protocols, Algorithms, and Source Code in C. New York: Wiley.

Schnell, R., Bachteler, T. and Reiher, J., 2009. Privacy-preserving record linkage using bloom filters. BMC Medical Informatics and Decision Making, 9(41), 1–11.

Schnell, R., Bachteler, T. and Reiher, J., 2010. Private record linkage with bloom filters. In: Proceedings of Statistics Canada Symposium, 26–29 October 2010. Ottawa: Statistics Canada, p 304–309.

Schnell, R., Bachteler, T. and Reiher, J., 2011. A Novel Error-Tolerant Anonymous Linking Code. Working Paper WP-GRLC-2011-02. Nuremberg: German Record Linkage Center.

Schnell, R., 2013. Privacy-preserving record linkage and privacy-preserving blocking for large files with cryptographic keys using multibit trees. In: Proceedings of the Joint Statistical Meetings, American Statistical Association, 3–8 August 2013, Quebec, Canada. Alexandria, VA: American Statistical Association, p 187–194.

Schnell, R., Hill, P. and Esser, E., 2013. Methoden der empirischen Sozialforschung (10th Edition). Munich: Oldenbourg.

Schnell, R., 2014. An efficient privacy-preserving record linkage technique for administrative data and censuses. Statistical Journal of the IAOS, 30, 263–270.

Schnell, R., Richter, A. and Borgs, C., 2014. Performance of different methods for privacy preserving record linkage with large scale medical data sets. Presentation at the International Health Data Linkage Conference, 28–30 April 2014, Vancouver, Canada.

Schulte-Nordholt, E., Hartgers, M. and Gircour, R. (Eds.), 2004. The Dutch Virtual Census of 2001: Analysis and Methodology. Voorburg/Heerlen: Statistics Netherlands. Available at: www.cbs.nl/NR/rdonlyres/D1716A60-0D13-4281-BED6-3607514888AD/0/b572001.pdf [accessed 2 December 2014].

Schulte-Nordholt, E., 2009. Data integration activities on the way to the Dutch Virtual Census of 2011. In: Proceedings of the Conference on Modernising Statistical Production, 2–4 November 2009, Stockholm, Sweden.

Smith, M. E. and Newcombe, H. B., 1975. Methods of computer linkage for hospital admission-separation records into cumulative health histories. Methods of Information in Medicine, 14(3), 118–125.

Smith, D. and Elliot, M. J., 2008. A measure of disclosure risk for tables of counts. Transactions on Data Privacy, 1(1), 34–52.

Smith, D. and Shlomo, N., 2014. Privacy preserving record linkage. Available at: www.cmist.manchester.ac.uk/medialibrary/archive-publications/reports/2014-01-Data_without_Boundaries_Report.pdf [accessed 22 December 2014].

Sorensen, H. T., Sabroe, S. and Olsen, J., 1996. A framework for evaluation of secondary data sources for epidemiological research. International Journal of Epidemiology, 25(2), 435–442.

StackOverflow, 2010. Jaro Winkler string comparator java code. Available at: http://stackoverflow.com/ questions/2848807/optimizing-jaro-winkler-algorithm [accessed 2 December 2014].

Stallings, W., 2011. Cryptography and Network Security: Principles and Practice (5th Edition). Boston, MA: Prentice Hall.

Statistics Finland, 2004. Use of Registers and Administrative Data Sources for Statistical Purposes: Best Practices of Statistics Finland. Helsinki: Tilastokeskus. Available at: http://unstats.un.org/unsd/ EconStatKB/Attachment172.aspx [accessed 2 December 2014].

Statistics New Zealand, 2006. Data integration manual. Technical Report, Wellington: Statistics New Zealand.

Statistics Sweden, 2001. The future development of the Swedish register system. R&D Report 2001:1, Statistics Sweden. Available at: www.scb.se/Grupp/Hitta_statistik/Forsta_Statistik/Metod/_ Dokument/RD2001_1_eng.pdf [accessed 2 December 2014].

Stefoski Mikeljevic, J., Johnston, C., Adamson, P. J., Wright, A., Bishop, J. A., Batman, P., Neal, R. D. and Forman, D., 2003. How complete has skin cancer registration been in the UK? A study from Yorkshire. European Journal of Cancer Prevention, 12(2), 125–133.

Steinmetzer, S. and Kroll, M., 2014. Automated cryptanalysis of Bloom filter encryptions of health data. In: Contribution to the 8th International Conference on Health Informatics, Lisbon 2015, 27 October 2014. Duisburg: University of Duisburg-Essen.

Steorts, R. C., Hall, R. and Fienberg, S. E., 2013. A Bayesian approach to graphical record linkage and de-duplication. Statistics Technical Report Draft (20 November 2013), Pittsburgh, PA: Carnegie-Mellon University.

Steorts, R. C., Ventura, S. L., Sadinle, M. and Fienberg, S. E., 2014. A comparison of blocking methods for record linkage. In: Domingo-Ferrer, J., editor. Privacy in Statistical Databases, Lecture Notes in Computer Science No 8744. Berlin: Springer, p 253–268.

Swamidass, S. J. and Baldi, P., 2007. Bounds and algorithms for fast exact searches of chemical finger-prints in linear and sublinear time. Journal of Chemical Information and Modeling, 47, 302–317.

Swiss Federal Statistical Office, 2012. The Swiss Census System: A comprehensive system of house-hold and person statistics. Paper presented at UNECE Conference of European Statisticians, Paris, 6–8 June 2012. Available at: www.unece.org/fileadmin/DAM/stats/documents/ece/ces/2012/55-SP_ Switzerland_-_the_swiss_census_system.pdf [accessed 2 December 2014].

Tancredi, A. and Liseo, B., 2011. A hierarchical Bayesian approach to matching and size population problems. Annals of Applied Statistics, 5(2B), 1553–1585.

Teppo, L., Pukkala, E. and Lehtonen, M., 1994. Data quality and quality control of a population-based cancer registry. Experience in Finland. Acta Oncologica, 33(4), 365–369.

Titterington, D. M., Smith, A. F. M. and Makov, U. E., 1988. Statistical Analysis of Finite Mixture Distributions. New York: Wiley.

Trinckes, J. J., 2013. The Definitive Guide to Complying with the HIPAA/HITECH Privacy and Security Rules. Boca Raton, FL: CRC Press.

Tromp, M., Ravelli, A. C., Meray, N., Reitsma, J. B. and Bonsel, G. J., 2008. An efficient validation method of probabilistic record linkage including readmissions and twins. Methods of Information in Medicine, 47(4), 356–363.

Tromp, M., Ravelli, A. C., Bonsel, G. J., Hasman, A. and Reitsma, J. B., 2011. Results from simulated data sets: Probabilistic record linkage outperforms deterministic record linkage. Journal of Clinical Epidemiology, 64(5), 565–572.

United Nations, 2008. Principles and Recommendations for Population and Housing Censuses. Statistical Papers, Series M, No.67/Rev.2. New York: United Nations.

United Nations Economic Commission for Europe, 2007. Register based statistics in Nordic countries. Available at: www.unece.org/fileadmin/DAM/stats/publications/Register_based_statistics_in_Nordic_ countries.pdf [accessed 2 December 2014].

United States Government Accountability Office, 2010. Key efforts to include hard-to-count populations went generally as planned; improvements could make the efforts more effective for next census. Report to Congressional Requesters. GAO-11-45. Available at: www.gao.gov/assets/320/313927.pdf [accessed 2 December 2014].

Universities of Leeds and Leicester, 2013. Paediatric intensive care audit network national report 2011–2013. Available at: http://www.picanet.org.uk/ [accessed 6 June 2015].

Vaidya, J. and Clifton, C., 2003. Privacy-preserving k-means clustering over vertically partitioned data. In: Proceedings of the 9th ACM SIGKDD International Conference on Knowledge Discovery and Data Mining. New York: ACM, p 206–215.

Valente, P., 2012. Overview of the 2010 round of population and housing censuses in the UNECE region. Paper submitted to the Seminar on Population and Housing Censuses at the 60th Plenary Session of the Conference of European Statisticians, 6–8 June 2012, Paris. Geneva: United Nations.

Vapnik, V., 2000. The Nature of Statistical Learning Theory (2nd Edition). Berlin: Springer.

Vatsalan, D., Christen, P. and Verykios, V. S., 2011. An efficient two-party protocol for approximate matching in private record linkage. In: Proceedings of the 9th Australasian Data Mining Conference – Volume 121. Ballarat, VIC: Australian Computer Society, p 125–136.

Vatsalan, D., Christen, P. and Verykios, V. S., 2013a. A taxonomy of privacy-preserving record linkage techniques. Information Systems, 38(6), 946–969.

Vatsalan, D., Christen, P. and Verykios, V. S., 2013b. Efficient two-party private blocking based on sorted nearest neighbourhood clustering. In: Proceedings of the 22nd ACM International Conference on Information and Knowledge Management. New York: ACM, p 1949–1958.

Vatsalan, D., Christen, P., O'Keefe, C. and Verykios, V. S., 2014. An evaluation framework for privacy-preserving record linkage. Journal of Privacy and Confidentiality, 6(1), 35–75.

Verykios, V. S. and Christen, P., 2013. Privacy-preserving record linkage. WIREs Data Mining and Knowledge Discovery, 3, 321–332.

Waien, S., 1997. Linking large administrative databases: A method for conducting emergency medical services cohort studies using existing data. Academic Emergency Medicine, 4(11), 1087–1095.

Wang, Y., Sharpe-Stimac, M., Cross, P. K., Druschel, C. M. and Hwang, S. A., 2005. Improving case ascertainment of a population-based birth defects registry in New York State using hospital discharge data. Birth Defects Research. Part A, Clinical and Molecular Teratology, 73(10), 663–668.

Weeks, A., Fallows, A., Broad, P., Merad, S. and Ashworth, K., 2013. Non-response weights for the UK Labour Force Survey? Results from the census non-response link study. Office for National Statistics, Newport. Available at: www.ons.gov.uk/ons/guide-method/method-quality/specific/labour-market/articles-and-reports/non-response-weights-for-the-uk-labour-force-survey.pdf [accessed 2 December 2014].

Westaby, S., Archer, N., Manning, N., Adwani, S., Grebenik, C., Ormerod, O., Pillai, R. and Wilson, N., 2007. Comparison of hospital episode statistics and central cardiac audit database in public reporting of congenital heart surgery mortality. BMJ, 335(7623), 759–764.

Wiklund, K. and Eklund, G., 1986. Reliability of record linkage in the Swedish Cancer-Environment Register. Acta Oncologica, 25(1), 11–14.

Willenborg, L. and De Waal, T., 2001. Elements of Statistical Disclosure Control, Lecture Notes in Statistics. New York: Springer.

Winkler, W. E., 1988. Using the EM algorithm for weight computation in the Fellegi-Sunter model of record linkage. In: Proceedings of the Section on Survey Research Methods. Alexandria, VA: American Statistical Association, p 667–671. Available at: https://www.amstat.org/sections/SRMS/Proceedings/ [accessed 26 June 2015].

Winkler, W. E., 1989a. Near automatic weight computation in the Fellegi-Sunter model of record linkage. In: Proceedings of the 5th Census Bureau Annual Research Conference. Washington, DC: US Department of Commerce, Bureau of the Census, p 145–155.

Winkler, W. E., 1989b. Frequency-based matching in the Fellegi-Sunter model of record linkage. In: Proceedings of the Section on Survey Research Methods, 4–6 January 1989, San Diego, CA. Alexandria, VA: American Statistical Association, p 778–783.

Winkler, W. E., 1990. String comparator metrics and enhanced decision rules in the Fellegi-Sunter model of record linkage. In: Proceedings of the Section on Survey Research Methods. Alexandria, VA: American Statistical Association, p 354–359. Available at: https://www.amstat.org/sections/SRMS/Proceedings/ [accessed 26 June 2015].

Winkler, W. E. and Scheuren, F., 1991. How computer matching error effects regression analysis: Exploratory and confirmatory analysis. Statistical Research Division Technical Report, Washington, DC: US Bureau of the Census.

Winkler, W. E., 1993a. Business name parsing and standardisation software. Unpublished Report, Washington, DC: Statistical Research Division, US Bureau of the Census.

Winkler, W. E., 1993b. Improved decision rules in the Fellegi-Sunter model of record linkage. In: Proceedings of the Section on Survey Research Methods. Alexandria, VA: American Statistical Association, p 274–279. Available at: https://www.amstat.org/sections/SRMS/Proceedings/ [accessed 26 June 2015].

Winkler, W. E., 1994. Advanced methods for record linkage. Statistical Research Report, Washington, DC: US Bureau of the Census.

Winkler, W. E., 1995. Matching and record linkage. In: Cox, B. G., Binder, D. A., Chinnappa, B. N., Christianson, A., Colledge, M. J. and Kott, P. S., editors. Business Survey Methods. New York: Wiley, p 355–384.

Winkler, W. E., 1999. The state of record linkage and current research problems. Available at: www.census.gov/srd/papers/pdf/rr99-04.pdf [accessed 17 December 2014].

Winkler, W. E., 2000. Machine learning, information retrieval, and record linkage. In: Proceedings of the Section on Survey Research Methods. Alexandria, VA: American Statistical Association, p 20–29. Available at: https://www.amstat.org/sections/SRMS/Proceedings/ [accessed 26 June 2015].

Winkler, W. E., 2002. Record linkage and Bayesian networks. In: Proceedings of the Section on Survey Research Methods. Alexandria, VA: American Statistical Association, CD-ROM. Available at: www.census.gov/srd/www/byyear.html [accessed 2 December 2014].

Winkler, W. E., 2003. A contingency table model for imputing data satisfying analytic constraints. In: Proceedings of the Section on Survey Research Methods. Alexandria, VA: American Statistical Association, CD-ROM. Available at: www.census.gov/srd/papers/pdf/rrs2003-07.pdf [accessed 2 December 2014].

Winkler, W. E., 2004. Approximate string comparator search strategies for very large administrative lists. In: Proceedings of the Section on Survey Research Methods. Alexandria, VA: American Statistical Association, CD-ROM. Available at: www.census.gov/srd/www/byyear.html [accessed 2 December 2014].

Winkler, W. E., 2006a. Overview of record linkage and current research directions. US Bureau of the Census, Statistical Research Division Report. Available at: www.census.gov/srd/papers/pdf/rrs2006-02.pdf [accessed 2 December 2014].

Winkler, W. E., 2006b. Automatic estimation of record linkage false match rates. In: Proceedings of the Section on Survey Research Methods. Alexandria, VA: American Statistical Association, CD-ROM. Available at: www.census.gov/srd/papers/pdf/rrs2007-05.pdf [accessed 2 December 2014].

Winkler, W. E., 2008. General methods and algorithms for imputing discrete data under a variety of constraints. Available at: www.census.gov/srd/papers/pdf/rrs2008-08.pdf [accessed 2 December 2014].

Winkler, W. E., 2009. Record linkage. In: Pfeffermann, D. and Rao, C. R., editors. Handbook of Statistics Vol. 29A, Sample Surveys: Design, Methods and Applications. Amsterdam: Elsevier, p 351–380.

Winkler, W. E., Yancey, W. E. and Porter, E. H., 2010. Fast record linkage of very large files in support of decennial and administrative records projects. In: Proceedings of the Section on Survey Research Methods, American Statistical Association, p 2120–2130. Available at: www.amstat.org/sections/srms/proceedings/y2010/Files/307067_57754.pdf [accessed 2 December 2014].

Winkler, W. E., 2011. Cleaning and using administrative lists: Methods and fast computational algorithms for record linkage and modelling/editing/imputation. In: Proceedings of the ESSnet Conference on Data Integration, Madrid, Spain, November 2011. Available at: www.ine.es/e/essnetdi_ws2011/ppts/Winkler.pdf [accessed 2 December 2014].

Winkler, W., 2013. Cleanup and statistical analysis of sets of national files. In: Proceedings of the Federal Committee on Statistical Methodology. Available at: https://fcsm.sites.usa.gov/reports/research/2013research/ [accessed 2 December 2014].

Wong, K.-S. and Kim, M. H., 2013. Privacy-preserving similarity coefficients for binary data. Computers and Mathematics with Applications, 65(9), 1280–1290.

World Health Organization, 2001. ICF: International Classification of Functioning, Disability and Health. Geneva: WHO.

World Health Organization, 2008. ICD-10: International Statistical Classification of Diseases and Related Health Problems (10th Revised Edition). Geneva: WHO.

Wright, J., 2010. Linking census records to death registrations. Australia Bureau of Statistics Report 131.0.55.030, Canberra, ACT: Australian Bureau of Statistics.

Yakout, M., Atallah, M. J. and Elmagarmid, A., 2009. Efficient private record linkage. In: Proceedings of the 25th International Conference on Data Engineering, 29 March – 2 April 2009, Shanghai, China. Los Alamitos, CA: IEEE Computer Society, p 1283–1286.

Yancey, W. E., 2004. Improving EM algorithm estimates for record linkage parameters. In: Joint Statistical Meetings – Section on Survey Research Methods.

Yancey, W. E., 2005. Evaluating string comparator performance for record linkage. Technical Report Statistical Research Report Series RRS2005/05, Washington, DC: US Bureau of the Census.

Yancey, W. E. and Winkler, W. E., 2006. BigMatch Software. Computer System. Available at: www.census.gov/srd/www/byyear.html [accessed 2 December 2014].

Yancey, W. E. and Winkler, W. E., 2009. BigMatch Software. Computer System. Available at: www.census.gov/srd/www/byyear.html [accessed 2 December 2014].

Yao, A. C., 1982. Protocols for secure computations. In: Proceedings of 23rd Symposium on Foundations of Computer Science (FOCS), 3–5 November 1982, Chicago, IL. Los Alamitos, CA: IEEE Computer Society, p 160–164.

Zhang, T. and Oles, F., 2001. Text categorization based on regularized linear classification methods. Information Retrieval, 4(1), 5–31.

Zhang, B. and Zhang, F., 2012. Secure similarity coefficients computation with malicious adversaries. In: Proceedings of the 4th International Conference on Intelligent Networking and Collaborative Systems (INCoS), 29 March – 2 April 2009, Shanghai, China. Los Alamitos, CA: IEEE Computer Society, p 303–310.

Zhu, V., Overhage, M., Egg, J., Downs, S. and Grannis, S., 2009. An empiric modification to the probabilistic record linkage algorithm using frequency-based weight scaling. Journal of the American Medical Informatics Association, 16(5), 738–745.

Zimmerman, P., 2014. Available at: http://www.philzimmermann.com [accessed 6 June 2015].

Zingmond, D., Ye, Z., Ettner, S. and Liu, H., 2004. Linking hospital discharge and death records-accuracy and sources of bias. Journal of Clinical Microbiology, 57(1), 21–29.

Index

Methodological Developments in Data Linkage, First Edition. Edited by Katie Harron, Harvey Goldstein and Chris Dibben.
© 2016 John Wiley & Sons, Ltd. Published 2016 by John Wiley & Sons, Ltd.

WILEY SERIES IN PROBABILITY AND STATISTICS

ESTABLISHED BY WALTER A. SHEWHART AND SAMUEL S. WILKS

Editors: *David J. Balding, Noel A. C. Cressie, Garrett M. Fitzmaurice, Geof H. Givens, Harvey Goldstein, Geert Molenberghs, David W. Scott, Adrian F. M. Smith, Ruey S. Tsay, Sanford Weisberg*
Editors Emeriti: *J. Stuart Hunter, Iain M. Johnstone, Joseph B. Kadane, Jozef L. Teugels*

The *Wiley Series in Probability and Statistics* is well established and authoritative. It covers many topics of current research interest in both pure and applied statistics and probability theory. Written by leading statisticians and institutions, the titles span both state-of-the-art developments in the field and classical methods.

Reflecting the wide range of current research in statistics, the series encompasses applied, methodological and theoretical statistics, ranging from applications and new techniques made possible by advances in computerized practice to rigorous treatment of theoretical approaches.

This series provides essential and invaluable reading for all statisticians, whether in academia, industry, government, or research.

† Now available in a lower priced paperback edition in the Wiley–Interscience Paperback Series.
* Now available in a lower priced paperback edition in the Wiley Classics Library.

BAJORSKI · Statistics for Imaging, Optics, and Photonics

BALAKRISHNAN and KOUTRAS · Runs and Scans with Applications

BALAKRISHNAN and NG · Precedence-Type Tests and Applications

BARNETT · Comparative Statistical Inference, *Third Edition*

BARNETT · Environmental Statistics

BARNETT and LEWIS · Outliers in Statistical Data, *Third Edition*

BARTHOLOMEW, KNOTT, and MOUSTAKI · Latent Variable Models and Factor
Analysis: A Unified Approach, *Third Edition*

BARTOSZYNSKI and NIEWIADOMSKA-BUGAJ · Probability and Statistical Inference, *Second Edition*

BASILEVSKY · Statistical Factor Analysis and Related Methods: Theory and Applications

BATES and WATTS · Nonlinear Regression Analysis and Its Applications

BECHHOFER, SANTNER, and GOLDSMAN · Design and Analysis of Experiments for
Statistical Selection, Screening, and Multiple Comparisons

BEH and LOMBARDO · Correspondence Analysis: Theory, Practice and New Strategies

BEIRLANT, GOEGEBEUR, SEGERS, TEUGELS, and DE WAAL · Statistics of
Extremes: Theory and Applications

BELSLEY Conditioning Diagnostics: Collinearity and Weak Data in Regression

† BELSLEY, KUH, and WELSCH · Regression Diagnostics: Identifying Influential Data
and Sources of Collinearity

BENDAT and PIERSOL · Random Data: Analysis and Measurement Procedures, *Fourth
Edition*

BERNARDO and SMITH · Bayesian Theory

BHAT and MILLER · Elements of Applied Stochastic Processes, *Third Edition*

BHATTACHARYA and WAYMIRE · Stochastic Processes with Applications

BIEMER, GROVES, LYBERG, MATHIOWETZ, and SUDMAN · Measurement Errors
in Surveys

BILLINGSLEY · Convergence of Probability Measures, *Second Edition*

BILLINGSLEY · Probability and Measure, *Anniversary Edition*

BIRKES and DODGE · Alternative Methods of Regression

BISGAARD and KULAHCI · Time Series Analysis and Forecasting by Example

BISWAS, DATTA, FINE, and SEGAL · Statistical Advances in the Biomedical Sciences:
Clinical Trials, Epidemiology, Survival Analysis, and Bioinformatics

BLISCHKE and MURTHY (editors) · Case Studies in Reliability and Maintenance

BLISCHKE and MURTHY · Reliability: Modeling, Prediction, and Optimization

BLOOMFIELD · Fourier Analysis of Time Series: An Introduction, *Second Edition*

BOLLEN · Structural Equations with Latent Variables

BOLLEN and CURRAN · Latent Curve Models: A Structural Equation Perspective

BONNINI, CORAIN, MAROZZI and SALMASO · Nonparametric Hypothesis Testing:
Rank and Permutation Methods with Applications in R

BOROVKOV · Ergodicity and Stability of Stochastic Processes

† Now available in a lower priced paperback edition in the Wiley–Interscience Paperback Series.

BOSQ and BLANKE · Inference and Prediction in Large Dimensions

BOULEAU · Numerical Methods for Stochastic Processes

* BOX and TIAO · Bayesian Inference in Statistical Analysis

BOX · Improving Almost Anything, *Revised Edition*

* BOX and DRAPER · Evolutionary Operation: A Statistical Method for Process Improvement

BOX and DRAPER · Response Surfaces, Mixtures, and Ridge Analyses, *Second Edition*

BOX, HUNTER, and HUNTER · Statistics for Experimenters: Design, Innovation, and Discovery, *Second Editon*

BOX, JENKINS, and REINSEL · Time Series Analysis: Forcasting and Control, *Fourth Edition*

BOX, LUCEÑO, and PANIAGUA-QUIÑONES · Statistical Control by Monitoring and Adjustment, *Second Edition*

* BROWN and HOLLANDER · Statistics: A Biomedical Introduction

CAIROLI and DALANG · Sequential Stochastic Optimization

CASTILLO, HADI, BALAKRISHNAN, and SARABIA · Extreme Value and Related Models with Applications in Engineering and Science

CHAN · Time Series: Applications to Finance with R and S-Plus^, *Second Edition*

CHARALAMBIDES · Combinatorial Methods in Discrete Distributions

CHATTERJEE and HADI · Regression Analysis by Example, *Fourth Edition*

CHATTERJEE and HADI · Sensitivity Analysis in Linear Regression

CHEN · The Fitness of Information: Quantitative Assessments of Critical Evidence

CHERNICK · Bootstrap Methods: A Guide for Practitioners and Researchers, *Second Edition*

CHERNICK and FRIIS · Introductory Biostatistics for the Health Sciences

CHILÈS and DELFINER · Geostatistics: Modeling Spatial Uncertainty, *Second Edition*

CHIU, STOYAN, KENDALL and MECKE · Stochastic Geometry and Its Applications, *Third Edition*

CHOW and LIU · Design and Analysis of Clinical Trials: Concepts and Methodologies, *Third Edition*

CLARKE · Linear Models: The Theory and Application of Analysis of Variance

CLARKE and DISNEY · Probability and Random Processes: A First Course with Applications, *Second Edition*

* COCHRAN and COX · Experimental Designs, *Second Edition*

COLLINS and LANZA · Latent Class and Latent Transition Analysis: With Applications in the Social, Behavioral, and Health Sciences

CONGDON · Applied Bayesian Modelling, *Second Edition*

CONGDON · Bayesian Models for Categorical Data

CONGDON · Bayesian Statistical Modelling, *Second Edition*

CONOVER · Practical Nonparametric Statistics, *Third Edition*

COOK · Regression Graphics

COOK and WEISBERG · An Introduction to Regression Graphics

* Now available in a lower priced paperback edition in the Wiley Classics Library.

* Now available in a lower priced paperback edition in the Wiley Classics Library.
† Now available in a lower priced paperback edition in the Wiley–Interscience Paperback Series.

EVANS, HASTINGS, and PEACOCK · Statistical Distributions, *Third Edition*

EVERITT, LANDAU, LEESE, and STAHL · Cluster Analysis, *Fifth Edition*

FEDERER and KING · Variations on Split Plot and Split Block Experiment Designs

FELLER · An Introduction to Probability Theory and Its Applications, Volume I, *Third Edition,* Revised; Volume II, *Second Edition*

FITZMAURICE, LAIRD, and WARE · Applied Longitudinal Analysis, *Second Edition*

* FLEISS · The Design and Analysis of Clinical Experiments

FLEISS · Statistical Methods for Rates and Proportions, Third Edition

† FLEMING and HARRINGTON · Counting Processes and Survival Analysis

FUJIKOSHI, ULYANOV, and SHIMIZU · Multivariate Statistics: High-Dimensional and Large-Sample Approximations

FULLER · Introduction to Statistical Time Series, Second Edition

† FULLER · Measurement Error Models

GALLANT · Nonlinear Statistical Models

GEISSER · Modes of Parametric Statistical Inference

GELMAN and MENG · Applied Bayesian Modeling and Causal Inference from ncomplete-Data Perspectives

GEWEKE · Contemporary Bayesian Econometrics and Statistics

GHOSH, MUKHOPADHYAY, and SEN · Sequential Estimation

GIESBRECHT and GUMPERTZ · Planning, Construction, and Statistical Analysis of Comparative Experiments

GIFI · Nonlinear Multivariate Analysis

GIVENS and HOETING · Computational Statistics

GLASSERMAN and YAO · Monotone Structure in Discrete-Event Systems

GNANADESIKAN · Methods for Statistical Data Analysis of Multivariate Observations, *Second Edition*

GOLDSTEIN · Multilevel Statistical Models, *Fourth Edition*

GOLDSTEIN and LEWIS · Assessment: Problems, Development, and Statistical Issues

GOLDSTEIN and WOOFF · Bayes Linear Statistics

GRAHAM · Markov Chains: Analytic and Monte Carlo Computations

GREENWOOD and NIKULIN · A Guide to Chi-Squared Testing

GROSS, SHORTLE, THOMPSON, and HARRIS · Fundamentals of Queueing Theory, *Fourth Edition*

GROSS, SHORTLE, THOMPSON, and HARRIS · Solutions Manual to Accompany Fundamentals of Queueing Theory, *Fourth Edition*

* HAHN and SHAPIRO · Statistical Models in Engineering

HAHN and MEEKER · Statistical Intervals: A Guide for Practitioners

HALD · A History of Probability and Statistics and their Applications Before 1750

† HAMPEL · Robust Statistics: The Approach Based on Influence Functions

HARTUNG, KNAPP, and SINHA · Statistical Meta-Analysis with Applications

HEIBERGER · Computation for the Analysis of Designed Experiments

* Now available in a lower priced paperback edition in the Wiley Classics Library.
† Now available in a lower priced paperback edition in the Wiley–Interscience Paperback Series.

---

* Now available in a lower priced paperback edition in the Wiley Classics Library.
† Now available in a lower priced paperback edition in the Wiley–Interscience Paperback Series.

JOHN · Statistical Methods in Engineering and Quality Assurance

JOHNSON · Multivariate Statistical Simulation

JOHNSON and BALAKRISHNAN · Advances in the Theory and Practice of Statistics: A Volume in Honor of Samuel Kotz

JOHNSON, KEMP, and KOTZ · Univariate Discrete Distributions, *Third Edition*

JOHNSON and KOTZ (editors) · Leading Personalities in Statistical Sciences: From the Seventeenth Century to the Present

JOHNSON, KOTZ, and BALAKRISHNAN · Continuous Univariate Distributions, Volume 1, *Second Edition*

JOHNSON, KOTZ, and BALAKRISHNAN · Continuous Univariate Distributions, Volume 2, *Second Edition*

JOHNSON, KOTZ, and BALAKRISHNAN · Discrete Multivariate Distributions

JUDGE, GRIFFITHS, HILL, LÜTKEPOHL, and LEE · The Theory and Practice of Econometrics, *Second Edition*

JUREK and MASON · Operator-Limit Distributions in Probability Theory

KADANE · Bayesian Methods and Ethics in a Clinical Trial Design

KADANE AND SCHUM · A Probabilistic Analysis of the Sacco and Vanzetti Evidence

KALBFLEISCH and PRENTICE · The Statistical Analysis of Failure Time Data, *Second Edition*

KARIYA and KURATA · Generalized Least Squares

KASS and VOS · Geometrical Foundations of Asymptotic Inference

† KAUFMAN and ROUSSEEUW · Finding Groups in Data: An Introduction to Cluster Analysis

KEDEM and FOKIANOS · Regression Models for Time Series Analysis

KENDALL, BARDEN, CARNE, and LE · Shape and Shape Theory

KHURI · Advanced Calculus with Applications in Statistics, *Second Edition*

KHURI, MATHEW, and SINHA · Statistical Tests for Mixed Linear Models

* KISH · Statistical Design for Research

KLEIBER and KOTZ · Statistical Size Distributions in Economics and Actuarial Sciences

KLEMELÄ · Smoothing of Multivariate Data: Density Estimation and Visualization

KLUGMAN, PANJER, and WILLMOT · Loss Models: From Data to Decisions, *Third Edition*

KLUGMAN, PANJER, and WILLMOT · Loss Models: Further Topics

KLUGMAN, PANJER, and WILLMOT · Solutions Manual to Accompany Loss Models: From Data to Decisions, *Third Edition*

KOSKI and NOBLE · Bayesian Networks: An Introduction

KOTZ, BALAKRISHNAN, and JOHNSON · Continuous Multivariate Distributions, Volume 1, *Second Edition*

KOTZ and JOHNSON (editors) · Encyclopedia of Statistical Sciences: Volumes 1 to 9 with Index

---

† Now available in a lower priced paperback edition in the Wiley–Interscience Paperback Series.
* Now available in a lower priced paperback edition in the Wiley Classics Library.

MARKOVICH · Nonparametric Analysis of Univariate Heavy-Tailed Data: Research and Practice

MARONNA, MARTIN and YOHAI · Robust Statistics: Theory and Methods

MASON, GUNST, and HESS · Statistical Design and Analysis of Experiments with Applications to Engineering and Science, *Second Edition*

McCULLOCH, SEARLE, and NEUHAUS · Generalized, Linear, and Mixed Models, *Second Edition*

McFADDEN · Management of Data in Clinical Trials, *Second Edition*

* McLACHLAN · Discriminant Analysis and Statistical Pattern Recognition

McLACHLAN, DO, and AMBROISE · Analyzing Microarray Gene Expression Data

McLACHLAN and KRISHNAN · The EM Algorithm and Extensions, *Second Edition*

McLACHLAN and PEEL · Finite Mixture Models

McNEIL · Epidemiological Research Methods

MEEKER and ESCOBAR · Statistical Methods for Reliability Data

MEERSCHAERT and SCHEFFLER · Limit Distributions for Sums of Independent Random Vectors: Heavy Tails in Theory and Practice

MENGERSEN, ROBERT, and TITTERINGTON · Mixtures: Estimation and Applications

MICKEY, DUNN, and CLARK · Applied Statistics: Analysis of Variance and Regression, *Third Edition*

* MILLER · Survival Analysis, *Second Edition*

MONTGOMERY, JENNINGS, and KULAHCI · Introduction to Time Series Analysis and Forecasting

MONTGOMERY, PECK, and VINING · Introduction to Linear Regression Analysis, *Fifth Edition*

MORGENTHALER and TUKEY · Configural Polysampling: A Route to Practical Robustness

MUIRHEAD · Aspects of Multivariate Statistical Theory

MULLER and STOYAN · Comparison Methods for Stochastic Models and Risks

MURTHY, XIE, and JIANG · Weibull Models

MYERS, MONTGOMERY, and ANDERSON-COOK · Response Surface Methodology: Process and Product Optimization Using Designed Experiments, *Third Edition*

MYERS, MONTGOMERY, VINING, and ROBINSON · Generalized Linear Models. With Applications in Engineering and the Sciences, *Second Edition*

NATVIG · Multistate Systems Reliability Theory With Applications

† NELSON · Accelerated Testing, Statistical Models, Test Plans, and Data Analyses

† NELSON · Applied Life Data Analysis

NEWMAN · Biostatistical Methods in Epidemiology

NG, TAIN, and TANG · Dirichlet Theory: Theory, Methods and Applications

OKABE, BOOTS, SUGIHARA, and CHIU · Spatial Tessellations: Concepts and Applications of Voronoi Diagrams, *Second Edition*

OLIVER and SMITH · Influence Diagrams, Belief Nets and Decision Analysis

---

* Now available in a lower priced paperback edition in the Wiley Classics Library.

† Now available in a lower priced paperback edition in the Wiley–Interscience Paperback Series.

* Now available in a lower priced paperback edition in the Wiley Classics Library.
† Now available in a lower priced paperback edition in the Wiley–Interscience Paperback Series.

ROYSTON and SAUERBREI · Multivariate Model Building: A Pragmatic Approach to Regression Analysis Based on Fractional Polynomials for Modeling Continuous Variables

* RUBIN · Multiple Imputation for Nonresponse in Surveys

RUBINSTEIN and KROESE · Simulation and the Monte Carlo Method, *Second Edition*

RUBINSTEIN and MELAMED · Modern Simulation and Modeling

RUBINSTEIN, RIDDER, and VAISMAN · Fast Sequential Monte Carlo Methods for Counting and Optimization

RYAN · Modern Engineering Statistics

RYAN · Modern Experimental Design

RYAN · Modern Regression Methods, *Second Edition*

RYAN · Sample Size Determination and Power

RYAN · Statistical Methods for Quality Improvement, *Third Edition*

SALEH · Theory of Preliminary Test and Stein-Type Estimation with Applications

SALTELLI, CHAN, and SCOTT (editors) · Sensitivity Analysis

SCHERER · Batch Effects and Noise in Microarray Experiments: Sources and Solutions

* SCHEFFE · The Analysis of Variance

SCHIMEK · Smoothing and Regression: Approaches, Computation, and Application

SCHOTT · Matrix Analysis for Statistics, *Second Edition*

SCHOUTENS · Levy Processes in Finance: Pricing Financial Derivatives

SCOTT · Multivariate Density Estimation: Theory, Practice, and Visualization

* SEARLE · Linear Models

† SEARLE · Linear Models for Unbalanced Data

† SEARLE · Matrix Algebra Useful for Statistics

† SEARLE, CASELLA, and McCULLOCH · Variance Components

SEARLE and WILLETT · Matrix Algebra for Applied Economics

SEBER · A Matrix Handbook For Statisticians

† SEBER · Multivariate Observations

SEBER and LEE · Linear Regression Analysis, Second Edition

† SEBER and WILD · Nonlinear Regression

SENNOTT · Stochastic Dynamic Programming and the Control of Queueing Systems

* SERFLING · Approximation Theorems of Mathematical Statistics

SHAFER and VOVK · Probability and Finance: It's Only a Game!

SHERMAN · Spatial Statistics and Spatio-Temporal Data: Covariance Functions and Directional Properties

SILVAPULLE and SEN · Constrained Statistical Inference: Inequality, Order, and Shape Restrictions

SINGPURWALLA · Reliability and Risk: A Bayesian Perspective

SMALL and MCLEISH · Hilbert Space Methods in Probability and Statistical Inference

SRIVASTAVA · Methods of Multivariate Statistics

---

* Now available in a lower priced paperback edition in the Wiley Classics Library.
† Now available in a lower priced paperback edition in the Wiley–Interscience Paperback Series.

---

† Now available in a lower priced paperback edition in the Wiley–Interscience Paperback Series.

* Now available in a lower priced paperback edition in the Wiley Classics Library.